Controversies in Orthopedic Surgery of The Upper Limb

E. Carlos Rodríguez-Merchán
Alonso Moreno-García
Editors

Controversies in Orthopedic Surgery of The Upper Limb

Springer

Editors
E. Carlos Rodríguez-Merchán
Department of Orthopedic Surgery
La Paz University Hospital-IdiPaz
Madrid, Spain

Alonso Moreno-García
Department of Orthopedic Surgery
La Paz University Hospital-IdiPaz
Madrid, Spain

ISBN 978-3-031-04906-4 ISBN 978-3-031-04907-1 (eBook)
https://doi.org/10.1007/978-3-031-04907-1

This Springer imprint is published by the registered company Springer Nature Switzerland AG
The registered company address is: Gewerbestrasse 11, 6330 Cham, Switzerland

Preface

In this book, we have reviewed and analyzed some important controversies in orthopedic surgery of the upper extremities. Seven chapters on shoulder problems have been included: displaced proximal humeral fractures in the elderly; acromioclavicular dislocations in adults; calcific tendinopathy of the rotator cuff in adults; recurrent anterior shoulder instability in adults; controversies in shoulder arthroplasty; clavicle fractures; and massive rotator cuff tears.

Two chapters have been devoted to humerus injuries: humeral shaft fixation in adults; and controversies in the management of intra-articular distal humerus fracture in adults. We have devoted four chapters to elbow pathology: controversies in the management of radial head fractures in adults; controversies in the surgical treatment of distal biceps tendon ruptures in adults; controversies in tennis elbow in adults; and controversies in elbow arthroplasty.

Wrist problems have been analyzed in five chapters: distal radius fractures in the elderly; scapholunate dissociation; wrist arthritis; controversies in carpal tunnel syndrome in adults; and problems of the distal radioulnar joint. Finally, two chapters on hand problems have been included: controversies in the treatment of fingertip amputations in adults; and metacarpophalangeal and proximal interphalangeal joint arthroplasty.

All the chapters have been written by experts in the corresponding topic; in which they have carried out a thorough review and analysis of the recent literature and have stated their points of view on topics of great current controversy. As editors of this book, we thank all the authors for their generous participation and hope that the contents of this book may be of use to orthopedic surgeons in general and especially to those dedicated to the surgery of upper limb injuries.

Madrid, Spain

E. Carlos Rodríguez-Merchán
Alonso Moreno-García

Contents

Displaced Proximal Humeral Fractures in the Elderly: Conservative Treatment Versus Open Reduction and Internal Fixation Versus Hemiarthroplasty Versus Reverse Shoulder Arthroplasty

1

Sarah Mills and Juan C. Rubio-Suárez

1.1 Introduction

Proximal humeral fractures (PHF) in the elderly are nowadays among the most frequent fractures. Their incidence is increasing fast associated with population aging. These fractures are related to osteoporosis or poor bone quality [1].

These fractures impair quality of life as they affect patients' independence, just after the event and even in the long term, when some patients still report some degree of disability [2].

Treatment for these fractures has been a matter of discussion in the last few years as it supposes a challenge. That is why many studies evaluating different techniques have been published. Surgical treatment is complex, but it was the preferred option some years ago. Due to the moderate-high rate of complications and unpredictable outcomes, numerous studies tried to evaluate clinical results and cost-effectiveness of the different therapeutic options available.

Although surgery has not proven superior clinical results (and it is, obviously, more expensive) when compared to conservative treatment in PHF in the elderly, in this chapter we will discuss the different surgical techniques that can be chosen.

1.2 Epidemiology, Pathoanatomy, and Fracture Classification

1.2.1 Epidemiology

PHF constitute 5–6% of all fractures in adults and are more frequent in women (2:1) [1]. In the last few years, their incidence increased simultaneously with osteoporosis' prevalence due to population aging. They are usually due to ground-level falls on an outstretched arm. Very often, these fractures are the first evidence of bone fragility. When present, secondary prevention of future fractures is mandatory. Risk factors for suffering a PHF, in addition to osteoporosis, are diabetes, epilepsy, or female gender.

The most common associated lesion is axillary nerve injury. Vascular injury is uncommon (<5%) and occurs more frequently in the elderly, associated with surgical neck fractures or subcoracoid dislocation of the humeral head. PHF

S. Mills (✉) · J. C. Rubio-Suárez
Department of Orthopedic Surgery, La Paz University Hospital, Madrid, Spain
e-mail: sarah.mills@salud.madrid.org

E. C. Rodríguez-Merchán, A. Moreno-Garcìa (eds.), *Controversies in Orthopedic Surgery of The Upper Limb*, https://doi.org/10.1007/978-3-031-04907-1_1

can present with concomitant chest wall injuries or other fractures due to the fall.

1.2.2 Pathoanatomy

Depending on fracture pattern and location, humeral head vascularization can be compromised. The principal blood supply depends on the posterior humeral circumflex artery. Vascularity of the humeral head is more likely to be intact if more than 8 mm of calcar is attached to the articular fragment.

Hertel described some criteria to predict ischemia in the humeral head (Table 1.1) [3]. It is very important to highlight that the presence of those factors does not predict avascular necrosis of the humeral head.

PHF can be displaced or not; when displaced, deforming forces are determined by:

- Pectoralis major that displaces shaft anteriorly and medially.
- Supraspinatus, infraspinatus, and teres minor that externally rotates greater tuberosity.
- Subscapularis internally rotates articular segment or lesser tuberosity.

1.2.3 Classification

AO/OTA classification can be used, but Neer classification is the most extended one. According to the later, fractures can occur at the surgical neck, anatomic neck, greater tuberosity (GT), and lesser tuberosity (LT), determining four principal fragments: GT, LT, articular fragment, and shaft. Neer classification is based on the anatomic relationship of the four parts [4].

Table 1.1 Hertel criteria for prediction of humeral head ischemia [3]

<8 mm of calcar attached to articular segment
Disrupted medial hinge
Increased fracture complexity
Displacement >10 mm
Angulation >45°

"A part" is considered only if one of the following:

- It is displaced more than 1 cm.
- It is angulated more than 45°.

Two parts surgical neck fractures are the most common. More complex fracture patterns are seen with increasing age.

1.3 Diagnosis: Clinical Presentation and Imaging

1.3.1 Clinical Presentation

Like other fractures, PHF I presents with pain, swelling, and decreased range of motion. On physical exam, we will typically find an extensive hematoma over the chest, arm, and forearm, known as Hennequin hematoma.

A comprehensive neurovascular exam must be performed, and axillary nerve examination should not be overlooked, by determining deltoid muscle function and lateral shoulder sensation. Arterial injuries are often masked by extensive collateral circulation that can preserve distal pulses, so a high grade of suspicion is needed.

1.3.2 Imaging

When a PHF is suspected, the following radiographs should be ordered:

- True AP radiograph – Grashey projection
- Scapular Y projection
- Axillary projection

CT scan is helpful in preoperative planning and when determining humeral head or GT tuberosity position when they are uncertain. It also serves to determine the presence of head-split fractures. MRI is helpful when a rotator cuff injury is suspected, but its use is not standardized.

1.4 Treatment

Treatment options for PHF in the elderly have been under debate in the last few years. Nonsurgical treatment was the preferred option before the arrival of new implants and techniques. Many recent studies investigate if this interest in surgical intervention is supported by evidence or it is only a fad due to the appearance of new techniques and implants. Shoulder arthroplasties as a therapeutic option for PHF appeared in the twenty-first century. After that, few studies investigated its effectiveness and outcomes.

Studies analyzing different techniques for PHF treatment show that there is no benefit of surgical intervention in displaced fractures in comparison to nonoperative treatment. In addition, all surgical techniques have more complications and are more expensive than conservative management [5–7]. Summarizing, published results do not support the increasing trend for surgery in elderly patients with PHF [8, 9].

1.4.1 Nonoperative Treatment

Nonoperative treatment consists of sling immobilization for 4–6 weeks, followed by progressive rehabilitation. Immediate physical therapy offers a faster recovery. The vast majority of PHF can be treated conservatively (Fig. 1.1).

- Minimally displaced surgical and anatomic neck fractures.
- GT fracture with <5 mm displacement.
- Patients who are unsuitable for surgery.
- In the last years, age was included as an indication for conservative treatment even in case of displaced and complex fractures.

1.4.2 Operative Treatment

Surgical treatment for displaced PHF in the elderly is a subject under debate. Different techniques and implants are available: angular-stable plates, nails, or arthroplasties. Their indications and characteristics are described in the following sections. However, to date, little evidence supports one technique over another. All of these techniques had been evaluated in randomized control trials (RCT) versus the nonoperative treatment, and no relevant differences were found in terms of clinical or functional outcomes [5, 8, 10].

1.4.2.1 Open Reduction and Internal Fixation (ORIF)

Angular stable plate with locking screws is a widely used treatment for PHF, and before the development of nails or arthroplasties, it was the gold-standard technique. Later studies showed a 30% rate of reinterventions due to complications [10].

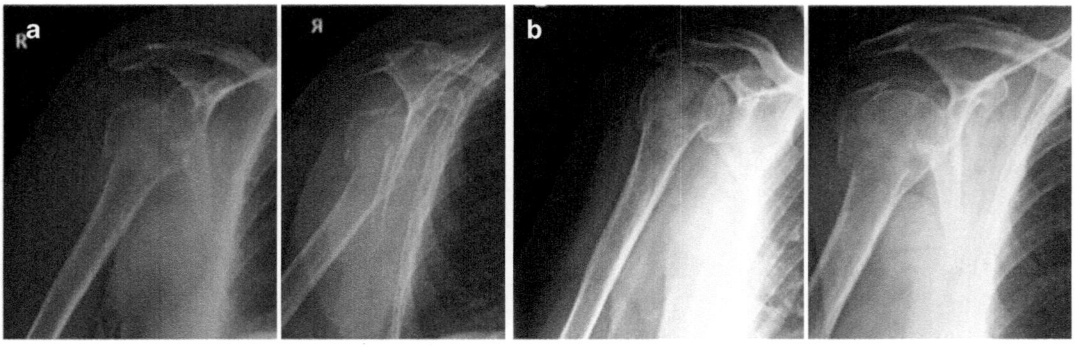

Fig. 1.1 84-year-old female with displaced proximal humeral fracture: (**a**) First X-ray evaluation after the fall. (**b**) Radiographical outcome: fracture healed after conservative treatment. Eight weeks follow-up

This technique is indicated if:

- GT is displaced >5 mm.
- Displaced 2-part fractures.
- 3- and 4-part fractures in younger patients.
- Head-splitting fractures in younger patients.

Better outcomes depend on some mechanical details, like the presence of medial support, which is necessary for fractures with posteromedial comminution, and calcar screw placement, which is critical to decreasing the risk of varus collapse of the articular fragment.

Technique

ORIF can be performed either by deltopectoral or lateral approach; this one has an increased risk for axillary nerve injury (Figs. 1.2 and 1.3).

- Nonabsorbable sutures are needed to isolate tuberosities and use them to reduce the fragments.
- The most common hardware used is a locking plate to fix the fracture once fragments are reduced.
  - The most frequent complication of this technique is screw cutout (14%). In osteoporotic bone, varus collapse is often seen, and it can be prevented with a screw placed inferomedial at calcar.
  - The plate must be placed lateral to the bicipital groove to avoid vascular injury (ascending branch of the anterior humeral circumflex artery).

Minimally invasive approaches were described to avoid soft tissue damage and healing problems due to periosteal stripping. These techniques present with two main disadvantages: a higher risk of axillary nerve injury and a more difficult fracture reduction maneuver [11].

Recent studies evaluate results for cemented augmentation locking screws. Results are promising, and hardware-related complications can be

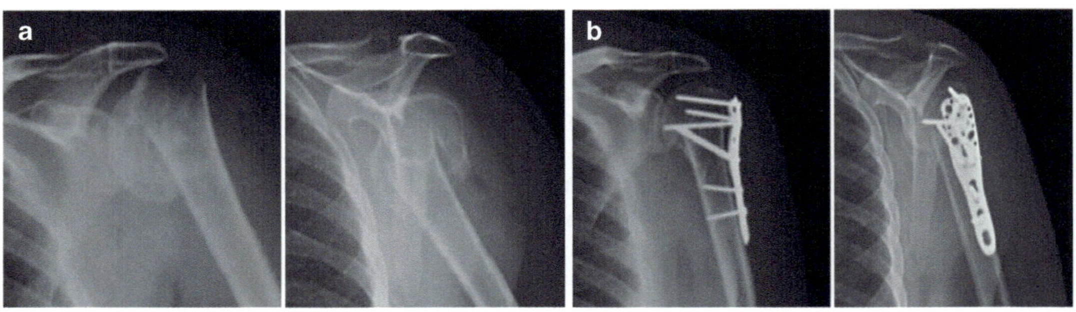

Fig. 1.2 (**a**) Displaced proximal humeral fracture in a 73-year-old female. (**b**) Radiographical outcome after treatment with open reduction and internal fixation with locking plate

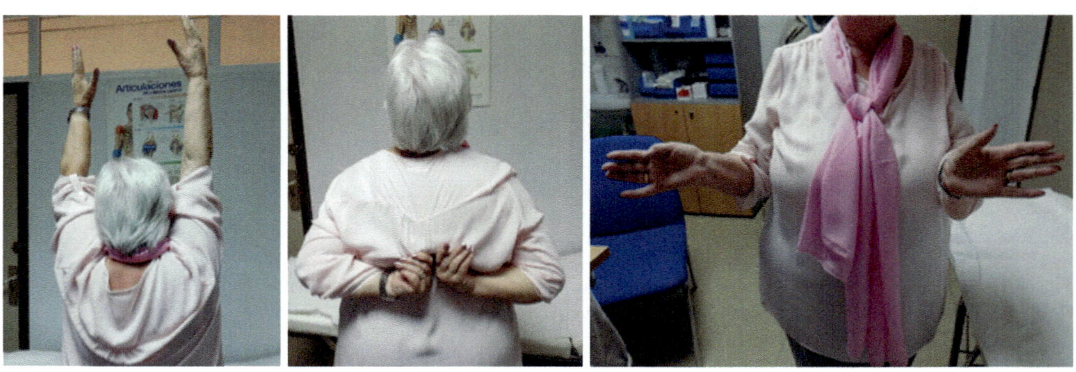

Fig. 1.3 Patient from Fig. 1.2, clinical outcome with full active range of motion after 15 months of follow-up and rehabilitation program

reduced drastically if this technique is employed. Neither clinical outcomes nor the need for revision surgery is modified; only the rate of implant-related failure and the global rate of complications were diminished. This technique also appears to help reduce the rate of avascular necrosis [12]. However, further studies are needed to achieve stronger evidence.

1.4.2.2 Intramedullary Nailing (IMN)

Intramedullary nailing can be used in surgical neck fractures or 3-part GT fractures in younger patients or patterns combined with shaft fractures. IMN can be performed in shorter surgical time, and there are no differences in complication rates when compared to ORIF with plates [13]. It offers less stability in torsion compared with plates, but no differences were found in fracture healing, nor ROM recovery compared to plating [14].

- The superior deltoid-splitting approach is used to insert the nail.
- The most common complications are rod migration and shoulder pain secondary to rotator cuff injury.
- Care should be taken when placing locking screws, as radial and musculocutaneous nerves can be injured.

1.4.2.3 Arthroplasty

Complex 3-part and 4-part fractures in the elderly are frequently impossible to fix due to comminution, poor bone quality, and high risk of mechanical and biological complications. For these cases, articular replacement seems to be a good solution.

Hemiarthroplasty (HA) was first employed in treating these fractures, but this technique is highly demandant, and good results are influenced by tuberosity healing, accurate size selection of the stem, and its final position. A functional rotator cuff is also needed for the proper functioning of a HA.

As results with plates and HA were inconsistent, reverse shoulder arthroplasty (RSA) emerged as an option to treat these complex fractures. Outcomes for RSA are less dependent on tuberosity healing and rotator cuff function/integrity compared to HA.

Age is a demonstrated predictor of outcome, so when choosing arthroplasty for treating a PHF, RSA is advisable over 70-year-old patients [15].

Hemiarthroplasty (HA)

The performance of a hemiarthroplasty is indicated in 4-part fractures, 3-part fractures with osteopenia, head-splitting, and severe articular fractures. HA is used in younger patients (40–65 y.o.) with complex fracture-dislocations or head-splitting component that may fail fixation.

- Recommended use of convertible stems in case reverse shoulder arthroplasty is needed.
- The deltopectoral approach is the most extended.
- Tuberosities must be sutured and passed through the prostheses' holes to improve stability.
- The height of the prosthesis is determined with the superior border of the pectoralis major tendon.
- Head to tuberosity distance (HTD) must be maintained (GT 8 mm below the articular surface) to respect external rotation kinematics.

Individualized assessment and preoperative planning are essential to succeed. Outcomes are better for younger patients and fractures treated acutely. It is very important to accurately choose the size of the prosthesis and to ensure the reattachment of the tuberosities to the stem/shaft [16].

Risk factors for a poor postoperative result are rotator cuff injuries, tuberosities malunion or nonunion, and age. Outcomes for this technique are not always satisfactory, and complications like significant postoperative pain, tuberosities' detachment, component malposition, instability, or rotator cuff tears are not uncommon (overall rate 35%) [16]. Healing of the tuberosities determines the success of this technique, and, when healing properly, better score punctuations and better ROM (in forward elevation and external rotation) are achieved [17]. Prosthesis has a mean survival time of 6.3 years [15].

When comparing HA with plating, better functional outcomes were registered with the use of

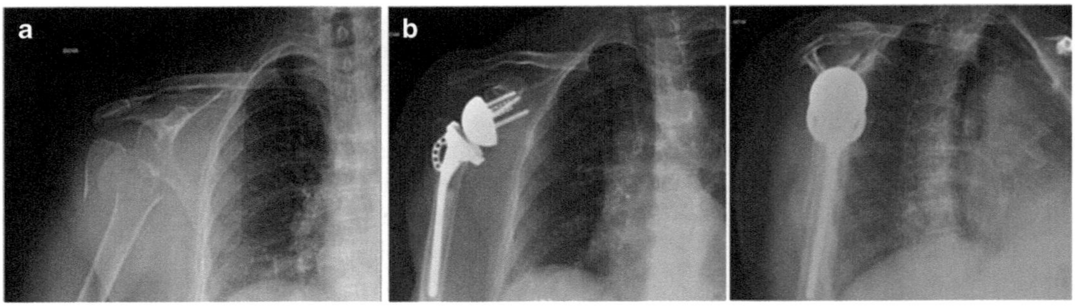

Fig. 1.4 (**a**) Female, 81-year-old, displaced proximal humeral 4-part fracture. (**b**) She was treated with reverse total shoulder arthroplasty

plates; however, HA had a lower rate of revision surgery and fewer surgical complications [18].

Due to poor results with HA, surgeons started using RSA to treat these complex fractures, which yielded better functional and patient-reported satisfaction scores when compared to HA. ROM in flexion after rehabilitation program was also better in RSA group, without differences for ROM in rotation. Both techniques have similar complication rates [17].

When analyzing the clinical and functional outcomes and comparing them with the nonoperative treatment, no differences were found, although the number of studies is scarce and evidence is low [5].

Reverse Shoulder Arthroplasty (RSA)

Reverse shoulder arthroplasty relies on deltoid muscle function instead of rotator cuff integrity or tuberosities position and healing. It is useful in low-demand elderly individuals with non-reconstructible tuberosities and poor bone stock or fracture-dislocations. Despite RSA can compensate for nonfunctioning rotator cuff, repairing tuberosities is recommended for an improved ROM.

Better outcomes if:

- Good glenoid bone stock is ensured.
- Restoration of humeral height and version. Poor results when retroversion of the humeral component is >40°.

The deltopectoral approach or the anterolateral deltoid splitting approach is the most frequently used.

Outcomes

The most reasonable options for treating PHF nowadays are RSA or nonoperative treatment. A randomized control trial (RCT) revealed that RSA has minimal benefits over conservative treatment in terms of pain perception [19]. RSA has been compared to ORIF too. Patient satisfaction and clinical outcomes resulted higher in the RSA group after two years of follow-up. Reverse total shoulder arthroplasty showed better ROM (except for internal rotation) and strength [10]. The complication rate for RSA is 8–11% [10, 17], with a 6% needing another surgery [10].

When compared to HA, RSA showed better results regarding patient satisfaction, outcome scores, and a higher range of motion (forward elevation). Healing of the tuberosities in RSA is irrelevant for score punctuation, and it is only relevant for recovery of external rotation (Fig. 1.4) [17].

1.5 Postoperative Rehabilitation

Rehabilitation is a very important part of the treatment of these fractures, and the best results are achieved when well established physical therapy protocols are followed. Stiffness is directly related to a long immobilization period.

- **Early passive range of motion.** As soon as the patient tolerates it
- **Active range of motion and progressive resistance**
- **Advance stretching and strengthening**

In minimally displaced fractures, an immediate rehabilitation program is an option, but. in displaced fractures, as is often the case in the elderly, immobilization for a small period is needed until the pain is relieved. It has been shown that stiffness related to immobilization, when it extends over 3 weeks, remains even after 2 years in the follow-up. The relevance of early rehabilitation has been widely proved, and it gains even more importance in the elderly. Adequate rehabilitation improves function and quality of life, and that is especially important in people that have poor neuromuscular status with bone fragility. Everything that compromises their independence can dramatically worsen their general health [2].

1.6 Outcomes Evaluation

Outcomes are generally evaluated with health questionnaires and functional scales, specifically conceived for upper limb affections.

1.6.1 Health Questionnaires

Scales as EQ-5D or 15D are the most frequently applied.

1.6.2 Functional Scales

Some examples are DASH score, Constant score, American Shoulder and Elbow Surgeons Standardized Shoulder Assessment Form (ASES), or Oxford shoulder score (OSS).

1.7 Overall Complications

- **Screw cutout:** The most frequent complication when locking plate fixation is used.
- **Avascular necrosis:** Better tolerated than in lower extremities. This complication is not related to risk factors for humeral head ischemia, nor type of fixation.
- **Nerve injury:**
  - **Axillary nerve:** Most common nerve injury (up to 60%)

    Deltoid-splitting approach
  - **Suprascapular nerve**
  - **Musculocutaneous nerve**
- **Malunion.**
- **Nonunion:** Risk increased with age and smoking. Nonunion of the tuberosities results in misfunctioning rotator cuff.
- **Rotator cuff injuries and dysfunction. Long head of biceps (LHB) tendon injuries.**
- **Missed posterior dislocation.** Maintain high suspicion in lesser tuberosity fractures.
- **Adhesive capsulitis.**
- **Posttraumatic arthritis.**
- **Infection.**

1.8 Mortality

Increased mortality has been related to different types of fractures: hip or periprosthetic fractures, vertebral fractures, distal femoral fracture, etc. [20]. All of them are often related somehow to a variable degree of frailness or comorbidities. Proximal humeral fractures are frequently associated with factors related to poor general health and morbidity, and also an increased mortality rate during the first year after the fracture has been described, especially in males and in those fractures treated surgically [21].

Registered one-year mortality rate after a PHF in people aged over 80 years old is 19.8%; the relative risk of dying after suffering a proximal humeral fracture was higher during the first 30 days after the incident (5 times higher) compared to the general population. Independent factors related to death were increased age, male sex (7 times higher), low bone mineral density, or concomitant fractures [21].

It is proposed that multidisciplinary teams (like in hip fractures in the elderly) may be advisable to treat these frail patients in order to reduce morbidity and mortality.

1.9 Conclusions

- Proximal humeral fractures represent 5% of all adult fractures and the second in frequency at the upper limb. They are related to osteoporosis, and almost 75% appear in people over 60 years of age. Its overall incidence is 40 in 100,000 patients, and, because of population aging and the increase of life expectancy, its incidence is predicted to triple in the next 10 years [19].
- These fractures impair quality of life and decrease patients' independence, so they have become a public health concern. Many studies have tried to establish protocols to improve their management.
- All therapeutic options available achieve pain relief (except in case of complications), but results are less predictable in terms of functional outcomes and range of motion. New implants and techniques were approved trying to fill this gap. Nevertheless, the gold-standard technique for treating PHF is still under debate. The implementation of different techniques and implants made necessary the development of studies, trying to determine whether to choose one over another, but the evidence is still scarce, and high-quality studies are still needed to establish more solid conclusions.
- Based on the evidence available, the trend is nonoperative treatment for PHF in the elderly, supported by moderate to high evidence. Current evidence shows that surgical treatment of displaced PHF in the elderly has no benefit compared to nonsurgical treatment. On these bases, surgical treatment must be very restrictive, and every case has to be individualized [9].
- In those cases in which surgery is needed, RSA seems to be the most adequate option. Elderly patients present with poor bone quality: it produces complex fracture patterns and also increases the risk of complications with ORIF. RSA showed better outcomes over the other surgical techniques (plates, nails, or hemiarthroplasty) in the elderly. All of them relieve pain, but RSA offers better results in terms of ROM and strength.
- RSA could be recommended in those cases of complex fractures with head split, head dislocation, or associated complex rotator cuff tears.
- The question now is "What do I choose? RSA or nonoperative treatment?" It is very important to individualize and study each patient's comorbidities and functional status. If surgery is chosen, we should remember that RSA offers a minimal advantage over conservative treatment and only in pain perception [19].

References

1. Palvanen M, Kannus P, Niemi S, Parkkari J. Update in the epidemiology of proximal humeral fractures. Clin Orthop Relat Res. 2006;442:87–92.
2. Hodgson SA, Mawson SJ, Saxton JM, Stanley D. Rehabilitation of two-part fractures of the neck of the humerus (two-year follow-up). J Shoulder Elb Surg. 2007;16:143–5.
3. Hertel R, Hempfing A, Stiehler M, Leunig M. Predictors of humeral head ischemia after intracapsular fracture of the proximal humerus. J Shoulder Elb Surg. 2004;13:427–33.
4. Neer CS. Four-segment classification of proximal humeral fractures: purpose and reliable use. J Shoulder Elb Surg. 2002;1:389–400.
5. Navarro CM, Brolund A, Ekholm C, et al. Treatment of humerus fractures in the elderly: a systematic review covering effectiveness, safety, economic aspects and current practice. PLoS One. 2018;13(12):e0207815.
6. Beks RB, Ochen Y, Frima H, et al. Operative versus nonoperative treatment of proximal humeral fractures: a systematic review, meta-analysis, and comparison of observational studies and randomized controlled trials. J Shoulder Elb Surg. 2018;27:1526–34.
7. Launonen AP, Lepola V, Flinkkilä T, Laitinen M, Paavola M, Malmivaara A. Treatment of proximal humerus fractures in the elderly. Acta Orthop. 2015;86:280–5.
8. Rangan A, Handoll H, Brealey S, et al. Surgical vs nonsurgical treatment of adults with displaced fractures of the proximal humerus the PROFHER randomized clinical trial. JAMA. 2015;313:1037–47.
9. Handoll H, Brealey S, Rangan A, et al. The ProFHer (PROximal fracture of the humerus: evaluation by randomisation) trial—a pragmatic multicentre randomized controlled trial evaluating the clinical effectiveness and cost-effectiveness of surgical compared with non-surgical treatment for proxi. Health Technol Assess (Rockv). 2015; https://doi.org/10.3310/hta19240.
10. Fraser AN, Bjørdal J, Wagle TM, et al. Reverse shoulder arthroplasty is superior to plate fixation at 2

years for displaced proximal humeral fractures in the elderly: a multicenter randomized controlled trial. J Bone Joint Surg Am. 2020;102:477–85.
11. Barco R, Barrientos I, Encinas C, Antuña SA. Minimally invasive poly-axial screw plating for three-part fractures of the proximal humerus. Injury. 2012;43(Suppl 2):7–11.
12. Foruria AM, Martinez-Catalan N, Valencia M, Morcillo D, Calvo E. Proximal humeral fracture locking plate fixation with anatomic reduction, and a short-and-cemented-screws configuration, dramatically reduces the implant related failure rate in elderly patients. JSES Int. 2021; https://doi.org/10.1016/j.jseint.2021.06.004.
13. Lekic N, Montero NM, Takemoto RC, Davidovitch RI, Egol KA. Treatment of two-part proximal humerus fractures: intramedullary nail compared to locked plating. HSS J. 2012;8:86–91.
14. Lee W, Park JY, Chun YM. Operative treatment of 2-part surgical neck fracture of the humerus: intramedullary nail versus locking compression plate with technical consideration. J Orthop Trauma. 2017;31:e270–4.
15. Robinson CM, Page RS, Hill RMF, Sanders DL, Court-Brown CM, Wakefield AE. Primary hemiarthroplasty for treatment of proximal humeral fractures. J Bone Joint Surg Am. 2003;85:1215–23.
16. Hartsock LA, Estes WJ, Murray CA, Friedman RJ. Shoulder hemiarthroplasty for proximal humeral fractures. Orthop Clin North Am. 1998;29:467–75.
17. Cuff DJ, Pupello DR. Comparison of hemiarthroplasty and reverse shoulder arthroplasty for the treatment of proximal humeral fractures in elderly patients. J Bone Joint Surg Am. 2013;95:2050–5.
18. Dai J, Chai Y, Wang C, Wen G. Meta-analysis comparing locking plate fixation with hemiarthroplasty for complex proximal humeral fractures. Eur J Orthop Surg Traumatol. 2014;24:305–13.
19. Lopiz Y, Alcobía-Díaz B, Galán-Olleros M, García-Fernández C, Picado AL, Marco F. Reverse shoulder arthroplasty versus nonoperative treatment for 3- or 4-part proximal humeral fractures in elderly patients: a prospective randomized controlled trial. J Shoulder Elb Surg. 2019;28:2259–71.
20. Merino-Rueda LR, Rubio-Sáez I, Mills S, Rubio-Suárez JC. Mortality of distal femur fractures in the elderly. Injury. 2021;52(Suppl 4):S71–5.
21. Bergdahl C, Wennergren D, Ekelund J, Möller M. Mortality after a proximal humeral fracture. Bone Joint J. 2020;102-B:1484–90.

Surgical Versus Conservative Interventions for Treating Acromioclavicular Dislocation of the Shoulder in Adults

2

Jorge de las Heras-Sotos, Alonso Moreno-García, and E. Carlos Rodríguez-Merchán

2.1 Introduction

Acromioclavicular joint (ACJ) dislocation is a frequent lesion, especially in young active patients. The main restrictors of the clavicle to avoid dislocation are the conoid and trapezoid ligaments that attach the clavicle to the coracoid (CC ligaments). In addition, the acromioclavicular joint has its own ligaments (AC ligaments: anterior, posterior, superior, and inferior) that contribute both to the vertical and the anteroposterior stability. Traditionally, minimal significance was given to the AC ligaments in relation to the pathoanatomy of these injury; however, recently, Kurata et al. found that the AC ligaments contribute significantly to AC joint stability, and superior displacement >50% of the AC joint can occur with AC ligament tears alone [1]. The trapezius and deltoid muscles, along with the deltotrapezoid fascia, contribute as well to the stabilization of the AC joint, in what Pastor et al. defined as a dynamic stabilization mechanism [2]. The AC joint serves as the link between the scapulothoracic, glenohumeral, and sternoclavicular joints and allows both gliding and rotational motion. It is usually injured after a lateral blow that drives the clavicle medially and superiorly, injuring the aforementioned ligaments and creating instability into the joint. In this chapter, we are going to review the best evidence available for the management of these injuries.

J. de las Heras-Sotos · A. Moreno-García
E. C. Rodríguez-Merchán (✉)
Department of Orthopedic Surgery, La Paz University Hospital-IdiPaz, Madrid, Spain

2.2 Epidemiology and Classification

Shoulder injuries are common, and the increased risk is mainly attributable to sport-related injuries. ACJ injury has been reported as the most common upper extremity injury in sports. In a recent study, the overall incidence was 2 per 10,000 person-years, being more common in young adults and males, although the risk for high-grade injuries was greater in older patients. ACJ injuries were related to sport activities and road traffic accidents [3]. In a study aimed to evaluate the incidence of ACJ injuries in a general population, Skjaker et al. reported that ACJ injuries constituted 11% of all shoulder injuries. Sports injuries accounted for 53%, compared to 27% in other shoulder injuries, and the most common sport associated with ACJ injuries was football [4].

The first classification of acute ACJ injuries was introduced by Tossy et al. They classified the injuries from grade I to III based on radiological examination and the degree of rupture of the supporting ligaments. Rockwood et al. established a more detailed classification that graded injuries from type I to VI [5]:

E. C. Rodríguez-Merchán, A. Moreno-Garcìa (eds.), *Controversies in Orthopedic Surgery of The Upper Limb*, https://doi.org/10.1007/978-3-031-04907-1_2

Type I: Incomplete injuries of the AC ligaments and no injury of the CC ligaments. There is pain at the AC joint but no displacement.

Type II: Complete injury of the AC ligaments with incomplete injury of the CC ligaments. There is upward displacement of the clavicle but not above the acromion (50% displacement) (Fig. 2.1).

Type III: Complete injury of both the AC and the CC ligaments. The clavicle is displaced upwards, with the lower cortex of the clavicle at the level of the superior cortex of the acromion (100% displacement) (Fig. 2.2).

Type IV: Complete injury of both AC and CC ligaments with posterior displacement of the clavicle, penetrating the trapezius muscle.

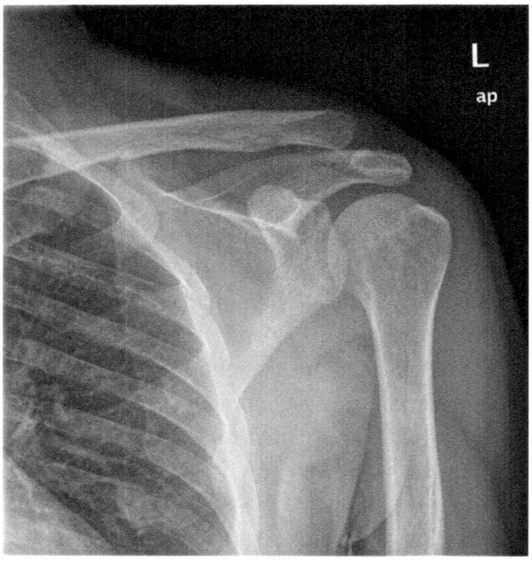

Fig. 2.1 Rockwood type II

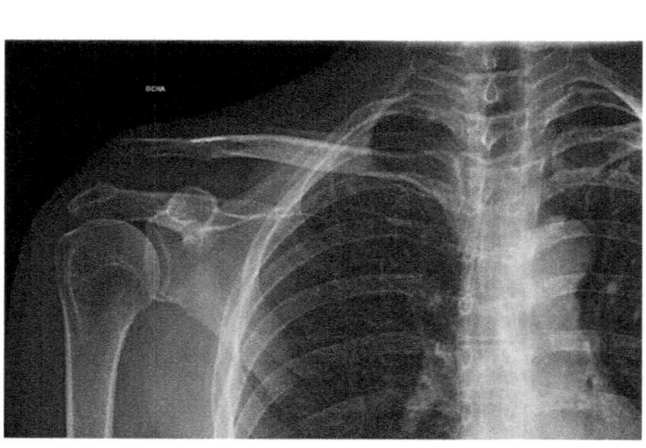

Fig. 2.2 Rockwood type III

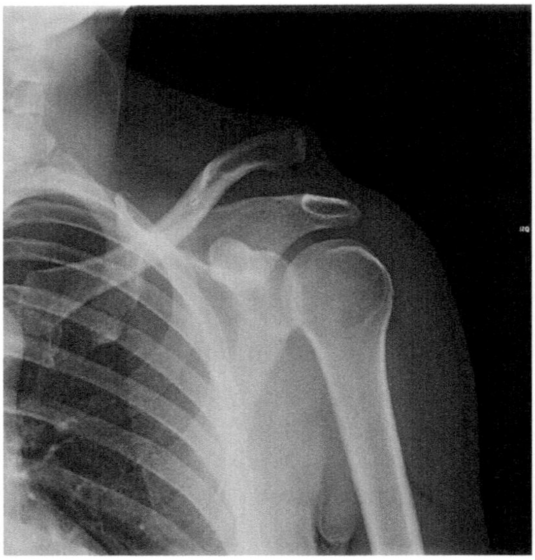

Fig. 2.3 Rockwood type V

Type V: Complete injury of both AC and CC ligaments with displacement of the clavicle above the acromion, significantly more than in type III, with disruption of the attachments of the deltoid and trapezius muscles (Fig. 2.3).

Type VI: Complete injury of both AC and CC ligaments with inferior displacement of the clavicle underneath the acromion and the coracoid process. This is a very rare entity.

2.3 Diagnosis

The clinical picture depends on the severity of the injury and the type of lesion. For **type I,** there is minimal to moderate local tenderness to palpation, mild swelling over the AC joint, and minimal pain with arm movements. In **type II**, the distal end of the clavicle may be slightly superior to the acromion, and there is usually a local ecchymosis. On clinical examination, anterior–posterior motion of the clavicle in the horizontal plane can present, but there should not be instability in the vertical plane. In **type III,** injuries and due to the severe ligamentous involvement, there is an inferior translation of the limb which produces the characteristic shoulder droop sign, the clavicle being prominent laterally. In this type of lesion, the AC joint can be reduced with upward pressure under the elbow or by having the patient actively shrug: the "shrug test." For **type IV**, we will find the same symptoms and findings as in type III, and in addition the examination of the injured shoulder from above reveals that the outline of the displaced clavicle is translated posteriorly compared with the uninjured shoulder. **Type V** is an exaggeration of the type III injury, and the distal end of the clavicle appears to be clearly displaced and tenting the skin. **Type VI** injuries are rare and frequently associated to severe concomitant injuries that the disruption of the AC joint may not be recognized initially. Characteristically, the superior aspect of the shoulder has a flat appearance, the acromion is prominent, and there is a step to the superior surface of the coracoid process.

Diagnostic imaging is essential for assessing the severity of ACJ separation. The AP view of the ACJ on radiographs with the patient in the sitting or standing position allows to assess the vertical translation of the clavicle with respect to the acromion. A projection-directed cephalad 10–15° (Zanca view) shows a clearer view and is preferred by some surgeons [6]. For the assessment of the horizontal translation, there is not a unanimous accepted method. Axial images, scapular Y views, or CT are used for that purpose [7]. Magnetic resonance imaging (MRI) is of special relevance when evaluating healed or reconstructed CC ligaments, through the evaluation of the signal intensities of the graft, tendon-bone interface, and neighboring bone [8].

2.4 Treatment and Results

Conservative treatment is the rule for ACJ injuries with no displacement or upward displacement of less than 50%. Regarding surgical treatment for ACJ dislocation, a recent review published by the Cochrane Library concludes that there is low-quality evidence that surgical treatment has no additional benefits in terms of function, return to former activities, and quality of life at 1 year compared with conservative treatment [9]. However, this review was based on low-quality evidence studies and outdated techniques, for what de Sa et al. "would caution readers against placing too much stock in the key findings of this Cochrane review" [10]. Nowadays, it is generally accepted that injuries grade IV to VI should be managed operatively, and controversy remains about optimal treatment of type III injuries.

In general, it is accepted that Rockwood **type I and II** injuries should be treated conservatively. Treatment of these injuries typically consists of analgesics, cryotherapy, and the use of a sling during 1–2 weeks. Early range of motion activities are permitted, and weaning of the sling as pain permits is advised [11].

Management of **type III** injuries is today a source of controversy. While many authors report excellent results with surgical treatment, although the evidence of many of these works is low, others like Schlegel et al., in a prospective study, report good results of conservative management [12]. A metanalysis published by Smith et al. concluded that there is a lack of well-designed studies to justify the optimum mode of treatment of grade III acromioclavicular dislocations [13]. In this situation, it is wise to recommend conservative management initially in type III injuries and only resorting to surgery when the trial of nonoperative management fails. An exception could be high-demand patients, athletes, and laborers in whom surgical treatment may be indicated firstly due to poor tolerance to ACJ instability.

Regarding **type IV, V, and VI** injuries, surgeons generally agree that active and fit-for-surgery patients may benefit from operative treatment. Again, there is a lack of well-designed controlled trials addressing this issue.

2.5 Surgical Treatment

The goal of surgical treatment is to restore bidirectional acromioclavicular joint stability by repairing or reconstructing the injured structures, either with or without use of arthroscopy, and respecting the local anatomy.

The timing to surgery is an important issue in surgical treatment of ACJ injuries. We know that the AC joint ligaments lose their potential to heal after 3 weeks following injury. In fact, after the studies of Maier et al., it is recommended to perform operative treatment as early as possible within a timeframe of 1 week after trauma to exploit the utmost biological healing potential of the injured ligaments. After their histological study, the authors' findings indicate that the human acromioclavicular ligament complex exhibits early and highly dynamic intrinsic responses to traumatic rupture [14]. When comparing the clinical and radiographic results and the complication rate between early and delayed surgical treatment of ACJ dislocation, Song et al. in a metanalysis showed that better functional outcomes and more satisfied reduction was achieved with early treatment. However, the authors acknowledged the need for high-quality evidence studies to support this assertion [15]. In agreement with basic science results and for clinical purposes, the separation line between acute and chronic cases is normally set at 3 weeks [6].

2.6 Acute Injuries

For the treatment of *acute cases*, less than 3 weeks from injury, several techniques have been published with the objective to achieve ACJ stabilization that will allow the healing of the injured ligaments. Historically, metal implants were used like the **Bosworth screw** from the clavicle to the coracoid process, introduced in 1941. It showed to be effective for the stabilization of the ACJ in injuries grade III, IV, and V. The need for a second surgery to remove the implant and higher patient satisfaction with newer suspensory devices has relegated the use of this technique. The **hook plate** was introduced later as an alternative implant, showing higher Constant scores and patient satisfaction when compared to the Bosworth screw (Fig. 2.4). It is a simple surgical technique, with minimally invasive access, allowing early resumption of normal activity. The hook plate fixation allows time for the native AC and CC ligaments to heal in place by reducing the AC joint and maintaining the reduction. Good clinical and radiological results have been published with its use. Kienast et al. reported 89% excellent and good results but with a complication rate of 10.6% [16]. Some authors have postulated the combination of hook plate fixation and CC repair. In this regard, Chen et al. reported fewer acromion complications and statistical differences in reduction maintenance [17]. When compared to suspensory devices, hook plate fixation shows poorer results as shown in a recent meta-analysis which reported that both techniques offered effective outcomes in relieving the pain although the suspensory technique showed an advantage over hook plate in terms of postoperative pain [18]. In a retrospective study, Unal et al. concluded that endo-button showed superior shoulder scores in the early stages when compared with hook plate fixation [19]. **Tension band wiring** method has also been used by some authors providing functionally satisfactory results, although high rate of complications has been reported with residual subluxation or loss of reduction in more than 45% of cases [20].

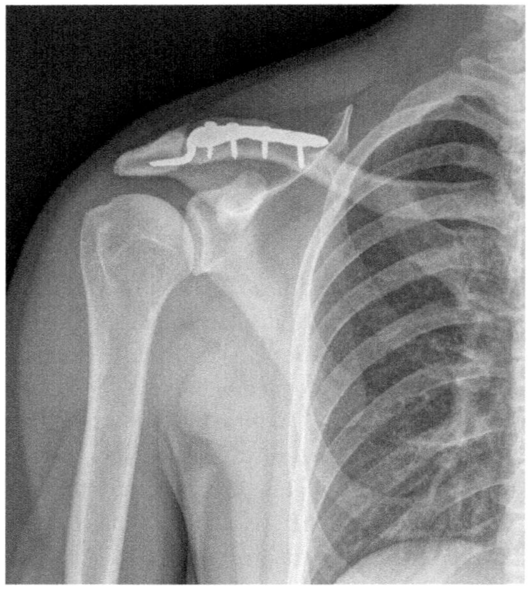

Fig. 2.4 Hook plate fixation

The **suspensory techniques** have gained increasing popularity in recent years for the treatment of acute ACJ injuries. The advantages of these novel techniques are the minimal invasive

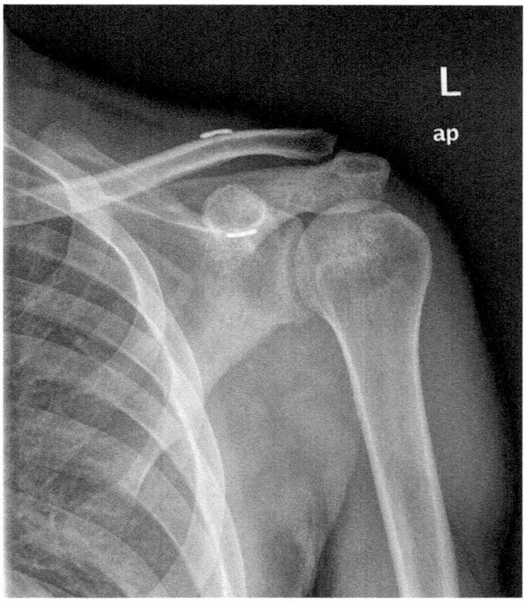

Fig. 2.5 DogBone suspensory technique

approach, the possibility of using arthroscopy, and there is no need for hardware removal. Several devices have been developed like the EndoButton, the TightRope, the DogBone, and the ZipTight, among others (Fig. 2.5). They all consist of metallic buttons placed on top of the clavicle and under the coracoid that are connected with a continuous loop of suture. They can be used as a single suspension device in a vertical placement, the device anchored at an isometric point of the CC ligament or in an anatomical manner with the use of two or more vertical stabilizers along the course of the CC ligaments, the latter allowing theoretically for a more physiological stabilization, restoring not only vertical but horizontal stability. Kurtoglu et al. presented recently their series of 25 patients treated with a suspensory loop device. The results were favorable in terms of functional recovery and pain relief. However, the major disadvantage found was radiological loss of AC joint reduction, which occurred in six cases [21]. In a study focusing on reduction loss after arthroscopic suspensory fixation of acute acromioclavicular dislocations, Çarkçi et al. found a 25% reduction loss of more than 3 mm. This loss did not create a statistically significant difference in Constant scores, but AC joint-specific tests, subjective evaluation, and aesthetic subjective satisfaction values were significantly impaired. The authors advocate that reduction maintaining is crucial for excellent functional and aesthetic results after fixation of the AC joint with a double-button device [22]. Özcafer et al. published their experience with the use of TightRope for the treatment of type V ACJ dislocations. In a series of 19 patients, the authors concluded that TightRope device can provide anatomical restoration in patients with acute type V ACJ dislocations without subluxation at the final follow-up examination at 1 year postop [23]. Wang et al. compared two popular suspensory devices, TightRope and EndoButton, in a retrospective case-control study. The authors concluded that there were no significant differences between the two groups regarding the Constant-Murley score and the coracoclavicular distance during the follow-up [24].

Biological augmentation is not advocated for acute injuries; however, some authors have developed techniques that use biological grafts that may be of interest in certain cases, like the one described by Ruzbarsky et al. of arthroscopic allograft CC ligament reconstruction [25].

Although the aforementioned techniques using metallic buttons have shown good clinical results, complication rates published are high, ranging from 20% to 44%. Another concern is the adverse clinical results by residual horizontal instability after CC ligament repair. Some authors have proposed the use of **suture anchors** on the coracoid to address vertical and horizontal stabilities simultaneously, advocating the use of small diameter tunnels to reduce the risk of fractures. Liu et al. reported on the use of CC ligament reconstruction using two suture anchors and ACJ augmentation using two strands of non-absorbable heavy sutures on high-grade AC dislocations. In their series of 29 patients, they obtained good clinical and functional results, with radiographs showing two partial loss of reduction, whereas no horizontal displacement was found, and one superficial wound infection and no neurovascular complications were recorded after a mean follow-up of 28 months [26]. Teixeira et al., in a recent publication, also stress the importance of addressing the horizontal instability of the ACJ when treating these injuries. The authors propose the achievement of additional horizontal stability through superior AC ligament repair using suture anchors [27]. Suture anchor fixation and double-button fixation technique have been recently compared by Topal et al., concluding that both techniques are reliable treatment methods that are not superior to one another and can yield excellent functional outcomes [28]. Hahem et al. have recently published an arthroscopically assisted coracoclavicular and horizontal acromioclavicular fixation technique in a modified figure-of-eight configuration using two strong FiberTape cerclage sutures [29].

The introduction of the arthroscopy for the treatment of ACJ injuries is nowadays well accepted, providing several advantages over open procedures. These techniques offer superior visualization of the base of the coracoid and require less soft tissue dissection and smaller incisions than open procedures. In addition, it allows the surgeon to identify and treat possible associated injuries within the glenohumeral joint and subacromial space. Arthroscopically assisted anatomic reconstruction using a suspensory device, with no need of a biological augmentation in acute injuries, was the consensus achieved by shoulder experts which has been recently published [6].

2.7 Chronic Injuries

If the initial trauma occurred more than 3 weeks before treatment, these cases should be considered chronic due to ligament limited healing capacity of both CC and AC ligaments from that point. The choice of treatment of chronic ACJ dislocation is controversial. In general, it is deemed necessary in chronic cases to perform arthroscopically assisted biologic reconstruction to recreate not only CC ligaments but also AC ligaments. Since less healing response is expected, the more surgical stability, increased by biological augmentation, is recommended. Biomechanical studies have demonstrated that combined AC and CC ligaments reconstruction provides better results than isolated CC reconstruction [30]. The transposition of the coracoacromial ligament from the acromion to the distal clavicle, keeping the coracoid insertion, was described by Weaver and Dunn in 1972. To improve mechanical stabilization, Weaver-Dunn procedure has been combined with suspensory button devices by other authors with good results [31]. Ranne et al. reported on the results of a series of 58 patients with chronic acromioclavicular separations treated with arthroscopic coracoclavicular ligament reconstructions using semitendinosus autografts. Constant and Simple Shoulder Test scores were determined before and 2 years after surgery, and general patient satisfaction also was assessed. In addition, the coracoclavicular distance was measured using anteroposterior radiographs taken 2 years after surgery. Eighty-five percent of the patients reported excellent subjective outcomes. Constant and Simple Shoulder Test scores showed significant improvement at 2 years postoperatively. The mean coracoclavicular distance increased from 10.5 ± 3.4 to 12.4 ± 3.9 mm ($P = 0.009$), two coracoid fractures were observed, one patient experienced a deep infection, and two patients had superficial postoperative infections. The authors conclude that coracoclavicular ligament reconstruction is a challenging procedure, but satisfactory results can be achieved with careful patient selection and good technique [32]. The use of synthetic ligament has been also described with favorable results [33], and some authors have introduced a technical variation that combines synthetic ligament reconstruction and anatomic allograft reconstruction of the CC ligaments. Yeranosian et al. reviewed the results of this combined technique on 10 patients with chronic ACJ dislocations, showing good clinical and functional results at a mean follow-up of 2 years. The authors concluded that this technique using a synthetic ligament along with an anatomic allograft coracoclavicular ligament reconstruction is a safe, effective alternative [34]. Romano et al. have recently reported on the use of a new device based on a permanent implantable Tube-Tape with integral eyelet which is looped around the coracoid, together with a titanium button for clavicle attachment, the Infinity-Lock Button

System. After a retrospective study of 15 patients, the authors concluded that this technique is effective for treatment of chronic grade III ACJ dislocation, resulting in elevated satisfaction ratings and predictable outcomes [35]. Cano-Martínez et al. also reported in the use of vertical and horizontal stabilization without biological augmentation. In a series of 21 patients after a mean follow-up of 49 months, the authors reported no significant differences with the uninjured shoulder of the Constant score and Acromioclavicular Joint Instability Scoring System. The radiological results were as well satisfactory [36].

Postoperatively, either for acute or chronic cases, a shoulder sling is recommended for immobilization for 3 weeks, with a limitation of range of motion with no activities of daily living for the first 6 weeks and a free range of motion 6 weeks after surgery [6].

2.8 Conclusions

Acromioclavicular joint (ACJ) dislocation is a frequent lesion, especially in young active patients and mainly attributable to sport-related injuries. The overall incidence is 2.0 per 10.000 person-years and constitutes 11% of all shoulder injuries. The most commonly used classification is the one from Rockwood that categorizes these injuries in type I to VI. The diagnosis is essentially based on plain X-ray, although CT is of use for the assessment of horizontal translation. Conservative treatment is the rule for ACJ injuries with no displacement or upward displacement of less than 50% (Rockwood type I and II). Management of type III injuries is today a source of controversy, but it is recommended conservative management initially and only resorting to surgery when the trial of nonoperative management fails. Regarding surgical treatment, arthroscopically assisted anatomic reconstruction using a suspensory device, with no need of a biological augmentation is the general recommendation, whereas biological reconstruction of coracoclavicular and acromioclavicular ligaments with tendon graft is advocated in chronic cases. Complications are not infrequent out of these techniques, and prospective well-designed studies are needed to standardize the operative approach of ACJ injuries.

References

1. Kurata S, Inoue K, Hasegawa H, Shimizu T, Iida A, Kawamura K, et al. The role of the acromioclavicular ligament in acromioclavicular joint stability: a cadaveric biomechanical study. Orthop J Sports Med. 2021;9(2):232596712098294.
2. Pastor MF, Averbeck AK, Welke B, Smith T, Claassen L, Wellmann M. The biomechanical influence of the deltotrapezoid fascia on horizontal and vertical acromioclavicular joint stability. Arch Orthop Trauma Surg. 2016;136:513–9.
3. Nordin JS, Olsson O, Lunsjö K. Acromioclavicular joint dislocations: incidence, injury profile, and patient characteristics from a prospective case series. JSES Int. 2020;4:246–50.
4. Skjaker SA, Enger M, Engebretsen L, Brox JI, Bøe B. Young men in sports are at highest risk of acromioclavicular joint injuries: a prospective cohort study. Knee Surg Sports Traumatol Arthrosc. 2021;29:2039–45.
5. Rockwood C, Williams G, Young D. Disorders of the acromioclavicular joint. In: Rockwood CA, editor. The shoulder. 3rd ed. Philadelphia, PA: WB Saunders; 2004. p. 521–95.
6. Rosso C, Martetschläger F, Saccomanno MF, Voss A, Lacheta L, Ângelo AC, et al. High degree of consensus achieved regarding diagnosis and treatment of acromioclavicular joint instability among ESA-ESSKA members. Knee Surg Sports Traumatol Arthrosc. 2021;29:2325–32.
7. Takase K, Hata Y, Morisawa Y, Goto M, Tanaka S, Hamada J, et al. Methods used to assess the severity of acromioclavicular joint separations in Japan: a survey. JSES Int. 2020;4:242–5.
8. Kani KK, Porrino JA, Mulcahy H, Chew FS. Surgical techniques for management of acromioclavicular joint separations: review and update for radiologists. Skelet Radiol. 2020;49:1195–206.
9. Tamaoki MJ, Lenza M, Matsunaga FT, Belloti JC, Matsumoto MH, Faloppa F. Surgical versus conservative interventions for treating acromioclavicular dislocation of the shoulder in adults. Cochrane Database Syst Rev. 2019;10:CD007429.
10. De SADL, Bhandari M. Cochrane in CORR: surgical versus conservative interventions for treating acromioclavicular dislocation of the shoulder in adults. Clin Orthop Relat Res. 2020;478:462–8.
11. Nolte PC, Lacheta L, Dekker TJ, Elrick BP, Millett PJ. Optimal management of acromioclavicular dislocation: current perspectives. Orthop Res Rev. 2020;12:27–44.

12. Schlegel TF, Burks RT, Marcus RL, Dunn HK. A prospective evaluation of untreated acute grade III acromioclavicular separations. Am J Sports Med. 2001;29:699–703.
13. Smith TO, Chester R, Pearse EO, Hing CB. Operative versus non-operative management following Rockwood grade III acromioclavicular separation: a meta-analysis of the current evidence base. J Orthop Traumatol. 2011;12:19–27.
14. Maier D, Tuecking L-R, Bernstein A, Lang G, Wagner FC, Jaeger M, et al. The acromioclavicular ligament shows an early and dynamic healing response following acute traumatic rupture. BMC Musculoskelet Disord. 2020;21(1):593.
15. Song T, Yan X, Ye T. Comparison of the outcome of early and delayed surgical treatment of complete acromioclavicular joint dislocation. Knee Surg Sports Traumatol Arthrosc. 2016;24:1943–50.
16. Kienast B, Thietje R, Queitsch C, Gille J, Schulz A, Meiners J. Mid-term results after operative treatment of Rockwood grade III-V acromioclavicular joint dislocations with an AC-hook-plate. Eur J Med Res. 2011;16(2):52.
17. Chen Y-T, Wu K-T, Jhan S-W, Hsu S-L, Liu H-C, Wang C-J, et al. Is coracoclavicular reconstruction necessary in hook plate fixation for acute unstable acromioclavicular dislocation? BMC Musculoskelet Disord. 2021;22(1):127.
18. Pan X, Lv R, Lv M, Zhang D. TightRope vs clavicular hook plate for Rockwood III–V acromioclavicular dislocations: a meta-analysis. Orthop Surg. 2020;12:1045–52.
19. Unal OK, Dagtas MZ. Comparison of the results of hook plate and endo-button used in the surgical treatment of acromioclavicular joint separation. Cureus. 2020;12(12):e11987.
20. Ozan F, Gök S, Okur KT, Altun İ, Kahraman M, Günay AE, et al. Midterm results of tension band wiring technique for acute Rockwood type III acromioclavicular joint dislocation. Cureus. 2020;12(12):e12203.
21. Kurtoglu A, Sukur E, Cicekli O, Daldal I, Kochai A, Sen Z, et al. Does the ZipTightTM effective to maintain reduction after the treatment of acute acromioclavicular joint dislocation? Medicine. 2020;99(9):e19387.
22. Çarkçı E, Polat AE, Gürpınar T. The frequency of reduction loss after arthroscopic fixation of acute acromioclavicular dislocations using a double-button device, and its effect on clinical and radiological results. J Orthop Surg Res. 2020;15(1):136.
23. Ozcafer R, Albayrak K, Lapcin O, Cetinkaya E, Arikan Y, Gul M. Early clinical and radiographic results of fixation with the TightRope device for Rockwood type V acromioclavicular joint dislocation: a retrospective review of 15 patients. Acta Orthop Traumatol Tur. 2020;54:473–7.
24. Wang Y-C, Yong MA, Wei-Zhong YU, Wang H. Surgical treatment of acute Rockwood III acromioclavicular dislocations—comparative study between two flip-button techniques. Sci Rep. 2020;10(1):4447.
25. Ruzbarsky JJ, Nolte P-C, Arner JW, Elrick BP, Tross A-K, Millett PJ. Arthroscopic acromioclavicular joint treatment with coracoclavicular fixation and allograft coracoclavicular ligament reconstruction for acute acromioclavicular dislocations. Arthrosc Tech. 2020;9:e1219–25.
26. Liu T, Bao F, Jiang T, Ji G, Li J, Jerosch J. Acromioclavicular joint separation: repair through suture anchors for coracoclavicular ligament and non-absorbable suture fixation for acromioclavicular joint. Orthop Surg. 2020;12:1362–71.
27. Teixeira Ramos J, Silva Gomes D, Quinaz Neto P, Sarmento M, Moura N, Cartucho A. Arthroscopic-assisted acromioclavicular joint dislocation repair: a modified technique for horizontal stabilization using suture anchors. Arthrosc Tech. 2021;10:e283–8.
28. Topal M, Köse A. Surgical management of Rockwood type 3 acromioclavicular joint injuries: a retrospective comparison of outcomes of suture anchor fixation and double-button fixation techniques. Medicine. 2020;99(21):e20312.
29. Hachem A, Rondanelli R, Costa G, Verdalet I, Ezzeddine H, Rius X. Arthroscopically assisted comprehensive double cerclage suture fixation technique for acute acromioclavicular joint separation. Arthrosc Tech. 2020;9:e1495–504.
30. Dyrna F, Imhoff FB, Haller B, Braun S, Obopilwe E, Apostolakos JM, et al. Primary stability of an acromioclavicular joint repair is affected by the type of additional reconstruction of the acromioclavicular capsule. Am J Sports Med. 2018;46:3471–9.
31. Galasso O, Tarducci L, de Benedetto M, Orlando N, Mercurio M, Gasparini G, et al. Modified Weaver-Dunn procedure for type 3 acromioclavicular joint dislocation: functional and radiological outcomes. Orthop J Sports Med. 2020;8(3):232596712090502.
32. Ranne JO, Kainonen TU, Lehtinen JT, Kanto KJ, Vastamäki HA, Kukkonen MK, et al. Arthroscopic coracoclavicular ligament reconstruction of chronic acromioclavicular dislocations using autogenous semitendinosus graft: a two-year follow-up study of 58 patients. Arthrosc Sports Med Rehab. 2020;2:e7–15.
33. Wood T, Rosell P, Clasper J. Preliminary results of the "surgiligtm" synthetic ligament in the management of chronic acromioclavicular joint disruption. J Royal Army Med Corps. 2009;155:191–3.
34. Yeranosian M, Rangarajan R, Bastian S, Blout C, Patel V, Lee B, et al. Anatomic reconstruction of acromioclavicular joint dislocations using allograft and synthetic ligament. JSES Int. 2020;4:515–8.
35. Romano AM, Casillo P, de Simone M, Nastrucci G, Risorto D, Susanna M, et al. The infinity-lock system for chronic grade III AC joint dislocation: a novel technique, rehabilitation protocol and short term results. J Clin Med. 2020;9(8):2519.
36. Cano-Martínez JA, Nicolás-Serrano G, Bento-Gerard J, Marín FP, Grau JA, Antón ML. Chronic acromioclavicular dislocations: multidirectional stabilization without grafting. JSES Int. 2020;4:519–31.

Calcific Tendinopathy of the Rotator Cuff in Adults: Operative Versus Nonoperative Management

3

E. Carlos Rodríguez-Merchán, Hortensia De la Corte-Rodríguez, Carlos A. Encinas-Ullán, and Primitivo Gómez-Cardero

3.1 Introduction

Rotator cuff calcific tendinitis (RCCT) is a frequent pathologic condition affecting the rotator cuff, principally happening in women in their forties [1–3]. Commonly, patients complain of a low-degree subacute shoulder pain augmenting during the night [3]. Plain radiography and ultrasound (US) are the imaging tests of choice [4], permitting easy identification of focal calcium depositions in the RC tendons, mainly in the supraspinatus (80%) and less commonly in the infraspinatus and subscapularis tendons (15% and 5% of all cases, respectively) [2].

Conversely, magnetic resonance imaging (MRI) is not usually indicated in this setting due to the well-known limitations of this imaging technique in the assessment of RCCT, even though it is considered the crucial imaging test to exclude other pathologic conditions of the shoulder [5–7]. RCCT is a self-limiting condition that can be completely asymptomatic in chronic stage and not in need of management. Nevertheless, in some cases, it can represent a painful and disabling condition, especially when considering the acute stage [3]. Discomfort intensity affects the selected management: conservative (rehabilitation medicine and oral anti-inflammatory medication) if pain is mild or more invasive (shock waves, surgery, and imaging-guided irrigation) when symptoms are more severe. Shock wave lithotripsy was shown to be not always resolving [8], and, at present, there is no standard of care for RCCT [1, 9].

Over the last years, US-guided percutaneous irrigation of calcific tendinopathy (US-PICT) has become more and more universally utilized [10] because of its minimal invasiveness compared to surgery and its radical impact on calcifications in comparison to shock waves, since mineralized deposits are disaggregated and removed outside the tendon [11, 12]. Moreover, it has been previously reported how US-PICT makes easier rapid shoulder function recovery and pain alleviation [13]. The technique is usually carried out with 16- to 21-gauge needles under local anesthesia. It is shown that even interventional or minor surgical techniques may be associated with a significant psychological burden in patients, possibly producing discomfort and anxiety [14].

The purpose of this chapter is to analyze recent literature evaluating the clinical outcomes of nonoperative and operative treatment for calcific tendinopathy of the shoulder.

E. C. Rodríguez-Merchán (✉) · C. A. Encinas-Ullán
P. Gómez-Cardero
Department of Orthopedic Surgery, "La Paz" University Hospital-IdiPaz, Madrid, Spain

H. De la Corte-Rodríguez
Department of Physical Medicine and Rehabilitation, "La Paz" University Hospital-IdiPaz, Madrid, Spain

E. C. Rodríguez-Merchán, A. Moreno-Garcìa (eds.), *Controversies in Orthopedic Surgery of The Upper Limb*, https://doi.org/10.1007/978-3-031-04907-1_3

3.2 Pathogenesis

In 2020 Cho et al. identified differentially expressed genes associated with extracellular matrix degradation and inflammatory regulation in calcific tendinopathy utilizing RNA sequencing [15]. They identified 202 differentially expressed genes (DEGs) between calcific and adjacent normal tendon tissues of rotator cuff using RNA sequencing-based transcriptome analysis. The DEGs were highly enriched in extracellular matrix (ECM) degradation and inflammation-related processes. Further, matrix metalloproteinase 9 (MMP9) and matrix metalloproteinase 13 (MMP13), two of the enzymes associated with ECM degradation, were encountered to be highly upregulated 25.85- and 19.40-fold, respectively, in the calcific tendon tissues compared to the adjacent normal tendon tissues. Histopathological analyses indicated collagen degradation and macrophage infiltration at the sites of calcific deposit in the rotator cuff tendon. This study could help to better understand the pathogenesis associated with calcific tendinopathy [15].

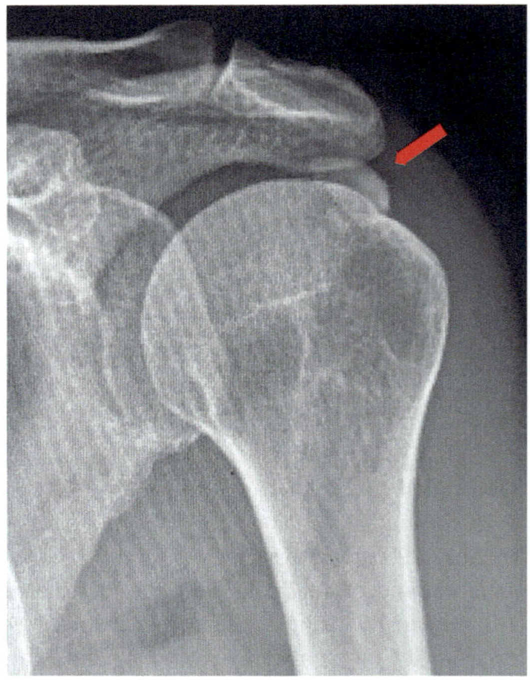

Fig. 3.1 Anteroposterior radiograph showing calcific tendinitis (arrow)

3.3 Imaging

RCCT has a typical imaging presentation: in most cases, calcific deposits appear as a dense opacity around the humeral head on conventional radiography (Fig. 3.1), as hyperechoic foci with or without acoustic shadow at ultrasound and as a signal void at magnetic resonance imaging (Fig. 3.2) [16]. Nonetheless, we have to take into account the possible unusual presentations of RCCT and the key imaging features to correctly differentiate RCCT from other RC conditions, such as calcific enthesopathy or RC tears. Other presentations of RCCT to be considered are intrabursal, intraosseous, and intramuscular migration of calcific deposits that may mimic infectious processes or malignancies. While intrabursal and intraosseous migration are quite common, intramuscular migration is an unusual evolution of RCCT. It is important also to know atypical regions affected by calcific tendinopathy as biceps brachii, pectoralis major, and deltoid tendons [16].

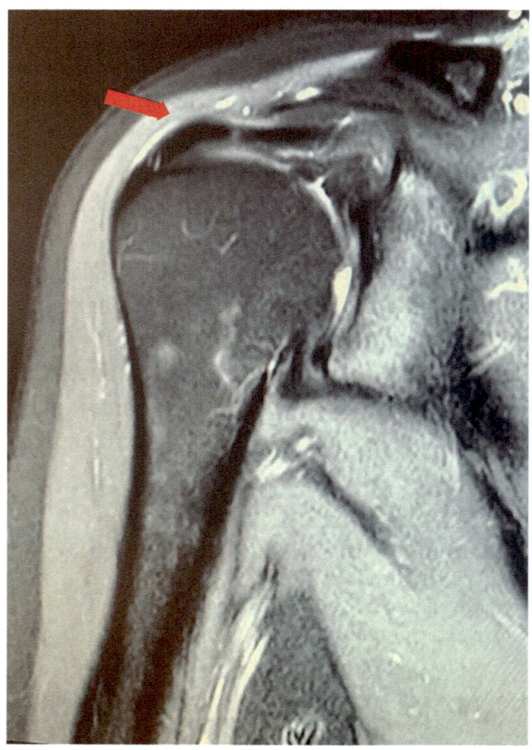

Fig. 3.2 Magnetic resonance imaging (MRI) showing calcific tendinitis (arrow)

An important question is to know whether MRI of the shoulder is ever appropriate in assessing patients with calcific tendinopathy of the rotator cuff. According to Beckmann et al., a shoulder MRI might be carried out for preoperative planning prior to surgical removal of calcium deposits, but even in this patient population, the prevalence of full-thickness rotator cuff tear is low [17].

In 2021, Laucis et al. compared the prevalence of rotator cuff (RC) tears on shoulder ultrasounds of patients with RC calcific tendinopathy (CaT) to that of a control group without CaT [18]. RC tears were diagnosed in 38% (19/50) of the control group (16 full-thickness) as compared to 22% (11/50) with CaT (6 full-thickness). The fewer full-thickness tears in the CaT group (12%, 6 of 50) compared to that in the control group (32%, 16 of 50) was statistically significant (P = 0.016, odds ratio 0.29). Only 7 of the 11 tears in the CaT group were in a calcium-containing tendon (3 full-thickness). The fewer calcium-containing tendon tears compared to tears in the control group was also statistically significant (P = 0.006, odds ratio 0.27). Moreover, the fewer full-thickness calcium-containing tendon tears (6%, 3/50) compared to full-thickness tears in the control group (32%, 16/50) were yet more statistically significant (P = 0.001, odds ratio 0.14). In patients with shoulder pain and CaT, Laucis et al. observed a decreased number of RC tears and especially calcium containing tendon tears, as compared to similar demographic patients with shoulder pain but without CaT [18].

In 2019, Beckman et al. compared the incidence of rotator cuff tears in the setting of calcific tendinopathy on MRI (a case controlled comparison) [19]. They found that patients presenting with indeterminate shoulder pain and rotator cuff calcific tendinopathy were not at augmented risk for having a rotator cuff tear compared with similar demographic patients without calcific tendinopathy presenting with shoulder pain. It appeared that calcific tendinopathy and rotator cuff tears likely arise from different pathological processes [19].

3.4 Treatment

According to Beckmann et al., in most cases, calcific tendinopathy is a self-limited process, typically resolving within a few weeks or months [17]. During this period, conservative treatment with nonsteroidal anti-inflammatory drugs, rehabilitation medicine, warm compresses, and possibly a corticosteroid injection into the subacromial bursa can be administered for symptomatic pain alleviation. Around 10% of patients with calcific tendinopathy will have protracted symptoms that are refractory to conservative treatment. Even in this population of patients with calcific tendinopathy and failed conservative treatment, the prevalence of full-thickness tear remains low. Extracorporeal shockwave therapy and ultrasound-guided needle techniques are efficacious in alleviating pain and resolving the calcium deposits in chronic calcific tendinopathy of the rotator cuff that has failed initial conservative management These treatments are minimally invasive and involve mostly minor complications of soreness, local bruising/ swelling, and subcutaneous hemorrhage, which happen in 10% of patients treated with ultrasound-guided needle techniques and 7%–19% of patients treated with extracorporeal shockwave therapy. Surgical removal of the calcium deposits of calcific tendinopathy is also efficacious in diminishing pain and ameliorating function by utilizing either arthroscopic or open techniques. Nonetheless, surgery is expensive and requires exposure to anesthesia and a longer recovery period compared with other less invasive treatments. For these reasons, surgery should be indicated in patients who have protracted, activity-limiting pain and have failed initial conservative and minimally invasive treatments. In this select population of patients with chronic calcific tendinopathy and prolonged refractory pain being considered for surgical removal of the calcifications, shoulder MRI may be warranted for preoperative planning [17].

3.4.1 Ultrasound-Guided Percutaneous Irrigation of Rotator Cuff Calcific Tendinopathy (US-PICT)

In 2020, Albano et al. assessed patients' experience of US-PICT. They found that US-PICT was a mildly painful, comfortable, and well-tolerated technique, regardless of any previous treatments. Patients' satisfaction was correlated with clinical benefit and full explanation of the technique and its complications [20].

3.4.1.1 US-Guided Percutaneous Irrigation of Calcific Tendinopathy of the Rotator Cuff in Patients with or Without Previous External Shockwave Therapy

In 2021, Lanza et al. compared the outcome of US-PICT of the rotator cuff in patients with or without previous external shockwave therapy (ESWT) [21]. They found that US-PICT of the rotator cuff was an efficacious technique to diminish shoulder pain and augment mobility in patients with calcific tendinopathy, both in short- and long-run time intervals. Previous unsuccessful ESWT did not affect the result of US-PICT.

3.4.1.2 Efficacy of Ultrasound-Guided Percutaneous Treatment of the Rotator Cuff Calcific Tendinopathy with Double Needle Technique

According to Saba et al., US-PICT with double needle was a dependable and reproducible procedure for treatment of the RCCT and their clinical symptoms, when conservative treatment was insufficient [22]. Only patients with calcification at least 5 mm in size with and with acute pain and functional limitation were selected. All patients had a shoulder radiograph to compare it with posttreatment. The patient was placed supine and disinfected profusely. Then percutaneous local anesthesia (Lidocaine 10 mg/mL) was carried out utilizing 25-gauge (G) needle, along the path chosen for the treatment and for both needles. Then, two 18 G needles were introduced into the calcification, with the first needle that must be inserted in a deep position. With a 20 mL syringe prefilled with saline and lidocaine (the irrigation of the calcification could be painful), pressure was applied to one of the two needles. It is possible to insert a 20 G needle into each needle to remove calcium that may obstruct needle tips. During the technique, the needle can also be moved to other areas to be treated, depending on the size and shape of the calcification. The duration of the treatment depended on the size and the hardness of the calcification. After the destruction of the calcification, the fragments pushed by the physiological solution were able to exit by from the other needle positioned inside the calcification creating a washing circuit. Finally, infiltration into the subacromial-subdeltoid bursa (SASD) with cortisone (Betamethasone dipropionate 1 mL) was performed [22].

3.4.1.3 US-PICT: Redefining Predictors of Treatment Outcome

In 2020, Vassalou et al., tried to identify prognostic factors affecting the clinical result in patients treated with rotator cuff US-PICT, by assessing the grade of calcium removal, the size and consistency of calcific deposits, and baseline level of shoulder pain and functionality [23]. The conclusion was that large calcifications and low-grade pain at baseline are correlated with short- and long-run pain amelioration. The grade of calcium removal did not impact pain or functional improvement beyond 1 week. Augmented calcification size, cystic appearance, and low-grade baseline pain predicted complete pain recovery at 1 year [23].

3.4.2 External Shock Wave Therapy (ESWT)

3.4.2.1 Focused, Radial, and Combined ESWT

A study with level 1 evidence (randomized control study) compared the clinical, functional, and ultrasonographic results of focused, radial, and combined ESWT in the management of calcific shoulder tendinopathy [24]. In the three studied groups, there was a significant amelioration in shoulder pain, active range of motion (ROM), and shoulder function by shoulder disability questionnaire (SDQ) at 1 week after the end of treatment and after 3 months follow-up. Furthermore, there was a significant sonographic reduction in calcification size in the three groups. At the end of the study, the best improvement as regards a decrease of calcification size was obtained in group III when compared with group I and group II. This study demonstrated clinical, functional, and sonographic improvement in all groups. The best therapy in calcific shoulder tendinopathy seemed to be combined focused and radial ESWT compared to interventions alone [24].

3.4.2.2 Effectiveness of Focused Shockwave Therapy Versus Radial Shockwave Therapy for Noncalcific Rotator Cuff Tendinopathies: A Randomized Clinical Trial

A randomized clinical trial, registered with ChiCTR1900022932, compared the effectiveness of focused shockwave therapy (F-SWT) versus radial shockwave therapy (R-SWT) for the treatment of noncalcific rotator cuff tendinopathies [25]. The conclusion was that both F-SWT and R-SWT were efficacious in patients with noncalcific rotator cuff tendinopathy. F-SWT proved to be significantly superior to R-SWT at long-run follow-up (more than 24 weeks).

3.4.3 Platelet-Rich Plasma (PRP)

In 2019, Kim et al. studied the effect of PRP on the degenerative rotator cuff tendinopathy according to the compositions [26]. They found that TGF-β1 and IL-1β among cellular components of PRP were related to clinical efficacy for RC tendinopathy, and concentration of IL-1β above 5.19 pg/mL and TGF-β1 above 61.79 μg/mL in PRP had better clinical results for RC tendinopathy than the exercise group. Patients were in supine position with their arms placed on the superior aspect of the iliac wing with the palm up and the elbow flexed. Kim et al. found the long head of biceps in the intertubercular groove transversely via ultrasound. After lining the probe along the long axis of biceps tendon, the probe was moved to the supraspinatus tendon in a parallel position. After finding the hypoechoic lesion, 2 mL of PRP solution was injected to the hypoechoic lesion of degenerative supraspinatus via 22-gauge syringe with peppering technique. Peppering technique was utilized to avoid tendon morphology disruption by injecting PRP into the tendon. The remaining 1 mL of PRP solution was used in analyzing the compositions of PRP [26].

3.4.4 Needle Aspiration

In 2020, Oudelaar et al. tried to identify prognostic factors for the effectiveness of needle aspiration of calcific deposits (NACD) for RCCT [27]. They found that a good initial response after NACD was associated with better results at 12 months. Patients with a longer duration of symptoms before NACD and patients who needed multiple procedures showed inferior results in terms of pain reduction and amelioration of quality of life. Smaller-size calcific deposits were associated with a less favorable result of shoulder function and quality of life scores and might therefore be less susceptible for NACD [27].

3.4.5 Dextrose Prolotherapy

In 2020, Catapano et al. systematically reviewed and assessed the efficacy and complication profile of prolotherapy using hyperosmolar dextrose solution injection for rotator cuff tendinopathy [28]. They found that prolotherapy with hyperosmolar dextrose solution was a potentially efficacious adjuvant intervention to rehabilitation medicine for patients with rotator cuff tendinopathy ranging from tendinosis to partial-thickness and small full-thickness tears. However, Catapano et al. stated that further studies were necessary to determine effects in subpopulations as well as optimal technique including dextrose concentration, volume, and location [28].

3.4.6 Sodium Thiosulfate

A study (clinical trial registration number NCT02538939) reported in 2020 assessed the tolerance and the feasibility of sodium thiosulfate (STS) lavage of calcific tendinopathy [29]. Overall, STS was well tolerated with no side effect occurring during the technique and the follow-up. Nonetheless, no significant effect on calcium disappearance could be shown compared with what is expected without STS. Darrieutort-Laffite et al. stated that new studies utilizing larger volume and repeated injections of STS were needed.

3.4.7 Surgical Treatment

Surgery should be reserved for patients who have protracted, activity-limiting pain and have failed initial conservative and minimally invasive treatments. In this select population of patients with chronic calcific tendinopathy and prolonged refractory pain being considered for surgical removal of the calcifications, shoulder MRI may be warranted for preoperative planning [30].

Surgical treatment is commonly considered if symptoms persist for more than 6 months after the start of nonoperative treatment [31]. Surgical intervention is undertaken in roughly 10% of patients, who have failed nonoperative treatment [32]. Operative management can be pursued via an arthroscopic or open approach. The open approach has been used historically but has a limited role with evolutions in arthroscopic techniques and training [31].

In the arthroscopic approach, calcium deposits are identified as a bulge within the tendon often with increased vascular patterns [33]. The tendon is commonly incised in a longitudinal manner to avoid rotator cuff tears and retraction and with the assistance of a cannula to minimize distribution of small calcification deposits [34, 35]. Effective needling of the calcification is confirmed when a snowstorm-like effect is seen in the space [34]. Additional shoulder pathologies can be addressed at the same time arthroscopically.

There have been sparse prospective randomized trials studying the effect of arthroscopic treatment on patient-reported results in patients with calcific tendinopathy of the shoulder. In a study by Sabeti et al. [36], the efficacy of arthroscopic treatment in 20 patients at 9 months after treatment was assessed. Constant and visual analog scale (VAS) pain scores significantly improved ($p < 0.01$). In a different study, Clement et al. [37] assessed the efficacy of arthroscopic treatment alone and arthroscopic treatment with subacromial decompression in 80 patients at 12 months after treatment. There was a statistically significant improvement in Constant and VAS pain scores for both groups ($p < 0.001$) but no statistical difference between them ($p > 0.05$).

Rompe et al. [38] and Rebuzzi et al. [39] investigated ESWT compared to arthroscopy for the treatment of calcific tendinopathy and found similar improvements between the two treatment methods. While arthroscopic treatment can provide patients relief, it is only recommended after failure of all other treatments given its invasiveness compared to ESWT and US-PICT. Controversy remains regarding the optimal methods for surgical management of calcific tendinitis. There is debate about removing all deposits versus leaving some deposits or whether or not the created tendon defect should be repaired.

In a study by Ark et al. [34], the authors concluded that complete removal of the deposits is not necessary after 12 of 14 patients obtained significant pain relief with residual calcium deposits evident on postoperative radiographs. Repair of the defects created from removal of the deposits was not performed. Alternatively, Jerosch et al. [40] suggested that complete removal of the deposits is necessary, but repair of defects afterward is not. In another study by Porcellini et al. [41], 63 patients who underwent arthroscopic debridement by one surgeon were analyzed. It was deemed that complete removal of the deposits and repair of the defects was appropriate. The authors stated that repair of the defects decreased the chance of further propagation of the tear and aids inpatient rehabilitation.

3.5 Comparative Studies

3.5.1 Operative Versus Nonoperative Management

According to Bechay et al., conservative treatment, ESWT, US-PICT, and operative management have all been found to be beneficial in the treatment of symptomatic calcific tendinopathy. Conservative management is very effective for most patients and should be the first line of treatment. In patients who fail conservative management, ESWT or US-PICT is often effective and should be the next step in treatment. Surgery should be reserved for patients who have failed these other modalities of treatment [30].

3.5.2 Radial ESWT Versus Ultrasound Therapy

Dedes et al. investigated the intensity of pain, the functionality of the upper limbs, and the quality of life of patients with rotator cuff tendinopathy by using two different therapeutic modalities, shockwave and ultrasound, whose results were evaluated pretreatment and posttreatment as well as after a 4-week follow-up [42]. The pain intensity was diminished, and both the functionality and quality of life were ameliorated after shockwave therapy posttreatment ($p < 0.001$) and at a 4-week follow-up ($p < 0.001$) compared with those found after the treatment. Similar improvements in all three parameters were also found after ultrasound treatment, but the results were not as pronounced as in the shockwave group. In conclusion, both radial shockwave and ultrasound therapies were found to be effective in the treatment of rotator cuff tendinopathy, the statistical analysis showing that radial shockwave therapy was superior to the ultrasound therapy posttreatment and at the 4-week follow-up [42].

3.5.3 Comparing Ultrasound-Guided Needling Combined with a Subacromial Corticosteroid Versus High-Energy ESWT

In a randomized controlled trial (level II of evidence), Louwerens et al. compared clinical and radiographic results after treatment with standardized high-energy ESWT and ultrasound-guided needling (UGN) in patients with symptomatic calcific tendinitis of the rotator cuff who were nonresponsive to conservative treatment [43]. Both techniques were successful in improving function and pain, with high satisfaction rates after 1-year follow-up. However, UGN was more effective in eliminating the calcific deposit, and the amount of additional treatments was greater in the ESWT group.

3.5.4 Comparison of Radial Extracorporeal Shockwave Therapy and Traditional Rehabilitation Medicine

A study investigated the efficacy of radial extracorporeal shockwave therapy (rESWT) in alleviating pain and ameliorating ROM and functionality besides conventional rehabilitation methods in the treatment of RCCT [44]. Duymaz and Sindel studied 80 patients (35 males, 45 females; mean age 53.3 years; range, 40–70 years) with chronic RCCT. Patients were randomly divided into two groups: rESWT group ($n = 40$) treated with conventional physiotherapy and rESWT and control group ($n = 40$) treated only with a conventional rehabilitation program. The traditional rehabilitation medicine program included ultrasound, transcutaneous electrical nerve stimulation, shoulder joint ROM and stretching exercises, and ice applications. All patients received a total of 20 treatments, 5 days a week for 4 weeks. rESWT was applied once a week for 4 weeks in total. Before and after treatment, all patients were assessed for age, height, weight, body mass index (BMI), pain intensity with a visual analog scale, shoulder ROM, and functional disability status with the shortened version of the Disabilities of the Arm, Shoulder and Hand questionnaire (QuickDASH). Mean BMI value of the participants was 26.1 kg/m^2. Although all parameters of the patients in both groups improved significantly, patients in the rESWT group had a statistically significant improvement in pain, ROM, and QuickDASH scores ($p < 0.001$, $p < 0.001$, and $p < 0.001$, respectively). The conclusion was that rESWT was an effective and noninvasive method of reducing pain and increasing ROM and functional status without the need for surgery [44].

3.6 Conclusions

In most cases, calcific tendinopathy is a self-limited process, typically resolving within a few weeks or months. During this period, conservative treatment with nonsteroidal anti-inflammatory drugs, rehabilitation medicine, warm compresses, and possibly a corticosteroid injection into the subacromial bursa can be administered for symptomatic pain alleviation. About 10% of patients with calcific tendinopathy will have protracted symptoms that are refractory to conservative treatment. Even in this population of patients with calcific tendinopathy and failed conservative management, the prevalence of full-thickness tear remains low. Extracorporeal shockwave therapy and ultrasound-guided needle techniques are efficacious in alleviating pain and resolving the calcium deposits in chronic calcific tendinopathy of the rotator cuff that has failed initial conservative treatment. These treatments are minimally invasive and involve mostly minor complications of soreness, local bruising/ swelling, and subcutaneous hemorrhage, which occur in 10% of patients treated with ultrasound-guided needle techniques and 7%–19% of patients treated with extracorporeal shockwave therapy. Surgical removal of the calcium deposits of calcific tendinopathy is also efficacious in decreasing pain and improving function by using either arthroscopic or open techniques. However, surgery comes at greater cost, exposure to anesthesia and a longer recovery period compared with other less-invasive treatments. For these reasons, surgery should be reserved for patients who have protracted, activity-limiting pain and have failed initial conservative and minimally invasive treatments.

References

1. Chianca V, Albano D, Messina M, Midiri F, Mauri G, Aliprandi A, et al. Rotator cuff calcific tendinopathy: from diagnosis to treatment. Acta Biomed. 2018;89(Suppl 1):186–96.
2. Uhthoff HK, Sarkar K. Calcifying tendinitis. Baillière's. Clin Rheumatol. 1989;3:567–81.
3. Mole D, Gonzalvez M, Roche O, Scarlat M. Introduction to calcifying tendinitis. In: Gazielly DF, Gleyze P, Thomas T, editors. The cuff. Paris: Elsevier; 1997. p. 141–3.
4. Sconfienza LM, Albano D, Allen G, Bazzocchi A, Bignotti B, Chianca V, et al. Clinical indications for musculoskeletal ultrasound updated in 2017 by European Society of Musculoskeletal Radiology (ESSR) consensus. Eur Radiol. 2018;28:5338–51.
5. Albano D, Chianca V, Zappia M, Russo R, Romano S, Sconfienza LM, et al. Imaging of usual and unusual complication of rotator cuff repair. J Comput Assist Tomogr. 2019;43:359–66.
6. Bellelli A, Silvestri E, Barile A, Albano D, Aliprandi A, Caudana R, et al. Position paper on magnetic resonance imaging protocols in the musculoskeletal system (excluding the spine) by the Italian College of Musculoskeletal Radiology. Radiol Med. 2019;124:522–38.
7. Albano D, Messina C, Sconfienza LM. Posterior shoulder instability: what to look for. Magn Reson Imaging Clin N Ame. 2020;28:211–21.
8. Hurt G, Baker CL Jr. Calcific tendinitis of the shoulder. Orthop Clin N Am. 2003;34:567–75.
9. Hsu CJ, Wang DY, Tseng KF, Fong YC, Hsu HC, Jim YF. Extracorporeal shock wave therapy for calcifying tendinitis of the shoulder. J Shoulder Elb Surg. 2008;17:55–9.
10. Silvestri E, Barile A, Albano D, Messina C, Orlandi D, Corazza A, et al. Interventional therapeutic procedures in the musculoskeletal system: an Italian survey by the Italian College of Musculoskeletal Radiology. Radiol Med. 2018;123:314–21.
11. Messina C, Sconfienza LM. Ultrasound-guided percutaneous irrigation of calcific tendinopathy. Semin Musculoskelet Radiol. 2016;20:409–13.

12. Albano D, Vicentin I, Messina C, Sconfienza LM. Post-surgical Achilles calcific tendinopathy treated with ultrasound guided percutaneous irrigation. Skelet Radiol. 2020;49:1475–80.
13. Serafini G, Sconfienza LM, Lacelli L, Silvestri E, Aliprandi A, Sardanelli F. Rotator cuff calcific tendonitis: short-term and 10-year outcomes after two-needle US guided percutaneous treatment–nonrandomized controlled trial. Radiology. 2009;252:157–64.
14. Verstraelen FU, Fievez E, Janssen L, Morrenhof W. Surgery for calcifying tendinitis of the shoulder: a systematic review. World J Orthop. 2017;8:424–30.
15. Cho N, Lee SG, Kim JO, Kim YA, Kim EM, Park C, et al. Identification of differentially expressed genes associated with extracellular matrix degradation and inflammatory regulation in calcific tendinopathy using RNA sequencing. Calcif Tissue Int. 2020;107:489–98.
16. Albano D, Coppola A, Gitto S, Rapisarda S, Messina C, Sconfienza LM. Imaging of calcific tendinopathy around the shoulder: usual and unusual presentations and common pitfalls. Radiol Med. 2021;126:608–19.
17. Beckmann NM. Editorial commentary: is magnetic resonance imaging of the shoulder ever appropriate in evaluating patients with calcific tendinopathy of the rotator cuff? Arthroscopy. 2020;36:991–2.
18. Laucis NC, Rosen KA, Thodge A, Leschied JR, Klochko CL, Soliman SB. Sonographic evaluation of the association between calcific tendinopathy and rotator cuff tear: a case-controlled comparison. Clin Rheumatol. 2021;40:2897–905.
19. Beckman NM, Tran MQ, Cai C. Incidence of rotator cuff tears in the setting of calcific tendinopathy on MRI: a case controlled comparison. Skelet Radiol. 2019;48:245–50.
20. Albano D, Gambino A, Messina C, Chianca V, Gitto S, Faenza S, et al. Ultrasound-guided percutaneous irrigation of rotator cuff calcific tendinopathy (US-PICT): patient experience. BioMed Res Intl. 2020:3086395.
21. Lanza E, Piccoli F, Intrieri C, Muglia R, Politi LS, Borroni M, et al. US-guided percutaneous irrigation of calcific tendinopathy of the rotator cuff in patients with or without previous external shockwave therapy. Radiol Med. 2021;126:117–23.
22. Saba L, De Filippo M, Saba F, Fellini F, Marcy PY, Dagan R, et al. Efficacy of ultrasound-guided percutaneous treatment of the rotator cuff calcific tendinopathy with double needle technique. J Orthop. 2020;20:195–7.
23. Vassalou EE, Klontzas ME, Plagou AP, Karantanas AH. Ultrasound-guided percutaneous irrigation of calcific tendinopathy: redefining predictors of treatment outcome. Eur Radiol. 2021;31:2634–43.
24. Al-Kahir MAB, El Khouly RM, Khodair SA, Elsergany MAAS, Hussein MI, Mowafi MEE. Focused, radial and combined shock wave therapy in treatment of calcific shoulder tendinopathy. Phys Sportsmed. 2021;49:480–7.
25. Li C, Li Z, Shi L, Wang P, Gao F, Sun W. Effectiveness of focused shockwave therapy versus radial shockwave therapy for noncalcific rotator cuff tendinopathies: a randomized clinical trial. Biomed Res Int. 2021;2021:6687094.
26. Kim SJ, Yeo SM, Noh SJ, Ha CW, Lee BC, Lee HS, et al. Effect of platelet-rich plasma on the degenerative rotator cuff tendinopathy according to the compositions. J Orthop Surg Res. 2019;14:408.
27. Oudelaar BW, Veld RHI, Schepers-Bok R, Ooms EM, Nelissen RGHH, Vochteloo AJH. Prognostic factors for the outcome of needle aspiration of calcific deposits for rotator cuff calcific tendinitis. Eur Radiol. 2020;30:4082–90.
28. Catapano M, Zhang K, Mittal M, Sangha H, Onishi K, de Sa D. Effectiveness of dextrose prolotherapy for rotator cuff tendinopathy: a systematic review. PM R. 2020;12:288–300.
29. Darrieurtort-Laffite C, Bertrand-Vasseur A, Garraud T, Planche L, Le Goff B. Tolerance and effect of sodium thiosulfate in calcific tendinitis of the rotator cuff. Clin Rheumatol. 2020;39:561–9.
30. Bechay J, Lawrence C, Namdari S. Calcific tendinopathy of the rotator cuff: a review of operative versus nonoperative management. Phys Sportsmed. 2020;48:241–6.
31. Sansone V, Maiorano E, Galluzzo A, Pascale V. Calcific tendinopathy of the shoulder: clinical perspectives into the mechanisms, pathogenesis, and treatment. Orthop Res Rev. 2018;10:63–72.
32. Lam F, Bhatia D, van Rooyen K, et al. Modern management of calcifying tendinitis of the shoulder. Curr Orthop. 2006;20:446–52.
33. ElShewy MT. Calcific tendinitis of the rotator cuff. World J Orthop. 2016;7(1):55.
34. Ark JW, Flock TJ, Flatow EL, Bigliani LU. Arthroscopic treatment of calcific tendinitis of the shoulder. Arthroscopy. 1992;8:183–8.
35. Seil R, Litzenburger H, Kohn D, Rupp S. Arthroscopic treatment of chronically painful calcifying tendinitis of the supraspinatus tendon. Arthroscopy. 2006;22:521–7.
36. Sabeti M, Schmidt M, Ziai P, Graf A, Nemecek E, Schueller-Weidekamm. C the intraoperative use of ultrasound facilitates significantly the arthroscopic debridement of calcific rotator cuff tendinitis. Arch Orthop Trauma Surg. 2014;134:651–6.
37. Clement N, Watts A, Phillips C, McBirnie JM. Short-term outcome after arthroscopic bursectomy debridement of rotator cuff calcific tendonopathy with and without subacromial decompression: a prospective randomized controlled trial. Arthroscopy. 2015;31:1680–7.
38. Rompe JD, Zoellner J, Nafe B. Shock wave therapy versus conventional surgery in the treatment of calcifying tendonitis of the shoulder. Clin Orthop Relat Res. 2001;387:72–82.
39. Rebuzzi E, Coletti N, Schiavetti S, Giusto F. Arthroscopy surgery versus shock wave therapy for chronic calcifying tendinitis of the shoulder. J Orthop Traumatol. 2008;9:179–85.

40. Jerosch J, Strauss JM, Schmiel S. Arthroscopic treatment of calcific tendonitis of the shoulder. Rev Cuba Ortop y Traumatol. 2017;31:118–30.
41. Porcellini G, Paladini P, Campi F, Paganelli M. Arthroscopic treatment of calcifying tendinitis of the shoulder : clinical and ultrasonographic follow-up findings at two to five years. J Shoulder Elb Surg. 2004;13:503–8.
42. Dedes V, Tzirogiannis K, Polikandrioti M, Dede AM, Nikolaidis C, Mitseas A, et al. Comparison of radial extracorporeal shockwave therapy versus ultrasound therapy in the treatment of rotator cuff tendinopathy. Folia Med. 2019;61:612–9.
43. Louwerens JKG, Sierevelt IN, Kramer ET, Boonstra R, van dem Bekerom MPJ, van Royen BJ, et al. Comparing ultrasound-guided needling combined with a subacromial corticosteroid injection versus high-energy extracorporeal shockwave therapy for calcific tendinitis of the rotator cuff: a randomized controlled trial. Arthroscopy. 2020:36:1823-33e1.
44. Duymaz T, Sindel D. Comparison of radial extracorporeal shock wave therapy and traditional physiotherapy in rotator cuff calcific tendinitis treatment. Arch Rheumatol. 2019;34:281–7.

Recurrent Anterior Shoulder Instability in Adults: Bankart or Latarjet?

4

Raul Barco and E. Carlos Rodríguez-Merchán

4.1 Introduction

Anterior shoulder dislocation is the most common major joint dislocation [1]. Anterior instability represents 90% of all shoulder dislocations [2]. Recurrence is frequent in the younger age groups in certain patterns of injury with bone loss and certain activities mostly overhead or contact sports. These populations represent a challenge to the treating surgeon.

In patients with recurrent shoulder dislocation, a surgical operation may be needed to improve shoulder function. The most reported shoulder surgeries for this problem are the arthroscopic Bankart repair and an open Latarjet procedure [1, 3].

The new technology of implants and techniques make Bankart repair of older studies (before 2000–2004) difficult to compare with more modern studies even though the surgical technique could be considered analogous [4].

It is undisputed that an arthroscopic Bankart repair has a few advantages with respect to the open Bankart technique, mostly less operative time, less morbidity, less postoperative pain, less hospitalization time, and less risk of complications [5].

Most surgeons will use arthroscopic techniques, in part influenced by the preferences of the patients, in part influenced by the exposure they have had during their training, in which they rarely see an open Bankart repair. However, recurrent instability is a frequent complication after an arthroscopic Bankart repair [6].

The Latarjet technique has been popular in France, where it was developed, not so much in the rest of the world. Its use has since expanded favored by the recognition of the importance of bone loss in the genesis of recurrences and its good outcomes in this setting when compared to other techniques [7].

Also, the development of arthroscopic techniques, new modes of fixation, and modifications of the Latarjet technique (including repair of glenohumeral ligaments) may modify the results of this technique and, perhaps, the rate of complications, so the debate is guaranteed to last a few more years [8]. The debate between the choices of techniques is based on the preference and skills of the surgeon more than in the published evidence [7].

It is almost unanimous that in the face of a critical glenoid bone defect (>25%) most surgeons will perform some kind of glenoid bone grafting, typically a Latarjet, but it is not clear what the attitude should be in defects under 25% in what has been termed ambiguously as subcritical or borderline bone defects or even in the absence of a glenoid bone defect [9].

R. Barco · E. C. Rodríguez-Merchán (✉)
Department of Orthopedic Surgery, La Paz University Hospital-IdiPaz, Madrid, Spain

E. C. Rodríguez-Merchán, A. Moreno-Garcìa (eds.), *Controversies in Orthopedic Surgery of The Upper Limb*, https://doi.org/10.1007/978-3-031-04907-1_4

Some surgeons will skew their decision based on the age and type of activity. It has been shown that, in the younger patients and those practicing throwing sports, anteroinferior shoulder instability is a frequent condition [10].

Patients older than 40 years were thought to have less recurrent instability after a Bankart repair, but recent long-term follow-up has shown increased recurrence rate when compared to Latarjet (9 vs 3; $P = 0.037$, in a cohort of 37 shoulders) and without the supposed benefit of decreasing the rate of arthropathy. The mechanism for arthropathy is unknown, but it has been correlated with the number of preoperative dislocations, the time of follow-up, and graft malposition or protruding implants [11].

The best procedure for recurrent anterior instability is yet controversial, and good results can be achieved with most techniques, but analysis of failures can help us guide our decision-making [12].

In this chapter, we will perform a review of available modern literature to try to determine which of the surgical techniques are recommended for treatment of anterior instability of the shoulder.

4.2 Bankart Procedure

4.2.1 Open Bankart Repair

According to Moroder et al. (2015), it was thought that neglected osseous glenoid defects was one of the causes for the high rates of recurrence published after long-term follow-up of open Bankart repair [13]. In a level IV study, the authors hypothesized that, in the absence of an important glenoid defect, an open Bankart repair would obtain a low rate of recurrence, so they examined 47 patients treated with an open Bankart repair. They obtained a double-contrast computed tomography scanning to exclude patients with a significant glenoid bone defect. Forty patients (85.1%) are available for evaluation after minimum follow-up of 20 years (maximum 25 years). Twenty-six (65%) were evaluated using a clinical exam and a bilateral radiograph of the shoulder, and the rest responded to a self-administered questionnaire and a telephone interview. Seven patients (17.5%) reported a recurrence, and in six of them it happened after being asymptomatic for more than 8 years. The mean Western Ontario Shoulder Instability Index (WOSI, See Appendix 1) score was 256.7 points, the mean Rowe score (Table 4.1) was 88.7 points, and the mean Subjective Shoulder Value (SSV) was 90.1%. When comparing it to the contralateral side, the mean range of motion of the operated shoulder was reduced in 4° of flexion, two levels of internal rotation, 5° of internal rotation, 5° of internal rotation in 90° of abduction, 7° of external rotation in neutral, and 7° of external rotation in 90° of abduction. The collective instability arthropathy index was 0.92 and 0.35 for the affected shoulder and the contralateral one, respectively. An open Bankart procedure obtained good results at 20 years of follow-up. However, the rate of recurrence was high, even after excluding patients with significant glenoid defects, and was associated with an increased shoulder-specific activity level [13].

Table 4.1 The Rowe score. The Rowe score was developed to assess postoperative function of the shoulder after instability repair

Function (/50 points)
No limitation in work and sports 50
No limitation in work, mild limitation in sports 35
Mild limitation in work above head and sports 20
Marked limitation and pain 0
Pain (/10 points)
None 10
Mild 5
Severe 0
Stability (/30 points)
No recurrence, subluxation, or apprehension 30
Apprehension when placing arm in certain positions 15
Subluxation (not requiring reduction) 10
Apprehension test positive or notion of instability 0
Mobility (/10 points)[a]
Normal mobility 10
<25% loss of normal ER, IR, and elevation 5
>25% loss of normal ER, IR, and elevation 0
Total (/100 points)
Excellent: 90–100 pts. Good: 75–89 pts. Average: 51–74 pts. Bad: <50 pts.

[a]*ER* External rotation, *IR* Internal rotation

According to Boshan et al., open Bankart repair shows a low rate of complications, and it still is an excellent surgical option for a selected group of patients with risk factors for failure after an arthroscopic Bankart repair, those being a previous history of recurrent instability or ligamentous laxity, concomitant glenoid or humeral bone defects, being a male, having a young age, and practicing contact sports. The authors highlight that controlling risk factors is especially important in patients that are not candidates for glenoid bone augmentation [2].

4.2.2 Arthroscopic Bankart Repair

Balg et al. described in 2007 the Instability Severity Index Score (Table 4.2). They found that a younger age, the use of the shoulder score for contact sports or overhead use, the use of the shoulder for sports competition activities, the association of hyperlaxity, and the presence of Hill-Sachs or glenoid erosion or avulsion were associated with increased failure rates after an arthroscopic Bankart repair [14].

Table 4.2 Instability Severity Index Score. Points are assigned according to the history and clinical exam of the patient and are summed up, the maximum score being 10 with an extreme risk of recurrence. The authors suggest that an isolated arthroscopic Bankart repair is recommended for those patients with less than 3 points

Prognostic factors		Points
Age at surgery (yrs)	≤20	2
	>20	0
Degree of sport participation (preoperative)		
Competitive		2
Recreational or none		0
Type of sport (preoperative)		
Contact or forced overhead		1
Other		0
Shoulder hyperlaxity		
Hyperlaxity (anterior/inferior)		1
Normal		0
Hill-Sachs lesion on AP radiograph		
Visible on external rotation		2
Not visible on external rotation		0
Glenoid loss of contour on AP radiograph		
Loss of contour		2
No lesion		0
Total (max. Points) 10		

Some controversy exists in the ability to predict failure by the ISIS score. Loppini et al. reported failure rates after an arthroscopic Bankart repair of 7% with ISIS scores <3, 14% with an ISIS of 4–6 (hazard ratio 2), and 45% when the ISIS>6 (hazard ratio 9) [15]. Accordingly, Thomazeau et al. published a recurrent rate after an isolated Bankart repair of 10% with an ISIS of <2 and of 35.6% when the ISIS was 3–4 [16]. On the other hand, other authors like Ruiz-Iban et al. found that an ISIS <7 was not predictive of failure, showing recurrence rates of 12.8% with an ISIS <3, 20% with an ISIS of 4–6, the difference not being significant [17, 18].

In 2014, Bouliane et al. evaluated if the ISIS and the WOSI scores could detect patients at risk of failure after an arthroscopic Bankart repair [19]. The authors registered the preoperative ISIS and WOSI scores of 110 patients (87 men, 79%) that underwent an arthroscopic Bankart repair for recurrent anterior glenohumeral instability. The mean age at the time of the intervention was 25.1 years (range 16–61). Patients were telephonically interviewed after 2 years of follow-up to determine if the patients had suffered a recurrent dislocation and to determine the rate of return to sport to preinjury levels. Six patients (5%) have an ISIS >6. One hundred patients (91% of the study population) were available for the interview. Six patients (6%) had a recurrent dislocation, and 28 (28%) did not go back to preinjury sports participation. No patient with dislocation had an ISIS >6. There were no differences in the mean WOSI scores of patients suffering a dislocation and those that did not. However, the ISIS was not associated to a return to preinjury activity [19].

In 2016, Aboalata et al. researched the long-term results of arthroscopic Bankart repair and the risk factors for failure in young patients [10]. They tested the hypotheses that the results of such intervention would be comparable to results of open repair published in the literature. They designed a level 4 evidence (case series) in 180 patients undergoing an arthroscopic Bankart pro-

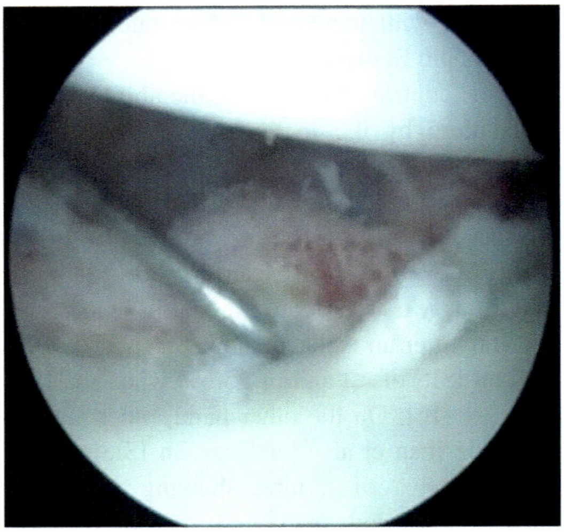

Fig. 4.1 Arthroscopic view of Bankart repair. A view of a Bankart repair performed with suture anchors and a mattress configuration repair is observed. The view is from the posterior portal of a right shoulder in the lateral decubitus position

cedure for recurrent instability that were followed-up for a minimum of 10 years (Fig. 4.1). Of those patients, 143 accepted the participation in this study. One hundred four patients where clinically evaluated using the ASES score, the Constant score, the AAOS score, the Rowe score, and the Dawson 12-pont questionnaire. The Samilson-Prieto classification was used to assess for arthropathy changes in the available radiographs of 100 patients. Additionally, 14 patients were assessed using a specific questionnaire and 24 patients after a telephone interview.

The global rate of redislocation was 18.18%. The rates of redislocation were different according for the different types of fixation: FASTak/Bio-FASTak, 15.1% (17/112); SureTac, 26.3% (5/19); and Panalok, 33.3% (4/12). Concomitant superior labral anterior to posterior (SLAP) repair did not influence the clinical results. The rate of redislocation was significantly altered by the age of the patient and the duration of postoperative rehabilitation. The rate of redislocation also tended toward an increase in cases of more than one dislocation event prior to the intervention. A severe dislocation arthropathy was present in 12% of the shoulders, and these degenerative changes were positively associated with the number of preoperative dislocations, the age of the patients, and the number of anchors. The rate of patient satisfaction with the procedure was 92.3%, and the return to sports was 49.5%. The authors concluded that the long-term results of arthroscopic Bankart repair were comparable to the published results of open Bankart repair with the added benefit of being able to treat concomitant lesions. The authors suggested that stabilization after a first dislocation event produced better clinical and radiological results than waiting for successive shoulder dislocations prior to the operation [10].

Other than recurrent dislocation, other forms of failure have been reported. A specific form of failure after Bankart repair using impacted glenoid anchors is the fracture of the anterior glenoid rim. In 2014, Park et al. reported the incidence of postoperative anterior glenoid rim fractures and the relationship of this fracture with the presence of osteolysis around the implants, the pattern of fracture, the number of anchors, and the amount of postoperative activity [20]. They reviewed the results of 570 patients undergoing an arthroscopic Bankart repair using anchors and found 9 patients, with at least 2-year follow-up, who required a revision for a glenoid rim fracture after a Bankart repair. The mean age of these patients was 28.8 years (range, 18–49) and a mean follow-up of 36.4 years. The mean time between the fracture and the index procedure was 27.3 months. The suture anchors used at the index operation were resorbable (poly-D-Lactic acid, PDLLA) without ceramic osteo-filler (seven cases) or metal (two cases). For revision surgery, PDLLA without ceramic osteo-filler suture anchors were used. Five patients including three and two with bioabsorbable and metal suture anchors, respectively, experienced glenoid rim fracture at more than 2 years postoperatively. Patients showing osteolysis around the initial suture anchor groups showed a higher incidence of glenoid rim fractures compared with the control group. The authors suggested that osteolysis around the anchors may predispose to a glenoid rim fracture, and the use of metal or bioabsorbable suture anchors without ceramic composite implants could be a stress riser at 2 years postoperatively [20].

The rate of recurrent instability may be unacceptable, more so in the event of associated lesions like humeral bone loss, glenoid bone loss, bad quality tissue, or very active young patients. To control some of these risk factors, associated techniques augmenting an arthroscopic Bankart repair have been developed. After elaboration of the ISIS score, Boileau has suggested the use of associated augmentation techniques after a Bankart repair and has suggested the use of an associated Trillat procedure in the presence of isolated hyperlaxity without significant bone loss, an associated remplissage in the presence of an isolated large Hill-Sachs, and an associated Bristow-Latarjet procedure in the presence of a glenoid or combined bone loss [21].

In 2016, Cho et al. compared in a case-control design study (level III evidence) the results of isolated arthroscopic Bankart repair with and without posterior capsulodesis for anterior shoulder instability with engaging Hill-Sachs lesions [22]. Thirty-five shoulders that underwent an isolated Bankart repair were prospectively evaluated and compared to another group of patients with a Bankart repair plus a remplissage (Fig. 4.2). The mean age at the time of surgery was 26.1 and 24.8 years for Bankart and Bankart + remplissage groups, respectively. Both Rowe and UCLA scores improved in both groups. The mean loss of external rotation was 3° and 8° for Bankart and Bankart + Remplissage groups, respectively. There was no loss of strength in any of the patients. The recurrence rate was 25.5% for the Bankart group and 5.4% in the Remplissage group. In conclusion, the addition of a posterior capsulodesis obtained good clinical results with a low recurrence rate at the expense of a minimal loss of external rotation without any loss of strength [22].

According to Camus et al., an arthroscopic remplissage in the presence of a Hill-Sachs lesion is one of the surgical options for the treatment of chronic anterior shoulder instability [23]. These authors performed a literature review comparing the results of isolated Bankart and Bankart with remplissage for patients with shoulder instability and an engaging Hill-Sachs lesion. Their hypothesis was that Bankart + remplissage patients would obtain superior results when compared to an isolated Bankart repair. They performed a meta-analysis of the literature (level III evidence). They identified three comparative studies including 146 patients, 74 of whom underwent an isolated Bankart repair and 72 underwent a Bankart repair with remplissage procedure. The authors found a significant risk of recurrent instability and dislocation after an isolated Bankart repair without differences in the rate of reoperation or the time of return to sport. Both Rowe and UCLA scores were inferior in the isolated Bankart repair group, and the authors concluded that the addition of a remplissage procedure in the presence of an engaging Hill-Sachs lesion and glenoid bone loss of less than 25% was supe-

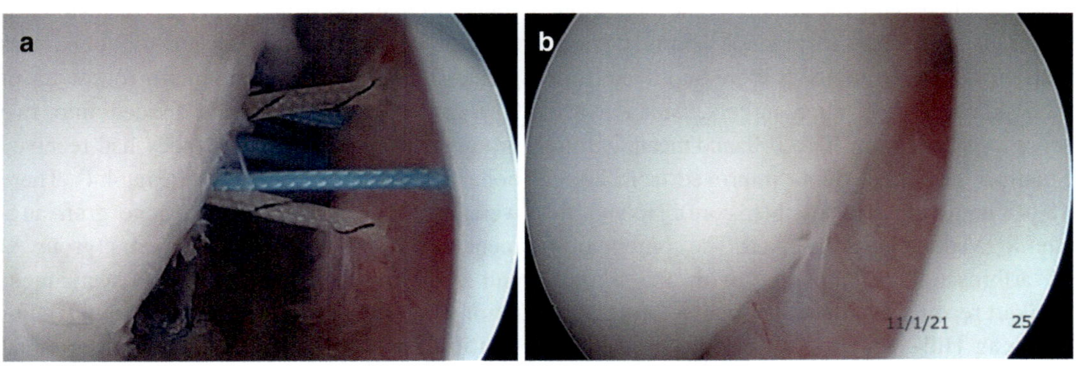

Fig. 4.2 Arthroscopic view of a remplissage repair in a right shoulder positioned in the lateral decubitus. The view is from the anterosuperior portal. A Hill-Sachs injury is viewed from the anterosuperior portal, and a remplissage procedure is being performed via use of suture anchors (**a**). After securing the knots on top of the infraspinatus, the capsulodesis effect is observed (**b**). This type of repair will prevent engagement of the Hill-Sachs injury

rior with regard to redislocation rate, recurrent instability, or functional scores [23].

In 2018, Lee et al. performed a retrospective case-control study (level III evidence) trying to identify risk factors for instability after an arthroscopic Bankart repair [24]. They performed a retrospective review of patients with anteroinferior shoulder instability that underwent a Bankart repair. Patients under 30 years with a minimum follow-up of 2 years were divided in two groups according to the presence of recurrent instability. An assessment of risk factors was performed using binary logistic regression analysis. Functional results were assessed by Row and Walch-Duplay scores. One hundred seventy shoulders (138 without recurrence, 32 with recurrent instability, 18.8% recurrent instability rate) were included. Both Rowe and Walch-Duplay scores were improved, although improvements were diminished in cases of recurrence. A high number of preoperative dislocations, an off-track Hill-Sachs lesion, and surgery after 6 months of the first episode showed a higher risk of recurrence [24].

In 2019, Brilakis et al. evaluated the long-term results of remplissage in addition to a an arthroscopic Bankart repair in cases of recurrent anterior shoulder instability with engaging Hill-Sachs without a critical glenoid bone defect in a level IV therapeutic case study [25]. Sixty-five patients with 30.1 years underwent the operation, and 51 (82%) were available for long-term evaluation (mean 8.1 years). Three patients suffered a new dislocation (5.6%). The rest of the patients were satisfied with the result of the operation, and 71% were able to practice sports without restriction. The mean ASES score improved from 72.5 points to 100 after surgery. Mean Rowe score improved from 40 to 100, and mean Oxford Shoulder Instability Score improved from 29 to 48 (48 being the best possible score). No significant ROM deficit was observed. The combination of arthroscopic remplissage with the classic Bankart repair was safe and effective for treating engaging Hill-Sachs lesions in patients without an inverted pear-shape glenoid (Fig. 4.3). The long-term results were good with a low rate if recurrence and no significant loss of eternal rotation [25].

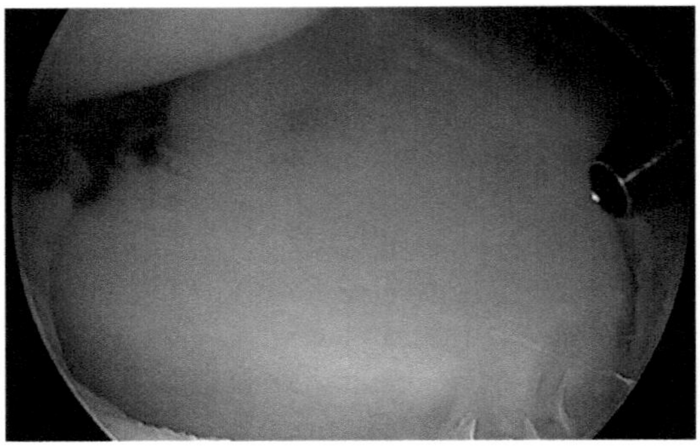

Fig. 4.3 Arthroscopic image of a glenoid with an inverted pear appearance. The scope is in the anterosuperior portal, and the Wissinger rod is being introduced from the posterior portal. Anteroinferior glenoid bone loss is observed. An inverted pear appearance usually represents a glenoid bone loss of approximately 25%

According to Iizawa et al., glenoid bone loss contributes to recurrent shoulder instability after an isolated arthroscopic Bankart repair. In the setting of significant glenoid bone loss, it seems that there is an increased failure rate. However, there is scarce data comparing augmentation using bone graft with non-augmentation for glenoid bone loss [26]. Iizawa et al. evaluated the clinical results of an arthroscopic Bankart repair with or without arthroscopic bone graft augmentation in a level 4 clinical evidence study. They tested the hypothesis that such bone graft augmentation techniques would restore shoulder stability and would produce excellent clinical results. Of the 552 patients treated for anterior glenohumeral instability with an arthroscopic Bankart repair, 68 patients met the inclusion criteria of presenting anterior glenoid bone loss greater than 20% and a minimum follow-up of 2 years. Patients were then divided into two groups depending on whether they had received bone graft augmentation or not (Fig. 4.4). There were 35 patients that received bone graft augmentation with a mean age of 21 years (group A) and 33 patients that did not receive bone augmentation with a mean age of 21 years (group B). For grafting, either autologous iliac bone or artificial bone made of hydroxyapatite was used (Fig. 4.4). Patients were evaluated with the rate of instability; the return to sport and the Rowe score were used. The mean Rowe score was 95 in group A

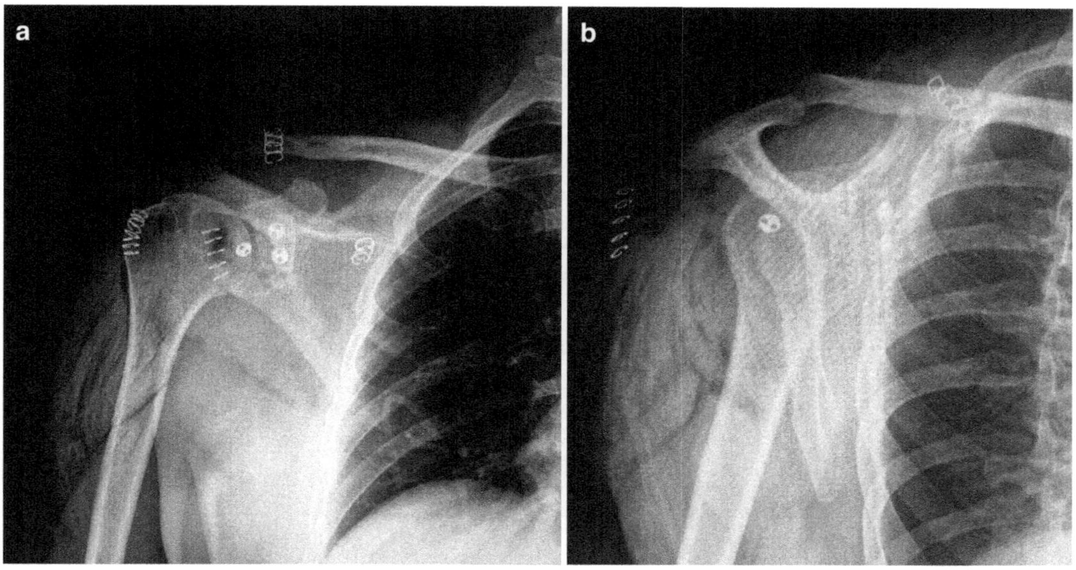

Fig. 4.4 Postoperative radiographs of a glenoid augmentation technique for instability using iliac crest bone graft fixed with a double suture-button technique. Anteroposterior (**a**) and lateral (**b**) views

and 69.7 on group B; the recurrence rate was 2.9% in group A and 48.5% in group B. Regarding collision athletes, 24 were in group A and 22 were in group B. Out of the patients with recurrence, 13 (59.1%) were contact athletes. Fifty percent of contact or collision athletes from both groups went back to practice their sport at the same preoperative level. Seven of the 11 patients in group B that went back to their preoperative sport suffered a recurrent dislocation. Nine athletes in group A and 3 in group B abandoned the sport for unrelated causes. In conclusion, in the presence of recurrent anterior instability of the shoulder with glenoid bone loss bone graft augmentation was beneficial when it was used in association with an arthroscopic Bankart repair, especially in athletes that practice collision sports [26].

4.3 Latarjet Procedure

Many authors have used anterior bone grafting technique, mostly Latarjet, to reconstruct anterior glenoid bone defects greater than 25% in what has been termed a critical defect with success. The presence of a combined Hill-Sachs injury has been shown to reduce the effective arc of motion of the shoulder free of instability and can influence the results of any technique, being a Bankart or a Latarjet procedure.

The initial concept of an engaging Hill-Sachs lesion was referred to as those lesions engaging with the arm at abduction and external rotation of 90° resembling a cocking phase of a throwing mechanism. It is obvious that all Hill-Sachs lesions were produced after a dislocation or subluxation event after engaging with the anterior glenoid rim, but after reduction the location of the Hill-Sachs lesion will influence the risk of dislocation. Medial Hill-Sachs injury will engage earlier than lateral Hill-Sachs lesions as they will reduce more the effective arc of motion of the shoulder. This evolution of concept was termed the glenoid track, resembling the track of motion the humeral head prints on the anterior glenoid as it is placed in a cocking position, and it is obviously affected by both the glenoid width and the location of the Hill-Sachs injury. As such, Hill-Sachs injuries are now classified as being on-track when they do not engage and off-track when they engage into the anterior glenoid rim. As such, some investigators will measure the glenoid track (the distance after calculating 83% of

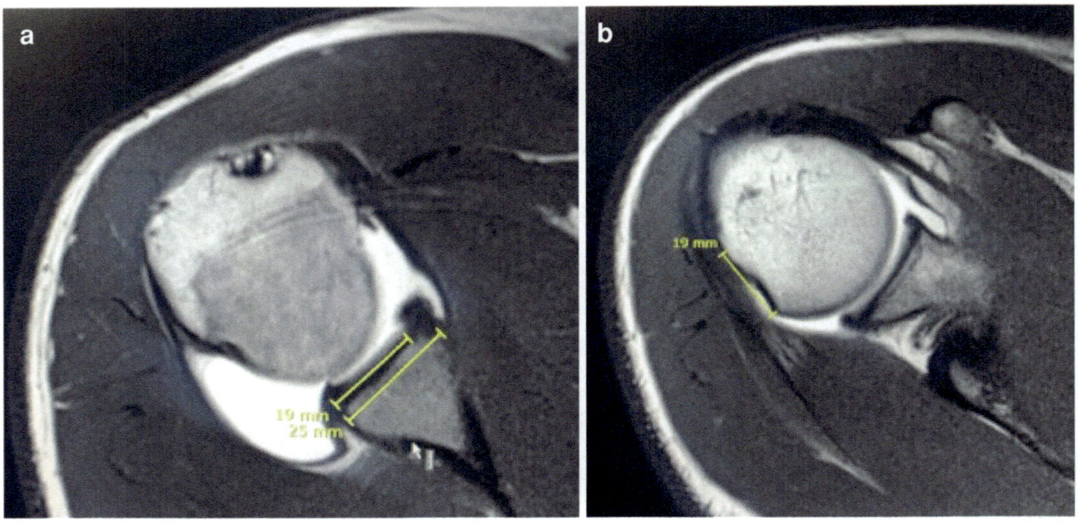

Fig. 4.5 The glenoid track concept can be calculated using a CT scan or, alternatively, in an appropriately performed MR scan. Typically, the width of the glenoid would be calculated on an "en face" view of the shoulder (in this case an axial cut) (**a**), and the Hill-Sachs interval (HIS) is calculated on an axial view (**b**). The glenoid has a 24% defect and a 20 mm diameter that multiplied by 83% gives a glenoid track of 15.7 mm. The HIS is 19 mm. Since the HIS is greater than the GT, this is considered an off-track Hill-Sachs injury

the native glenoid and subtracting the current glenoid defect), the Hill Sachs interval which is the distance from the insertion of the rotator cuff to the medial border of the Hill Sachs. If the HSI > GT, the lesion is considered as being off-track and has a greater risk of incurring into engagement during activities with external rotation of the shoulder. If the HSI < GT, the lesion is on-track (Fig. 4.5).

Some authors have used this preoperative tool to assess the risk of recurrence and, even in the presence of anterior glenoid bone defects <25%, will use an anterior bone augmentation in cases with an off-track Hill-Sachs injury to alter the relation of the glenoid track and the Hill-Sachs interval to make this an on-track injury (Fig. 4.6).

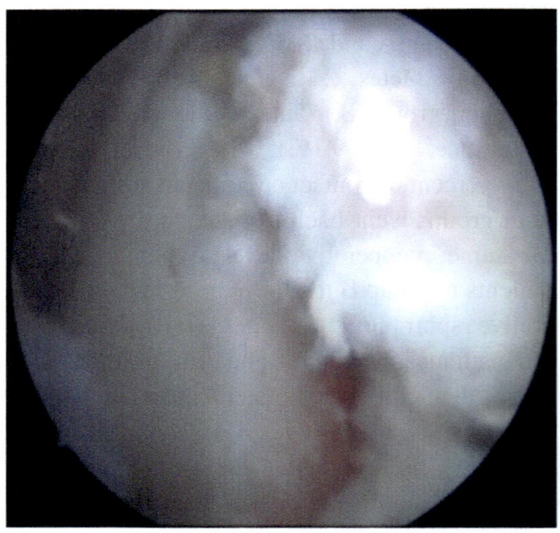

Fig. 4.6 An arthroscopic view from the anterosuperior portal of an arthroscopic Latarjet procedure using the classic arthroscopic techniques fixed with 2 screws

This concept has been clinically validated by Shaha et al. [27]. They studied 57 shoulders treated with an isolated, primary arthroscopic Bankart reconstruction with a mean patient age of 25.5 years, and a mean follow-up was of 48.3 months. Preoperative magnetic resonance imaging was used to determine glenoid bone loss and Hill-Sachs lesion size and location and to measure the glenoid track to classify the shoulders as on-track or off-track. They reported 10 recurrences (18%). Of the 49 on-track patients, 4 (8%) had treatment that failed compared with 6 (75%) of 8 off-track patients (p = 0.0001). Six (60%) of 10 patients with recurrence of instability were off-track compared with 2 (4%) of 47 patients in the stable group (p = 0.0001). The positive predictive value of an off-track measurement was 75% compared with 44% for the predictive value of glenoid bone loss of >20% highlighting the importance of the Hill-Sachs lesion, the interplay of the humeral and glenoid defect at some point of the arc of motion, and the ability to predict the risk of recurrence [27].

This concept highlights the importance of appropriately sizing of the anterior bone defect in the presence of critical glenoid bone defects in the presence of medial Hill-Sachs lesions (large HSI). Latarjet may only correct for certain combined defects and can be prone to failure in cases of smaller coracoids or very medial Hill-Sachs injuries. In these cases, the use of larger glenoid bone grafts or the association of a remplissage procedure must be pondered and points out that preoperative assessment of the coracoid dimensions will now have a role in the preoperative assessment and decision-making of the unstable shoulder with combined bone defects.

Calvo et al. in a level-IV evidence case-control study reported in the rates of recurrent instability according to the glenoid track concept using the arthroscopic classic Latarjet procedure [28]. A postoperative computed tomography scan and a clinical evaluation, including the Rowe and Western Ontario Shoulder Instability scores, were performed at a minimum 1- and 2-year follow-up, respectively. Postoperatively, 2 groups of patients were obtained: (1) patients with postoperative persistent off-track Hill-Sachs lesions and (2) patients with postoperative on-track Hill-Sachs lesions. Clinical and imaging data were compared between the 2 groups. A total of 51 patients (n = 51 shoulders), with a mean age of 29.8 ± 8.4 years (range, 15–50 years), met the inclusion criteria. Six shoulders (11.8%) still showed off-track Hill-Sachs lesions despite Latarjet surgery. There were no postoperative dislocations, but three patients reported subluxations. The subluxation rate was significantly higher in the postoperative persistent off-track Hill-Sachs lesions (2 [33%] vs 1 [2.2%]; $P = 0.033$). There was a wider preoperative HSI (29.8 ± 2.4 mm vs. 22.9 ± 3.5 mm; $P < 0.001$) and a larger preoperative ΔHSI-GT (12.2 ± 3.8 mm vs 4.82 ± 3.2 mm; $P < 0.001$) in the persistent off-track Hill-Sachs lesions. A receiver operating characteristic curve was performed based on preoperative ΔHSI-GT values. A preoperative ΔHSI-GT value ≥7.45 mm predicted a persistent off-track Hill-Sachs lesions after Latarjet surgery (sensitivity, 100%; specificity, 87%; positive predictive value, 50%; and negative predictive value, 100%). Six patients (11.8%) retained an OFF-HS and had a statistically significantly higher failure rate after Latarjet surgery compared with those with postoperative on-track Hill-Sachs lesions [28].

4.3.1 Modified Open Latarjet

According to Yang et al., recurrent anterior shoulder dislocation in the setting of an engaging Hill-Sachs lesion is frequent. The Latarjet procedure has been well described to restore shoulder stability in patients with glenoid bone loss >25%. However, the treatment of those patients with a combined humoral head and mild glenoid bone loss (<25%) is yet not clear [29]. A level-III cohort study assessed the results of the modified Latarjet procedure for patients with combined defects of the humeral head and anterior glenoid. They also compared the results of patients with <25% of glenoid bone loss with those having >25% glenoid bone loss (Fig. 4.5). The hypothesis was that both groups would have similar recurrence rates and subjective results. A modified Latarjet procedure was performed in 40 patients with recurrent anterior shoulder instability. An engaging Hill-Sachs by arthroscopic examination was confirmed, and glenoid bone loss <25% formed group A. A second group of 12 patients with glenoid bone loss >25% and an engaging Hill-Sachs lesion formed Group B. At a mean follow-up of 3.5 years, patients were evaluated with the Instability Severity Index Score (ISIS), the Beighton score, and the use of 3D imaging to assess bone loss (Fig. 4.7). To assess postoperative results, the authors used the Single Assessment Numeric Evaluation (SANE), Western Ontario Shoulder Instability Index (WOSI), recurrence rate, radiographs, ROM, and dynamometer strength. The main glenoid bone loss was 15% in Group A and 34% in Group B. Both groups had comparable WOSI scores (356 vs. 475). The SANE score was better in

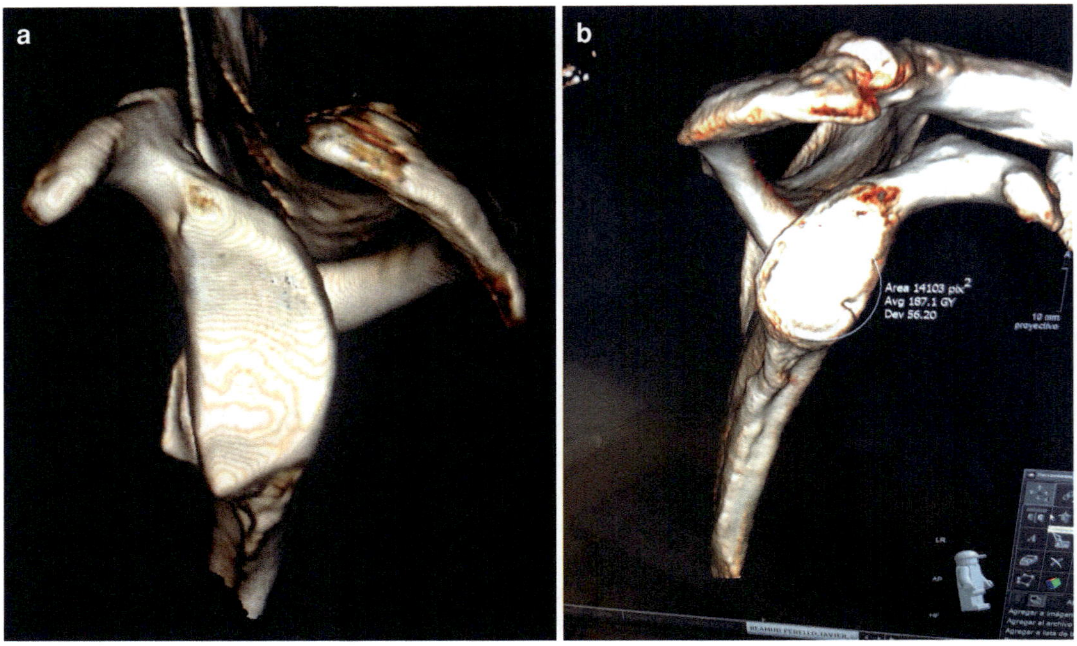

Fig. 4.7 Glenoid defects are best studied using 3d-CT reconstructions in the "en face" view. Two examples can be observed: a patient with a critical glenoid bone defect <25% (**a**) and a patient with a subcritical bone defect (**b**)

Group A (86 versus 77), and Group B suffered a greater loss of external rotation (9.2° versus 15.8°) and weaker thumbs-down abduction and external rotation strength. Strength in abduction and external rotation and subscapularis achieved at least 75% of the contralateral shoulder. Graft resorption was similar in both groups (32% versus 33%). The global rate of recurrent instability for the study defined as any subluxation or dislocation was 15%, the rates being similar for both groups (15% versus 17%). The rate of complications was 25% for both groups. The modified Latarjet procedure produced satisfactory results in patients with combined bone loss that usually suffered greater recurrence rates after traditional arthroscopic stabilization procedures. Previous surgical attempts and a higher Beighton score negatively influenced the results after a modified Latarjet. Additionally, it was observed that a higher number of surgical stabilization procedures and a higher Beighton score could predict the WOSI score [29].

4.3.2 Arthroscopic Latarjet

In 2014, Dumont et al. described the results of the arthroscopic Latarjet technique combining the benefits of arthroscopic surgery with the low rate of recurrent instability associated with the procedure (Fig. 4.7). Additionally, up to that date, only short-term results of arthroscopic Latarjet had been published. They described the results of a series of cases (level-IV evidence) to evaluate the results after a minimum follow-up of 5 years after an arthroscopic Latarjet technique using two screws for fixation. Patients reported if they had suffered a dislocation or a subluxation or a new surgery, and they completed the WOSI score. A total of 62 of 87 patients were contacted for evaluation at a mean follow-up of 76.4 months. No patient suffered a new dislocation after surgery, and one patient reported subluxations after surgery for a total rate of 1.59% of recurrent instability with a mean WOSI score of 90.6% [30].

4.3.3 Open Latarjet Vs. Arthroscopic Latarjet

In 2017, Kordasiewicz et al. compared the short-term clinical results of open and arthroscopic Latarjet in patients with anterior shoulder instability. They tested the hypothesis that the arthroscopic technique would be comparable to the open technique. In a Level- III evidence study, they analyzed the clinical results of patients operated with the Latarjet technique [31]. Consecutive patients operated between 2006 and 2011 comprised the open group and patient operated after 2011 comprised the arthroscopic group. They were able to evaluate 48 out of 55 (87%) shoulders in the open group and 62 of 64 (97%) shoulders in the arthroscopic group. Patients' results were evaluated using the Walch-Duplay score, the Rowe score, and a self-reported subjective score on satisfaction and function of the shoulder. CT scan evaluation was used to assess graft healing. The surgical time was 10 min less in the arthroscopic group (110 min versus 120 min). The number of intraoperative complications was six in the open group and five in the arthroscopic group, and results were comparable in both groups without significant differences with a satisfaction rate of 96.8% in open and 91.9% in the arthroscopic group. The subjective shoulder function score was 92.2% in open and 90% in arthroscopic group, the Rowe score was 87.8 in the open 78.9 in the arthroscopic group, the Walch-Duplay score was 83.9 and 91.9% in the arthroscopic group, and the presence of subjective apprehension was 28.7% in the open group and 50% in the arthroscopic group. The range of motion was similar in both groups with external rotation with the arm at the side being greater in the arthroscopic group (14° versus 7°). Three cases of recurrent instability were reported in the open group for a rate of 6.2% and 4.8% in the arthroscopic group. Revision surgery was performed in four patients in the open group and six in the arthroscope group. The radiographic evaluation showed significant less problems of bone healing after arthroscopic surgery (5%). However, partial osteolysis of the proximal part of the bone block was significantly more frequent using the arthroscopic technique. The authors concluded that arthroscopic stabilization showed satisfactory results and were comparable to the open procedure [31].

A recent meta-analysis by Hurley et al. reported the results of shoulder anterior instability with significant glenoid bone loss [32]. Even though open Latarjet is the standard treatment, the use of arthroscopic techniques is increasing, and the authors underwent this investigation to provide insight as to which technique gave better results.

They included six studies with 896 patients with a similar recurrent instability rate (2% vs 2.4%, open versus arthroscopic, respectively), revision procedures (2.4 vs. 5.4%), and total rate of complications (13.8 vs. 11.9%). However, the open procedure had a lower rate of persistent apprehension (10.2% vs. 35.7%). After achieving the learning curve, the operative time was similar for both procedures. Although technically difficult, the arthroscopic technique proved to be a valuable and safe alternative at the cost of a steep learning curve. The authors suggested that only centers with a greater caseload and expert arthroscopists should perform the arthroscopic technique (Fig. 4.8) [32].

4.3.4 Latarjet vs. Anterior Glenoid Reconstruction Using Fresh Distal Tibia Allograft (DTA)

Early results of fresh distal tibial allograft (DTA) reported by Frank et al. suggested encouraging early results for the treatment of recurrent shoulder instability but lacked a comparison with the Latarjet procedure. The authors performed a cohort study (level III evidence) in which they compared the clinical results of patients undergoing DTA or Latarjet. They reviewed patients with a minimum glenoid bone loss greater than 15% that underwent either a DTA or Latarjet procedure after a minimal follow-up of 2 year [33]. Patients undergoing DTA were matched 1:1 with the Latarjet procedure with regard to age, BMI, contact sports, and previous number of operations. Patients were evaluated before and after the

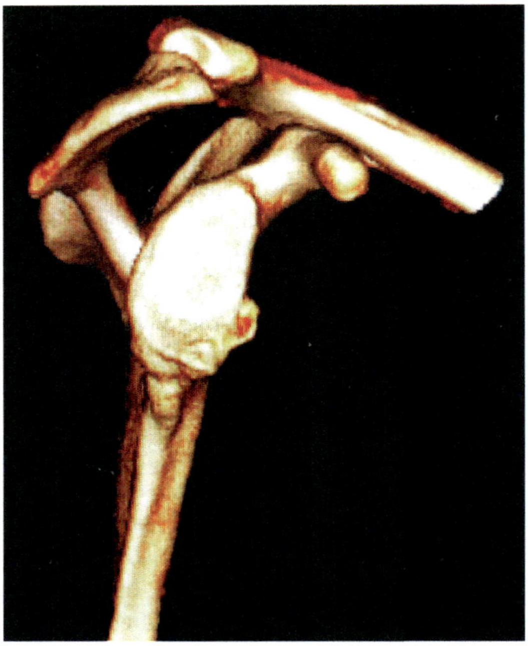

Fig. 4.8 One-year follow-up computer tomography (CT) scan after an arthroscopic Latarjet. Partial graft resorption following Wolff law is observed. As this case was fixed using a FiberTape cerclage fixation system, no problem with implant protrusion or hardware problems are observed

operation with a clinical exam and SST, VAS, ASES score, WOSI score, and SANE score. They analyzed the complications, the reoperations, and the number of episodes of recurrent instability. They reviewed 100 patients (50 Latarjet and 50 DTA) with a mean age of 25.6 years and a mean follow-up of 45 months. Thirty-two patients (64%) in each group had had a previous operation of the shoulder. Patients undergoing a DSA had a significantly greater bone loss than patients undergoing the Latarjet procedure (28.6% vs. 22.4%). Patients in both groups experienced significant improvements for all scores after surgery. No differences were found in VAS (0.67 vs. 1.83), ASES (91.06 vs. 89.74), Western Ontario Shoulder Instability Index (74.30 vs. 89.69), or Single Assessment Numeric Evaluation (80.68 vs. 90.08). However, Latarjet patients had a higher SSV score. Ten complications were reported, 5 for each group with 3 reinterventions in each group, for a total recurrent instability rate of 1%. Fresh DTA reconstruction was effective in restoring clinical stability in recurrent shoulder instability, but longer-term follow-up is required to test if these results are maintained over time [33].

4.3.5 Latarjet After Failed Arthroscopic Bankart Repair

Given that the complication profile is different between a Bankart repair and a Latarjet procedure, some surgeons make the decision of performing a primary Bankart repair and will leave Latarjet as a bailout surgery in case of recurrent instability after a failed Bankart repair. Werthel et al. tried to determine if the outcome of primary Latarjet and secondary Latarjet after a failed primary arthroscopic Bankart repair was equivalent [34]. They developed a level III cohort study in which the authors reviewed two cohorts of patients: primary Latarjet versus secondary Latarjet after a failed primary Bankart repair in a multicentric study. They analyzed the rate of recurrent instability, reoperation rate, the complications, the pain, the Walch-Duplay score, and the SST. Three hundred and eight patients participated in the study. Seventy-two patients (23.4%) did not answer and were considered lost to follow-up, so 236 patients were available for analysis. The mean follow-up was 3.4 years, and there were 20 patients in group 1 and 216 patients in group 2. Recurrent instability was similar for both groups (5% in group 1 versus 2.3% in group 2) and revision surgery (0% in group 1 and 2.3% in group 2). Group 1 patients had significant worse pain results (2.56 vs. 1.2) and patient-reported outcomes (Walch-Duplay 52 vs. 72.2 and SST 9.3 vs 10.7) than patients undergoing a primary Latarjet technique. The authors stated that the assumption that a failed Bankart repair could be revised to a Latarjet procedure with a similar result is incorrect and highlighted the importance of performing the right intervention at the right time [34].

4.4 Comparative Studies: Bankart Vs. Latarjet

4.4.1 Arthroscopic Bankart vs. Open Bristow-Latarjet

In 2014, Zarezade et al. compared an arthroscopic Bankart procedure and an open Latarjet procedure [1]. Patients were evaluated after surgery using Rowe, UCLA, and Constant scores. Six patients (16.22%) had a Rowe score of less than 75 points: one having undergone a Latarjet procedure and five undergoing a Bankart repair (5.26 vs. 27.78). Nine patients (24.32%) showed a moderate improvement, six Latarjet and three Bankart surgeries. Twenty-two patients showed a great improvement in the Rowe score, including 12 Latarjet and 10 Bankart (63.16 vs. 55.56). Both techniques were similar although some of the variables like the level of performance, the pain level, the use of analgesia, and the range of internal rotation were improved with the Latarjet technique. The authors concluded that the Latarjet was the preferable technique if there was no contraindication for its use [1].

An et al. performed a systematic review and meta-analysis to compare the results of a Bankart repair against the Latarjet technique [35]. They identified eight studies with 795 shoulders: 416 undergoing an open or arthroscopic Bankart repair and 379 undergoing an open Latarjet. They included primary and revision surgeries. The authors reported that the Latarjet procedure was associated with a significant decreased rate of recurrent instability and redislocation without significant differences in the rate of complications between both techniques. The Latarjet procedure showed a higher Rowe score and had decreased loss of external rotation and concluded it was viable alternative, and probably superior to a Bankart repair due to its increased restoration of stability without an increase in the rate of complications [35].

In 2018, Jeon et al. compared in a cohort study (level-III evidence) the clinical result and recurrence rate between a Bankart repair and a Latarjet procedure in patients with a subcritical glenoid bone defect (glenoid bone loss between 15 and 20%) [9]. They reviewed 149 patients (118 Bankart and 31 Latarjet) with a mean follow-up of 28.9 months and a mean age at the time of the index operation of 28.9 years. Rowe and UCLA scores improved from 42 and 22. 9 preoperatively to 90 and 32.5 postoperatively in the Bankart group and from 31 and 22.3 points to 91.1 and 32.3 in the Latarjet group, respectively. In the final evaluation, no differences were found between groups in Rowe or UCLA scores. The mean loss of motion in flexion, external rotation in abduction, and internal rotation was 3°, 11.6°, and 0.6 of vertebral bodies in the Bankart group and 3.7°, 10.3°, and 0.9 spinal segments in the Latarjet group, respectively. However, the loss of external rotation was greater in the Bankart group when compared with the Latarjet group (13.3° vs. 7.3°), and the recurrence rate was lower in the Bankart group when compared to the Latarjet group (22.9% vs. 6.5%). Both techniques showed improved clinical results and pain relief in patients with a borderline glenoid bone loss. However, the Latarjet procedure showed fewer recurrences (6.5% vs. 22.9%) and less decrease of external rotation (7.3° vs. 13.3°), and the authors stated that Latarjet could be a more reliable operation in patients with a borderline glenoid bone defect [9].

4.4.2 Arthroscopic Bankart vs. Open Bristow-Latarjet in Patients Older than 40

In 2020, Ernstbrunner et al. analyzed in a level-III evidence cohort study comparing the long-term results of an arthroscopic Bankart repair and the Latarjet technique in patients older than 40 [11]. They reported the results on 35 patients (36 shoulders) with a mean age at the time of the operation of 47 years and a mean follow-up of 13.2 years. The clinical and radiographic results were compared with those of a prior study including 39 patients (40 shoulders) of a similar age that had been treated using an open Latarjet technique. Six shoulders (17%) suffered a recurrent dislocation at a mean of 5.3 years after the index operation, and three additional shoulders suffered subluxation (8%), and three more experience persistent apprehension (8%). Revision surgery was performed in 8 patients (22%), consisting of 2 Bankart surgeries and 6 open Latarjet procedures. The relative Constant score and the SSV increased at final follow-up. Stabilization arthropathy was advanced in 16 shoulders (47%) and had progressed by at least 2 grades in 21 patients (62%). In the Bankart group, there were higher rates of redislocation and subluxation than in the open Latarjet (9 versus 3); also, the mean final SSV was significantly decreased in the Bankart group (86% versus 91%). There were no significant differences in between the two groups in the final rates of advanced arthropathy (16 versus 14) and revision (8 versus 7). This study shows that Latarjet is a more reliable operation regarding restoration of stability when compared to an arthroscopic Bankart repair. It is noteworthy to point out that the rates of arthropathy are not different in this age group as some surgeons have the initial thought that Latarjet may be more prone to arthropathy than the Bankart procedure [11].

4.4.3 Arthroscopic Bankart Repair with Remplissage vs. Open Latarjet

In 2018, Bah et al. compared short-term shoulder stability after an arthroscopic Bankart with remplissage and open Latarjet in patients with recurrent instability with a large Hill-Sachs lesion with the hypothesis that the recurrence rate would be higher after the Bankart-remplissage procedure [36]. They performed a retrospective comparative study in two hospitals recruiting patients with chronic anterior instability with a large Hill-Sachs defect in a Level-II evidence study comparing 43 patients treated with an arthroscopic Bankart repair and remplissage with 53 patients treated with an open Latarjet technique. Both groups were similar in age at the time of surgery and length of follow-up. All patients were evaluated by independent observers in which they assessed the number of recurrences, the range of motion, and functional scores including the subjective shoulder value (SSV), the Walch-Duplay score, and the Rowe score. The mean time to follow up was 47.3 months. The rate of recurrence at last follow-up was not significantly different between both groups (9.3% vs. 11.2%). The Bankart group showed higher loss of external rotation, and a higher proportion of patients had residual pain (21% vs. 9%). The SSV, the Walch-Duplay, and Rowe scores were similar for both groups. This study highlights that augmentation of a Bankart procedure will reduce the short-term radiolocation rate of an arthroscopic procedure and will perform similarly to a Latarjet procedure. It remains to be seen if the long-term results will reproduce this initial data. However, loss of external rotation and residual pain were significantly higher with the Bankart and remplissage technique, and patients should be counseled in this regard [36].

4.4.4 Arthroscopic Bankart Repair vs. Open Latarjet vs. Capsular Shift

In a level-III therapeutic study published by Xu et al. in 2019, the authors explored the hypothesis that the result of open traditional techniques and modern arthroscopic techniques would be similar [12]. They retrospectively analyzed 168 patients with recurrent anterior shoulder instability with a mean age of 30.8 years in which they compared three techniques: a Bankart arthroscopic repair in 33 men and 20 women, an open Latarjet in 34 men and 18 women, and a capsular shift in 31 men 14 women. They analyzed the ISIS, the Rowe score and the SSV at the mean follow-up of 67.6 months.

The preoperative ISIS score was higher than three, with a mean preoperative score of 6.4 points. All three techniques were effective in improving the function of the shoulder and reducing symptoms although the Latarjet was the best with regard to subjective perception of the shoulder. The Rowe scores were 92.3, 96.2, and 93.2 for arthroscopic Bankart, open Latarjet, and capsular shift, respectively. There were no differences with regard to functional scores; however, the Latarjet group was superior to the other groups in SSV and subjective shoulder value for sports (SSV sports) practice. There were two recurrences in both the Bankert group and capsular shift group and no recurrences in the open Latarjet group. The authors concluded that the latter was the most effective technique in reducing recurrences and achieved higher stability although all surgeries increased the preoperative function and improved pain [12].

4.5 Conclusions

A systematic review has shown that open Latarjet is better than open Bankart achieving less recurrences with a similar rate of complications. In another study, patients operated with the Latarjet technique showed less recurrences and higher Rowe scores when compared with an arthroscopic Bankart repair. One publication supported better results for return to sport and subjective perception of the shoulder in patients undergoing an arthroscopic Bankart repair.

In the presence of a critical bone defect, most authors support the use of some bony reconstruction, mostly Latarjet. In a study comparing borderline glenoid bone defects (15–20%) and glenoid bone loss, both techniques were effective in reducing pain and clinical symptoms, but the Latarjet showed less recurrences and less loss of external rotation than arthroscopic Bankart. It is yet to be cleared if that benefit is maintained in glenoid bone loss <15%.

In patients older than 40 years, both Bankart and Latarjet have been effective, but Latarjet achieves less recurrences, and the degree of shoulder arthropathy was not decreased using an arthroscopic Bankart repair.

In patients with recurrent anterior shoulder instability and a significant Hill-Sachs lesion, both an arthroscopic Bankart repair with remplissage and open Latarjet are safe and effective with similar recurrent rates, but loss of external rotation and residual pain were more frequent with the Bankart and remplissage group.

Another study compared an arthroscopic Bankart against open Latarjet and open capsular shift and highlighted the benefits of each procedure but showed that Latarjet was most effective in reducing recurrence.

Additional long-term data is needed to assess the effectiveness of these techniques, and more comparative studies are warranted to tailor the best treatment for each patient. As highlighted in the introduction, listening to the patient's wants and needs, performing a meticulous clinical exam, and having a candid discussion about the results and complications of the available techniques will generally produce a satisfactory result. Preoperative tools for assessing the risk of recurrence are available and may be helpful in guiding the clinical decision-making. Different augmentation techniques can be used to reduce the rate of recurrent dislocation.

Appendix 1: WOSI Score

The WOSI score is a patient-reported outcome score using 21 items pertaining to 4 domains (physical symptoms, emotion, lifestyle and sports recreation, and work) with 0 being the best possible score (no instability related symptoms or limitations and 2100 being the worst possible score). Some authors will express it as a percentage. The WOSI score can be accessed in its English version in the following publication:

The Development and Evaluation of a Disease-Specific Quality of Life Measurement Tool for Shoulder Instability The Western Ontario Shoulder Instability Index (WOSI)Am J Sports Med November 1998 vol. 26 no. 6 764-772 Alexandra Kirkley, MD, FRCSC*, Sharon Griffin, CSS, Heidi McLintock, BSc, PT, MSc and, Linda Ng, BSc, PT.

References

1. Zarezade A, Dehghani M, Rozati AR, Banadaki HS, Shekarchizade N. Comparison of Bristow procedure and Bankart arthroscopic method as the treatment of recurrent shoulder instability. Adv Biomed Res. 2014;3:256.
2. Bokshan SL, Marcaccio SE, Lemme NJ, Owens BD. Open Bankart repair for anterior shoulder instability. Oper Tech Orthop. 2020;30:100822.

3. Blonna D, Bellato E, Caranzano F, Assom M, Rossi R, Castoldi F. Arthroscopic Bankart repair versus open Bristow-Latarjet for shoulder instability: a matched-pair multicenter study focused on return to sport. Am J Sports Med. 2016;44:3198–205.
4. Gao B, DeFroda S, Bokshan S, Ready LV, Sullivan K, Etzel C, Owens BD. Arthroscopic versus open Bankart repairs in recurrent anterior shoulder instability: a systematic review of the association between publication date and postoperative recurrent instability in systematic reviews. Arthroscopy. 2020;36: 862–71.
5. Uchiyama Y, Handa A, Shimpuku E, Omi H, Hashimoto H, Imai T, Watanabe M. Open Bankart repair plus inferior capsular shift versus arthroscopic Bankart repair without augmentations for traumatic anterior shoulder instability: a prospective study. J Orthop Surg. 2017;25:1–8.
6. Pogorzelski J, Fritz EM, Horan MP, Katthagen JC, Provencher MT, Millett PJ. Failure following arthroscopic Bankart repair for traumatic anteroinferior instability of the shoulder: is a glenoid labral articular disruption (GLAD) lesion a risk factor for recurrent instability? J Shoulder Elb Surg. 2018;27:e235–42.
7. Bessiere C, Trojani C, Carles M, Mehta SS, Boileau P. The open Latarjet procedure is more reliable in terms of shoulder stability than arthroscopic Bankart repair. Clin Orthop Relat Res. 2014;472:2345–51.
8. Hachem AI, Costa DOG, Rondanelli SR, Rius X, Barco R. Latarjet cerclage: the metal-free fixation. Arthrosc Tech. 2020;9:e1397–408.
9. Jeon YS, Jeong HY, Lee DK, Rhee YG. Borderline glenoid bone defect in anterior shoulder instability: Latarjet procedure versus Bankart repair. Am J Sports Med. 2018;46:2170–6.
10. Aboalata M, Plath JE, Seppel G, Juretzko J, Vogt S, Imhoff AB. Results of arthroscopic Bankart repair for anterior-inferior shoulder instability at 13-year hollow-up. Am J Sports Med. 2016;45:782–7.
11. Ernstbrunner L, De Nard B, Olthof M, Beeler S, Bouaicha S, Gerber C, Wieser K. Long-term results of the arthroscopic Bankart repair for recurrent anterior shoulder instability in patients older than 40 years: a comparison with the open Latarjet procedure. Am J Sports Med. 2020;48:2090–6.
12. Xu Y, Wu K, Ma Q, Zhang L, Zhang Y, Xu W, Guo JJ. Comparison of clinical and patient-reported outcomes of three procedures for recurrent anterior shoulder instability: arthroscopic Bankart repair, capsular shift, and open Latarjet. J Orthop Surg Res. 2019;14:326.
13. Moroder P, Odorizzi M, Pizzinini S, Demetz E, Resch H, Moroder P. Open Bankart repair for the treatment of anterior shoulder instability without substantial osseous glenoid defects: results after a minimum follow-up of twenty years. J Bone Joint Surg Am. 2015;97:1398–405.
14. Balg F, Boileau P. The instability severity index score. A simple pre-operative score to select patients for arthroscopic or open shoulder stabilisation. J Bone Joint Surg Br. 2007;89:1470–7.
15. Loppini M, Delle Rose G, Borroni M, et al. Is the instability severity index score a valid tool for predicting failure afterprimary arthroscopic stabilization for anterior glenohumeral instability? Arthroscopy. 2019;35:361–6.
16. Thomazeau H, Courage O, Barth J, Pélégri C, Charousset C, Lespagnol F, Nourissat G, Audebert S, Guillo S, Toussaint B, Lafosse L, Bradel J, Veillard D, Boileau P. French arthroscopy society. Can we improve the indication for Bankart arthroscopic repair? A preliminary clinical study using the ISIS score. Orthop Traumatol Surg Res. 2010;96(8 Suppl):S77–83.
17. Ruiz Ibán MA, Asenjo Gismero CV, Moros Marco S, Ruiz Díaz R, Del Olmo HT, Del Monte BG, García Navlet M, Ávila Lafuente JL, Díaz HJ. Instability severity index score values below 7 do not predict recurrence after arthroscopic Bankart repair. Knee Surg Sports Traumatol Arthrosc. 2019;27:3905–11.
18. Dekker TJ, Peebles LA, Bernhardson AS, et al. Limited predictive value of the instability severity index score: evaluation of 217 consecutive cases of recurrent anterior shoulder instability. Arthroscopy. 2021;37:1381–91.
19. Bouliane M, Saliken D, Beaupre LA, Silveira A, Saraswat MK, Sheps DM. Evaluation of the instability severity index score and the Western Ontario shoulder instability index as predictors of failure following arthroscopic Bankart repair. Bone Joint J. 2014;96-B:1688–92.
20. Park J-Y, Lee S-J, Oh S-K, Oh KS, Noh YM, Suh K-T. Glenoid rim fracture through anchor points after arthroscopic Bankart repair for shoulder instability. Int Orthop (SICOT). 2015;39:241–8.
21. Boeileau P, Lemmex DB. Editorial commentary: which patients are likely to undergo redislocation after an arthroscopic Bankart repair? Preoperative instability severity index scoring over 3 points-the game is vver! Arthroscopy. 2019;35:367–71.
22. Cho NS, Yoo JH, Juh HS, Rhee YG. Anterior shoulder instability with engaging Hill–Sachs defects: a comparison of arthroscopic Bankart repair with and without posterior capsulodesis. Knee Surg Sports Traumatol Arthrosc 2016;24:3801-3808.
23. Camus D, Domos P, Berard E, Toulemonde J, Mansat P, Bonnevialle N. Isolated arthroscopic Bankart repair vs. Bankart repair with "remplissage" for anterior shoulder instability with engaging hill-Sachs lesion: a meta-analysis. Orthop Traumatol Surg Res. 2018;104:803–9.
24. Lee SH, Lim KH, Kim JW. Risk factors for recurrence of anterior-inferior instability of the shoulder after arthroscopic Bankart repair in patients younger than 30 years. Arthroscopy. 2018;34:2530–6.
25. Brilakis E, Avramidis G, Malahias MA, Stathellis A, Deligeorgis A, Chiotis I, Mataragas E, Chronopoulos E, Antonogiannakis E. Long-term outcome of arthroscopic remplissage in addition to the classic

Bankart repair for the management of recurrent anterior shoulder instability with engaging Hill–Sachs lesions. Knee Surg Sports Traumatol Arthrosc. 2019;27:305–13.
26. Iizawa N, Yoneda M, Yamada S, Mizuno N, Goto K, Iwashita S, Mae T, Hashiguchi H, Takai S. Benefits of bone graft augmentation to arthroscopic Bankart repair for recurrent anterior shoulder instability with glenoid bone loss. Knee Surg Sports Traumatol Arthrosc. 2020;28:2325–33.
27. Shaha JS, Cook JB, Rowles DJ, Bottoni CR, Shaha SH, Tokish JM. Clinical validation of the glenoid track concept in anterior glenohumeral instability. J Bone Joint Surg Am. 2016;98:1918–23.
28. Calvo E, Luengo G, Morcillo D, Foruria AM, Valencia M. Revision arthroscopic Bankart repair versus arthroscopic Latarjet for failed primary arthroscopic stabilization with subcritical bone loss. Orthop J Sports Med. 2021;9:23259671211001809.
29. Yang JS, Mazzocca AD, Cote MP, Edgar CM, Arciero RA. Recurrent anterior shoulder instability with combined bone loss: treatment and results with the modified Latarjet procedure. Am J Sports Med. 2016;44:922–32.
30. Dumont GD, Fogerty S, Rosso C, Lafosse L. The arthroscopic Latarjet procedure for anterior shoulder instability: 5-year minimum follow-up. Am J Sports Med. 2014;42:2560–6.
31. Kordasiewicz B, Małachowski K, Kicinski M, Chaberek S, Pomianowski S. Comparative study of open and arthroscopic coracoid transfer for shoulder anterior instability (Latarjet)—clinical results at short term follow-up. Int Orthop (SICOT). 2017;41:1023–33.
32. Hurley ET, Fat DL, Farrington SK, Mullet H. Open versus arthroscopic Latarjet procedure for anterior shoulder instability: a systematic review and meta-analysis. Am J Sports Med. 2019;47:1248–53.
33. Frank RM, Romeo AA, Richardson C, Sumner S, Verma NN, Cole BJ, Nicholson GP, Provencher MT. Outcomes of Latarjet versus distal tibia allograft for anterior shoulder instability repair: a matched cohort analysis. Am J Sports Med. 2018;46:1030–8.
34. Werthel J-D, Sabatier V, Schoch B, Amsallem L, Vigan M, Hardy A. Outcomes of the Latarjet procedure for the treatment of chronic anterior shoulder instability: patients with prior arthroscopic Bankart repair versus primary cases. Am J Sports Med. 2020;48:27–32.
35. An VVG, Sivakumar BS, Phan K, Trantalis J. A systematic review and meta-analysis of clinical and patient-reported outcomes following two procedures for recurrent traumatic anterior instability of the shoulder: Latarjet procedure vs. Bankart repair. J Shoulder Elbow Surg. 2016;25:853–63.
36. Bah A, Lateur GM, Kouevidjin BT, Bassinga JYS, Issa M, Jaafar A, Beaudouin E. Chronic anterior shoulder instability with significant Hill–Sachs lesion: Arthroscopic Bankart with remplissage versus open Latarjet procedure. Orthop Traumatol Surg Res. 2018;104:17–22.

5 Controversies in Shoulder Arthroplasty

Julián Fernández-González, Alberto Del Olmo-Galeano, Julián Del Rio-Hortelano, and David Martínez-Vélez

5.1 Introduction

The shoulder has become the third most frequently replaced joint, after the hip and knee. Since Neer's early designs used for fractures, shoulder prostheses have evolved to accommodate the proximal humeral anatomy, including humeral head size and height, version, tilt, and restoring distances from the center of the humeral head to the diaphysis, both in anteroposterior and lateromedial directions. This has been possible thanks to the variability in the modularity between the head and the humeral stem.

Another evolutionary aspect since the Neer prostheses is the progressive decrease of cemented fixation in favor of the uncemented one, based either on the search for biological integration or on the idea of preserving the greatest amount of bone, preferring short stem or stemless implants.

However, the most important step in the evolution of shoulder arthroplasty was undoubtedly the introduction of the reverse total shoulder prosthesis. Since its initial indication in rotator cuff arthropathy, obtaining satisfactory and reliable results in terms of pain relief and especially in terms of function, its use has been extended to other indications, most notably proximal humerus fractures, evolved primary osteoarthritis, tumors and revisions of failed osteosynthesis, hemiarthroplasties, and total arthroplasties.

The reverse prosthesis has undergone important changes since its first designs with the aim of minimizing the complications initially observed. Probably, the most important complication was scapular erosion (notching) that led to early loosening of the glenoid component. This has been notably corrected with changes introduced in the different designs, mainly in terms of the inclination of the humeral cut and greater lateralization of the center of rotation of the glenosphere.

In line with this, we are entering a new stage that aims to achieve a better placement of the prostheses, particularly of the glenoid component regarding its orientation and the need to provide bone graft or augmented implants to obtain a better function as well as a greater longevity of the implant.

The objective of this chapter is to address the fundamental concepts in shoulder arthroplasty and the controversial points that arise today within its indications and the different kinds of arthroplasties.

The chapter is structured in sections organized by pathologies, followed by the most frequent complications found with arthroplasty. There is also a section of special relevance nowadays which addresses the treatment of glenoid bone defects.

J. Fernández-González (✉) · A. Del Olmo-Galeano · J. Del Rio-Hortelano · D. Martínez-Vélez
Department of Orthopedic Surgery, La Princesa University Hospital, Madrid, Spain

E. C. Rodríguez-Merchán, A. Moreno-Garcìa (eds.), *Controversies in Orthopedic Surgery of The Upper Limb*, https://doi.org/10.1007/978-3-031-04907-1_5

5.2 Rotator Cuff Arthropathy

Rotator cuff arthropathy has always been the primary indication for RSA (Fig. 5.1). Reverse prostheses arose from the need to restore mobility of the shoulder of patients with associated massive and irreparable injuries of the rotator cuff in which anatomical prostheses, generally large-headed hemiarthroplasties, dramatically relieved pain but did not improve the absence of active mobility; that is, the patient persisted with the known pseudoparalytic shoulder.

Although there were previous designs, it was the design by Paul Grammont that brought the most important advancement in what this type of prosthesis is today. The Grammont prosthesis introduced two key features: a large hemispherical glenoid component of two sizes (36 and 42 mm) without neck, and a small humeral cup oriented almost horizontally (155°), covering less than half of the hemisphere. With this, a medialization of the center of rotation of the new implants was obtained, as the base of the hemisphere is in contact with the glenoid, and therefore it is possible to reduce the force exerted upon the glenoid implant (a reason for failure of TSA) [1]. Also with these two sizes, an attempt was made to improve the range of motion of the prosthesis and its stability.

Moreover, the deltoid, a fundamental muscle in this prosthesis, recovered its tension, achieving the recovery of the mobility of the shoulder, but only in anteflexion and abduction. Rotations will depend on the state of the rest of the rotator cuff, and today it is essential that at least the teres minor muscle is well preserved to maintain an acceptable active external rotation. Internal rotation is preserved by the integrity of the pectoralis major if the subscapularis is affected. The design of the reverse prosthesis, determined by its own nature, allows less mobility in rotation than that of the anatomical ones.

The reverse prosthesis is not fully constrained but responds to the semiconstrained type and therefore is susceptible to being unstable if one does not

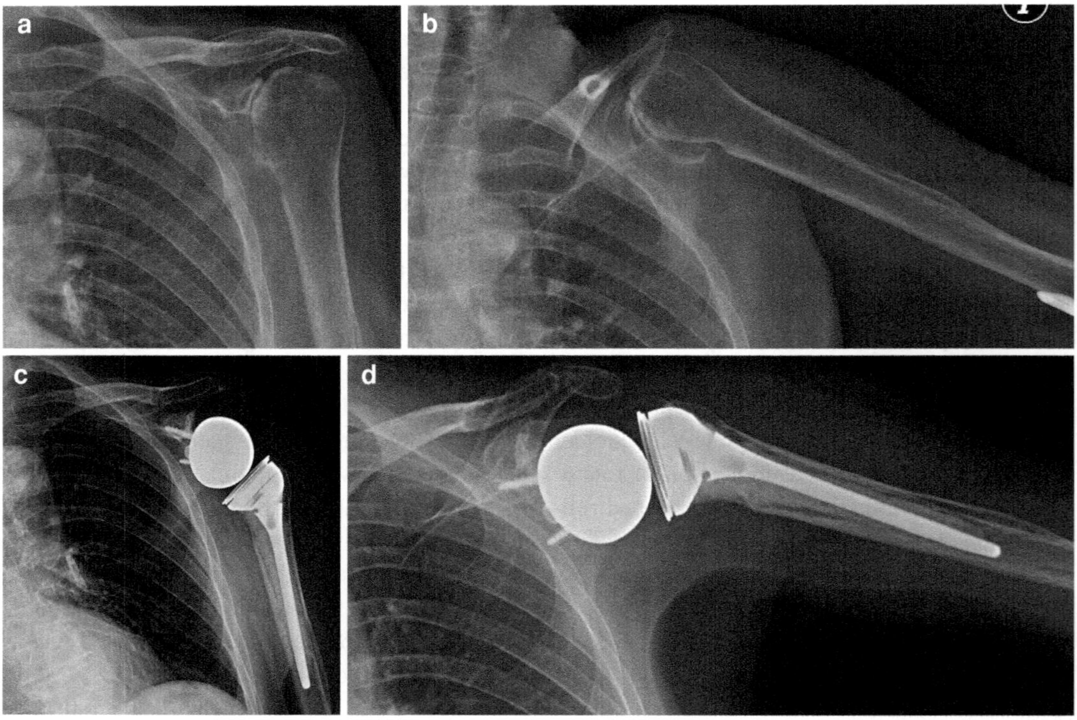

Fig. 5.1 An 80-year-old woman presented with severe shoulder pain and disability. X-ray images showed a characteristic rotator cuff arthropathy with degenerative changes in the glenohumeral joint and acromial bone thinning (**a** and **b**). RSA was performed, lending the patient pain-free and with great function (**c** and **d**)

perform a good surgical technique and there is not a minimum of preserved soft tissues [1].

The first complications, in addition to the deficit of internal rotation, were the erosion of the scapular neck and the wear of the polyethylene due to the impact of the polyethylene against the neck of the scapula (known as notching—up to 62%) [2]. This happened prematurely in the first designs, since up to 68% of the patients who presented this notching already had radiological changes at the end of the first year after implantation. Nonetheless, authors such as Werner et al. [3] saw that few cases progressed over time after that first year, which differed from the work of Lévigne et al. [2], in which a higher percentage progressed over time. Notching progress has been associated with a worse clinical outcome, especially in Nerot's cases 3 and 4 [2].

Other complications that appeared with the first designs in a significant percentage were instability and infection. These last two complications have decreased notably in recent years owing to a better surgical technique and better management of the soft tissues.

5.2.1 Young Patients

An important fact to take into account, especially in young patients, is the case in which an active external rotation defect is identified preoperatively in the clinical examination and confirmed with a MRI (identifying absence of infraspinatus and teres minor). In these patients, a latissimus dorsi transfer should be considered and anticipated before the surgery according to the L'Episcopo technique, well described in different articles, to restore lost external rotation [4]. Some articles propose the transfer of the lower portion of the trapezius, as an alternative to the above [5].

Trying to reduce scapular notching has been the subject of many compute-modeling studies. This has been achieved by:

- Reducing the humeral neck—shaft angle (less than 155 degrees)
- A greater lateralization and inferior tilt of the glenoid component

5.2.2 Humeral Cut Neck-Shaft Angle of Less than 155 Degrees

Studies have shown that a humeral cut neck-shaft angle of less than 155 degrees (non-anatomic Grammont's prosthesis) and a lateralization of the glenosphere of at least 2–4 mm were able to reduce the incidence of scapular erosion [6]. However, this can lead to differences in the range of motion. Computer-modeling studies have demonstrated that an angulation of 135° improves mobility in adduction but decreases it in abduction, as opposed to what happens with a humeral cut of 155° although what both types of cut achieve in the end is an equal range of motion in the abduction-adduction axis. There are also changes in the rotation, shown in Table 5.1 [6–8].

5.2.3 Studies that Compare the RSA with or Without Lateralization with Bone Graft

Clinical studies that compare the RSA with or without lateralization with bone graft, and in terms of mobility, show mixed results. Collin et al. observed that in the case of prostheses with graft, they obtained significantly better movement in anterior flexion but not in rotations [9].

Table 5.1 Influence of the humeral neck shaft angle cut in range of motion based in computer-modeling studies [6–8]

	Humeral neck shaft angle cut 155°	Humeral neck shaft angle cut 135°
Abduction	Improved	
Adduction		Improved
External rotation at 10° abduction		Improved
Internal rotation 10° abduction		Improved
External rotation 90° abduction		Reduced
Extension		Improved
Forward flexion	Equal	Equal
Total ABD + ADD	Same ROM	Same ROM

ROM Range of motion, *ABD* Abduction, *ADD* Adduction

On the contrary, Greiner et al. in a prospective study, although with a small sample, did not observe that the use of the bone graft lead to better anterior flexion, but they did observe better external rotation and without significant differences in the Constant-Murley score [10]. Athwal et al. in a retrospective study also found no differences in terms of range of mobility, strength, and Constant-Murley score [11]. In these three studies, they did not find a significantly better external rotation with the graft, contrary to what was expected when using a glenosphere component without lateralization [9–11].

5.2.4 Degree of Lowering of the Center of Rotation

Another issue for debate is the degree of lowering of the center of rotation. It is accepted that greater distalization leads to better mobility by achieving greater deltoid tension. However, there are studies that show that this also leads to complications such as nerve injuries, often underdiagnosed postoperatively, especially of the axillary nerve in its anterior branch, up to 25.8% [12], and a higher percentage of acromion or scapular spine fractures and reoperations [13].

5.2.5 Size of the Glenosphere

Regarding the size of the glenosphere, Mollon et al. observed greater active abduction and anterior flexion in patients with a 42 mm glenosphere than with a 38 mm glenosphere, and this effect was more significant in women [14]. However, Torrens et al. with a larger glenosphere showed a significant decrease in notching but no differences in functional scales [15]. A later study by Muller et al. with a longer follow-up of 5 years, but fewer patients, noted with a 44 mm glenosphere a greater external rotation of 12° on average compared to a 36 mm glenosphere. However, the authors are not certain that this translates to a clinical benefit for the patient [16]. They also observed that patients with a 44 mm glenosphere had greater strength in abduction (they explain this finding based on the fact that the deltoid muscle and external rotator muscles improve their power by increasing their length when using a larger glenosphere), but they did not find differences in terms of stability between both diameters.

5.3 Glenohumeral Osteoarthritis

Glenohumeral osteoarthritis in patients over 60 years has been successfully treated in recent decades with a total shoulder arthroplasty with good results in terms of pain relief and function. The state of the rotator cuff is mainly what dictates the indication of a total anatomical shoulder arthroplasty (TSA) versus the reverse (RSA). Nowadays it is accepted that the state of chondral and bone wear of the glenoid cavity must also be taken into account.

Hemiarthroplasty (HA) has few indications in cases of glenohumeral osteoarthritis, since the glenoid cavity is affected in most cases, and the immediate functional results in terms of pain relief are much better with TSA, although traditionally it was said that the results were comparable after 1 year of follow-up. In our experience, during the first year after a HA, the patient does not perceive any improvement in his symptoms and in his quality of life. For this reason, our view is that a patient over 60 years with glenohumeral osteoarthritis and with good rotator cuff status is a candidate for a total anatomical arthroplasty and rarely for a hemiarthroplasty.

5.3.1 Comparison Between HA and TSA

Supporting our own experience, there are studies that compare HA and TSA, such as that of Bartelt et al. that find greater pain relief, greater range of motion, and longer survival with TSA than with HA. In another work, Dillon et al. observed a greater risk of revision in patients undergoing HA than in TSA [17]. However, longer-term studies such as the one of Denard et al. observed a 10-year survival rate of the glenoids of 62.5% [18]. Therefore, the choice of a TSA or a HA should be made according to the patient characteristics, taking into account age, activity carried out, state of the glenoid, and knowing the disadvantages of each technique. It has already been indicated that after a year the results are almost equal; however, more pain relief and better function have always been observed in TSA, although not being significant (Figs. 5.2 and 5.3).

5.3.2 Thinned Supraspinatus Tendon with a Partial Tear

Nevertheless, there is a point of controversy in patients with glenohumeral osteoarthritis who present a thinned supraspinatus tendon with a partial tear. If many years ago they were candidates for a TSA, today there is a tendency to perform a RSA. This change in the indication is due to the risk of an early tear of the rotator cuff which, in addition to the clear immediate functional impairment perceived by the patient, will also cause loosening of the glenoid component of

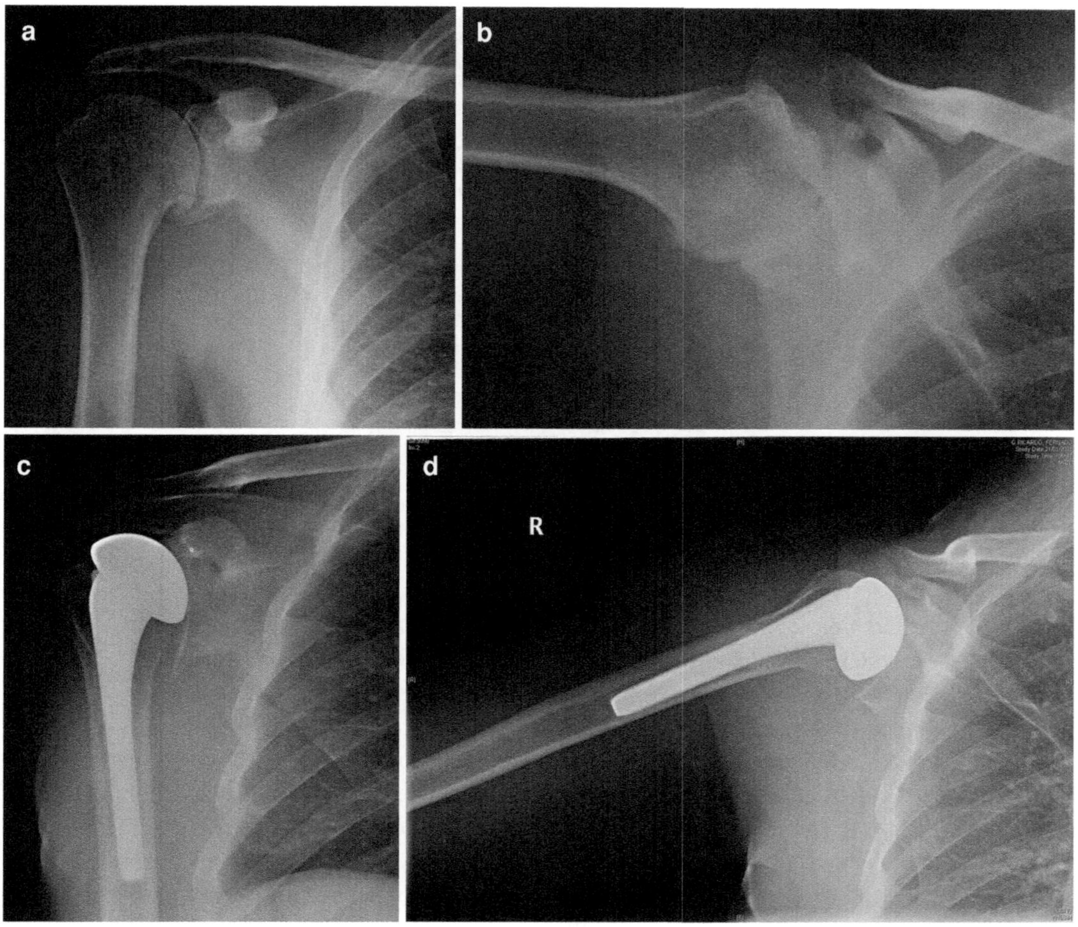

Fig. 5.2 Preoperative X-ray images of a 48-year-old male with glenohumeral osteoarthritis in his right shoulder (**a** and **b**). A hemiarthroplasty was performed after extensive soft tissues release and glenoid microfractures in some of its surface. The inferior glenoid osteophyte was not adequately removed (**c**) and (**d**). Despite the X-ray's appearance, the patient is pain-free after 4 years and with great mobility (abduction of 160° and complete rotations). A hemiarthroplasty was used because of his age, and adequate release and balance of soft tissues was essential to achieve this good clinical result

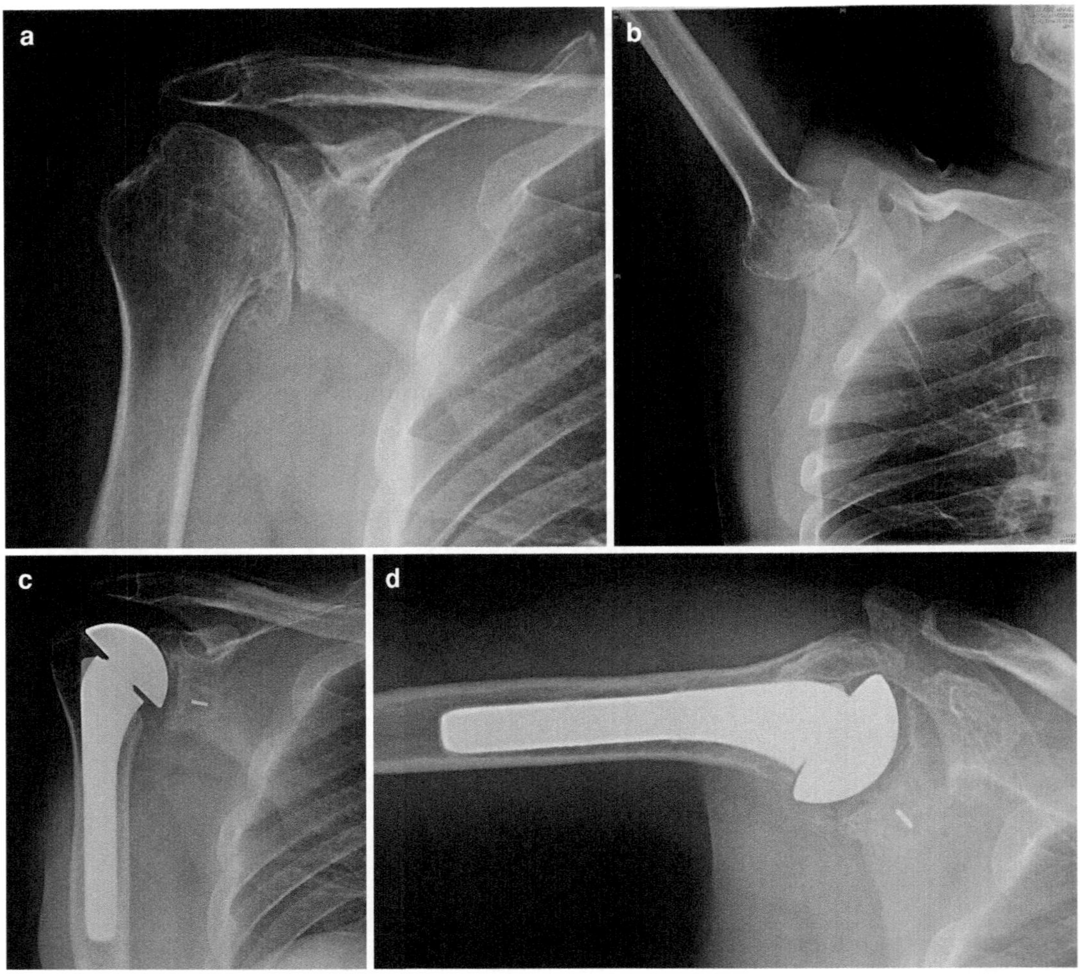

Fig. 5.3 Preoperative X-ray images of a 60-year-old man with right shoulder osteoarthritis (**a** and **b**). TSA was performed, with a keeled glenoid component (**c** and **d**), and after 4 years the patient shows a nearly complete range of motion and absence of any clinical symptoms

the TSA in a short time due to the well-known rocking-horse effect. Likewise, the non-cemented fixation of the glenoid component, as well as the lower shear forces to which this component is subjected, favors the choice of the RSA.

In these cases of osteoarthritis with thinning of the supraspinatus tendon, the infraspinatus and teres minor tendons are usually well preserved, so the RSA will lead to very satisfactory results in terms of anterior elevation and external rotation. The only drawback of the RSA is the loss of internal rotation suffered by most patients compared to the TSA that must be previously explained to the patient but which they normally accept for the benefits obtained in exchange.

5.3.3 Young Patients with Glenohumeral Osteoarthritis

Another point of debate is young patients with glenohumeral osteoarthritis in whom conservative treatment or arthroscopic debridement surgery have failed. Arthroscopic debridement to relieve pain and improve function, with or without capsular release, has been used in patients with osteoarthritis who are poor candidates for arthroplasty due to their young age or their high level of activity. Arthroscopic debridement may be successful to relief pain, stiffness, or mechanical symptoms, and it can be useful until the implantation of a prosthesis [19]. However, high failure rates have been recorded of up to 30%, so arthroscopy may be indicated in patients under 47 years, while above that age it is usually doomed to failure [20]. Treatment consists of what has been described as "the comprehensive arthroscopic management" (CAM) which, in addition to the extraction of loose bodies, regularization of chondral lesions, synovectomies, tenotomy or tenodesis of the long head of the biceps, and capsule release, includes an osteoplasty of the humeral head, removal of the anterior osteophyte, and decompression of the axillary nerve [19, 20]. Microfractures can also be associated with high-grade lesions [20]. As previously mentioned, Mitchell et al. observed after 5 years of follow-up that 26% progressed to arthroplasty, and, in a more recent work, they observed a progression to arthroplasty of 15.8% and that the cases with a type B2 or C Walch glenoid defect, age over 50 years, and greater signs of osteoarthritis in the Kellgren-Lawrence classification are those with the worst prognosis [19]. In these patients, in whom arthroscopic techniques fail, there are several arthroplasty options, from resurfacing arthroplasty to RSA.

5.3.4 Resurfacing Arthroplasty (Stemless Shoulder Arthroplasty)

Resurfacing arthroplasty (stemless shoulder arthroplasty), either partial or total, seeks to reestablish the tilt and version of the humeral head, as well as to maintain the offset of the humeral head with respect to the medullary canal. Partial resurfacing arthroplasty is indicated in cases of injuries to the humeral head with good condition of the glenoid articular cartilage, such as cases of non-advanced osteonecrosis. Total resurfacing is recommended in patients with rheumatoid arthritis, arthropathy secondary to instability, advanced osteonecrosis, and primary osteoarthritis. However, there are few published studies, one by Bailie et al. of 36 patients with a mean age less than 55 years with little follow-up, in which at 3 years only one patient required revision to a TSA [21].

5.3.5 Primary Osteoarthritis Patients with Joint Impingement, Posterior Erosion, and Posterior Subluxation of the Humeral Head

There is a group of primary osteoarthritis patients with joint impingement, posterior erosion, and posterior subluxation of the humeral head for which there are several techniques and surgical gestures intended to avoid a poor functional result or complications such as mobilization of the glenoid component or instability [22]:

- Corrective eccentric reaming
- Posterior bone grafting
- Augmented glenoid implants
- Glenoid reconstruction with a reverse prosthesis

The appearance of bone defects found in glenohumeral osteoarthritis is of such an importance that it will be treated thoroughly later in this chapter.

The cause of the posterior erosion and posterior subluxation of the head is uncertain. While Neer considered that the posterior subluxation was a consequence of the posterior erosion, Walch thinks that an excessive retroversion (>15°) is the primary cause and one that could be treated initially to avoid this situation [23]. This subluxation would be dynamic, only occurring in certain positions at first but eventually becoming permanent over time. Treatment in these cases is controversial and will be discussed later in the section on glenoid bone defects.

5.3.6 Reverse Prosthesis in Young Patients

Reverse prosthesis in young patients with glenohumeral osteoarthritis should be the last option of treatment. Clear indications of RSA in these patients are a history of several rotator cuff surgeries that lead to its irreparability in which osteoarthritis conditions contraindicate a tendon transfer, great patient comorbidity, and large bone defects such as those observed in certain cases of rheumatoid arthritis and of course in revisions of failed prostheses. However, studies show that the RSA in these young patients does not provide the same satisfaction as in older patients.

5.4 Failed Anatomic Shoulder Arthroplasties

Undoubtedly, an anatomic shoulder arthroplasty correctly indicated obtains satisfactory results in terms of pain relief and function. However, they can fail due to the increased life expectancy of patients, along with the overuse they receive due to the good clinical condition they render the patients in.

Revision of shoulder arthroplasty offers unpredictable results depending on the state of bone stock and the rotator cuff that these patients present. Currently, the good results obtained with the RSA in primary processes have led to its use in patients in whom their prior prostheses failed, achieving acceptable clinical results (Fig. 5.4).

We can find different situations of failure of an anatomic shoulder arthroplasty:

- Failure of an HA placed either in a fracture, in an osteonecrotic bone, or in a primary or secondary osteoarthritis with glenoid chondral erosion
- Failure of a TSA due to injury of the rotator cuff or to mobilization of the glenoid component, poor positioning, or infection

The revision of these prostheses is not easy. Patient characteristics and the state of the soft and bone tissues that accompany the prosthesis must be assessed. As for the patient considerations, we should identify the patient with pain that affects his daily life and that requires the use of analgesics daily. His medical history and information about the first surgery should be assessed to rule out an infectious cause of the problem. In this case, a blood test that includes ESR and CPR would be advised and, in cases where the implant has been in place for more than a year, a gallium scan. There is also the possibility of aspiration of joint fluid under ultrasound control. The germs most frequently implicated in these slow course infections are *Propionibacterium acnes* and, less frequently, *Staphylococcus epidermidis*.

Regarding imaging tests, changes in simple x-rays such as elevation of the humeral head or clear radiolucent lines around the components are signs of possible component mobilization. CT can aid us to evaluate the state of the rotator cuff and, particularly, the bone stock of the glenoid cavity.

In the literature, it is the glenoid component that has most frequently been described as the mobilized element and causing revision surgery. However, more recently, other causes of failure have been proposed, and it is no longer seen by some authors as the fundamental cause of revision. As we already said, the symptoms of the patient together with the simple radiological changes alert us of a possible mobilization of the glenoid component (changes in position or, more importantly, increase in radiolucencies around the pegs or keel, depending on the case). In these cases, the options range from removing the glenoid component (described in the literature even by arthroscopic means) to leaving the glenoid uncovered until a new glenoid component is implanted by open surgery and to the most frequent option, which is to perform the revision in one time, keeping in mind the frequent need to provide a structural graft. Currently, the revision would probably imply utilizing RSA.

The existing studies in the literature show a wide range of results. Placing a RSA after a TSA has been associated with decreased mobility, especially internal rotation, and acromion stress fractures. Melis et al. reported a satisfaction rate of 86% despite requiring subsequent surgeries in 21% of the cases [24].

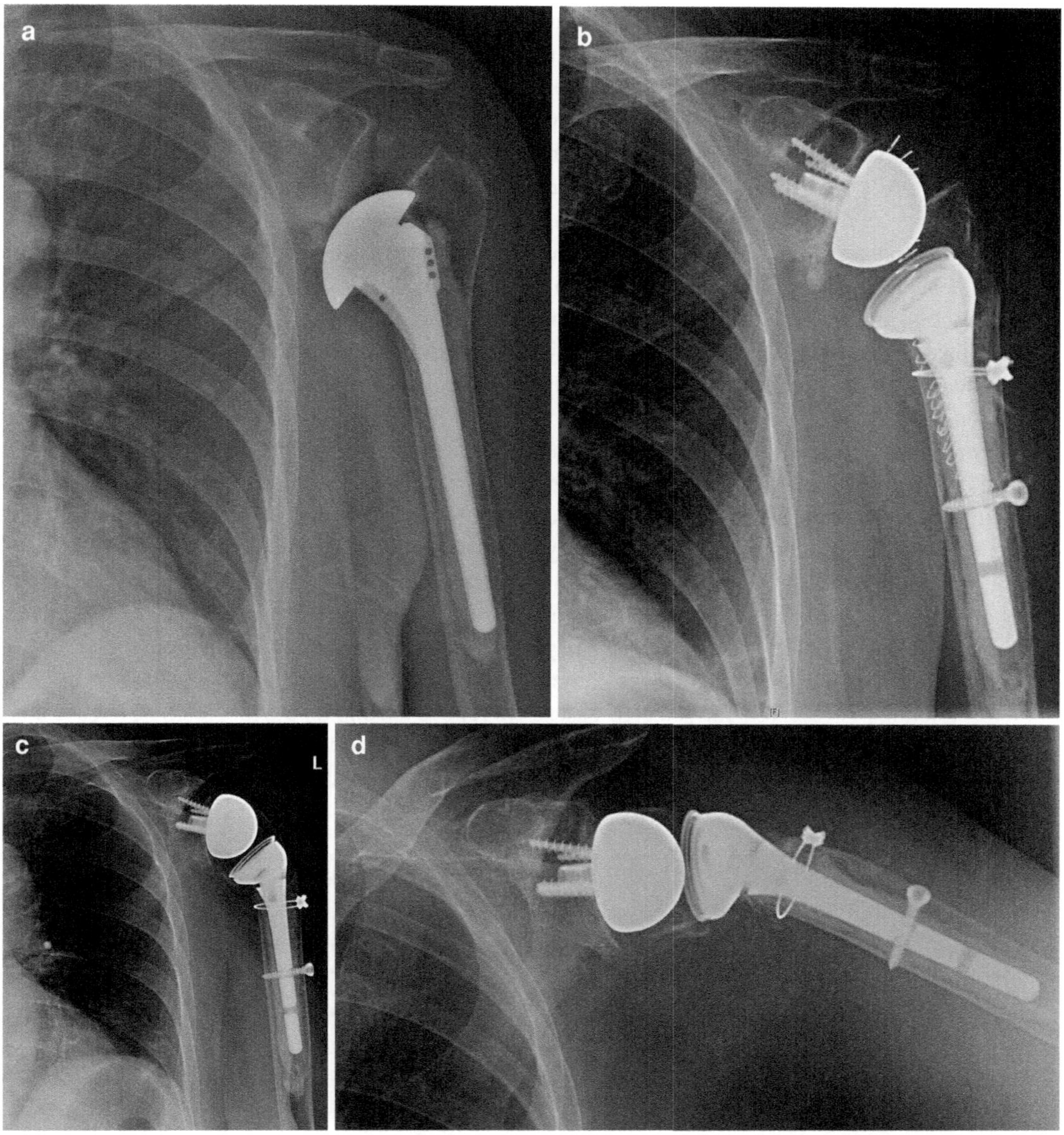

Fig. 5.4 A 72-year-old woman with a painful hemiarthroplasty (**a**). Revision was done with RSA. It was necessary to perform a proximal osteotomy to remove part of the cemented cap. The RSA was then fixed cementless thanks to the possibility of fixation with screws (**b**). After 4 years, the patient has improved in range of motion, with 130 degrees of abduction, good external rotation, and limited internal rotation up to level L5 (**c** and **d**)

5.5 Proximal Humeral Fractures

Proximal humeral fractures in patients over 70 years are adequately managed in 85% of cases with conservative treatment. Although a recent Cochrane study concludes that there are no differences in the outcome of surgical versus conservative treatment in displaced surgical neck fractures, it is accepted in most studies that displaced fractures with 3 or 4 fragments in people over 70 years and without medical conditions that contraindicate surgery, reverse arthroplasty, or osteosynthesis are nowadays an indication, and rarely a hemiarthroplasty can also be utilized [25].

The alternative to RSA in these displaced fractures is the osteosynthesis with a locking plate, which in many centers is accepted as an indication up to 75 years of age, at least in countries with greater longevity and good quality of life of their patients. However, fracture–dislocation in patients over 70 years of age is a clear indication for RSA and rarely for osteosynthesis, due to the technical difficulty of the surgery and the probable complications, mainly the necrosis of the humeral head. Necrosis usually leads to prominence of the screws of the implant causing pain or functional disability, forcing a second surgery more laborious and difficult with the only possible option of RSA.

As mentioned, fractures of the proximal humerus treated by hemiarthroplasty are in clear regression owing to the better results obtained with a RSA, largely due to the fact that they depend less on integration of the tuberosities for an acceptable functional result. For this reason, in most countries, the use of the reverse arthroplasty is preferred, and hemiarthroplasty in proximal humerus fractures is reserved for selected cases like fractures involving the humeral head (split-fractures) in young patients (Fig. 5.5).

Regarding the fixation of the tuberosities, especially of the greater one, there are no controversies about reattaching them, if possible, to achieve a better function of the reverse prosthesis in terms of mobility in anterior flexion and external rotation. A systematic review of the use of reverse prostheses in acute fractures, comparing those placed with or without reattachment of the tuberosities, corroborates the above, observing greater mobility in anterior flexion (126° vs. 112°) and in external rotation (24° vs. 15°) when they had been reattached [26].

Another interesting aspect would be to know the most adequate degree of version of the implant; however, from our point of view, the same indications as those of degenerative cases should be followed. The glenoid component should not be placed in a retroversion of more than 10° due to the risk of instability, and, as for the humeral component, it would be advisable around 10°–20° of retroversion as we previously mentioned, in order to relieve tension on the tuberosities, to ease their reattachment, and at the same time to obtain adequate internal and external rotation. However, in

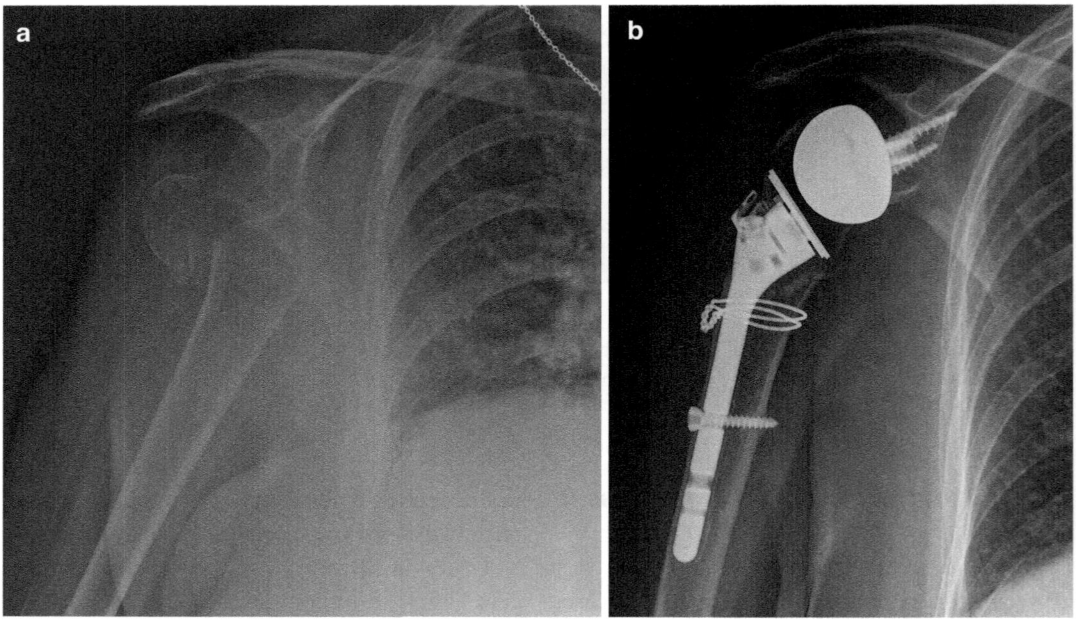

Fig. 5.5 Preoperative X-ray image of an 83-year-old female who sustained a fracture-dislocation of the proximal humerus after a fall at home (**a**). RSA was performed with good results in terms of pain and especially restoring ROM, obtaining complete abduction and external rotation thanks to the reattachment and integration of the greater tuberosity (**b**)

one study by Favre et al., they advised placing the implant in a neutral position or in slight anteversion, to achieve greater stability without losing external rotation [27].

In a systematic review carried out in our Service of 5 prospective clinical trials (not yet published), comparing reverse prosthesis (RSA) versus conservative treatment, osteosynthesis (ORIF), and hemiarthroplasty (HA) [28–32], it was observed that RSA offers better functionality than the other techniques on the Constant-Murley functional scale (a difference in the mean value of 11.44 points was observed (99% CI, [5.75–17.13], $p < 0.001$)). Regarding the functional scales used (DASH, Oxford Shoulder Score, UCLA), significant differences were obtained in favor of the RSA with respect to the HA and ORIF techniques but not to the conservative treatment, on a single study. Despite finding significant pain relief in participants treated with RSA in one of the studies, this did not translate into a higher quality of life (no significant differences found for the EQ-5D, SF-12, and WOOS scales). Two studies showed a greater range of motion in anterior flexion and abduction, but not in internal or external rotation, in participants with RSA compared to those treated with HA. Comparison with ORIF and conservative management regarding range of motion was not available.

In the radiological evaluation, 19 cases of scapular erosion were described (12.3%) [(8 in grade 2 of the Nerot-Sirveaux classification (Bradley, 2018)] and 53 cases of resorption or malunion of the tuberosities (34%) among the 154 participants who underwent RSA in 4 different studies, with no impact on functional results. Two studies reported 33 cases (37%) of periarticular ossification in 89 people who underwent RSA, with no clinical impact either. However, in the other techniques, a greater proportion of radiographic complications were described: greater proportion of resorption/malunion of the tuberosities in those treated with HA and cases of rotator cuff tear and avascular necrosis in the ORIF and conservative groups.

RSA seems to lead to fewer complications, with a relative risk (RR) of 0.48 (95% CI, [0.25–0.93], $p = 0.03$), after the results of three studies with a maximum follow-up of 49 months.

In conclusion, from these studies, we can infer that patients with RSA seem to be more satisfied, although only one of two studies found significant differences in this regard. Likewise, these studies showed better functional results of reverse prostheses in patients between 70 and 80 years of age, when compared to osteosynthesis and hemiarthroplasty. Nonetheless, a significant fact to keep in mind is that as patients get older, especially over 80 years, the results with RSA are equal to those obtained with conservative treatment. Moreover, we were surprised to find a normal distribution in the results of patients who underwent a RSA and a bimodal distribution of results in patients with HA (i.e., a proportion of patients with good results as well as a higher proportion of very poor results). These poor results of HA have not been reported with the reverse prosthesis [28–32].

Comparing the functional results and complications of RSA in proximal humerus fractures versus degenerative pathology, there is a study that compares 108 vs. 1876, respectively, and finds several remarkable facts [33]:

- At 1 year, both groups are equal from the functional point of view, in terms of mobility and in terms of the scores on the functional scales.
- Postoperative complications are less frequent in the group of fractures (4.6% vs. 7.15), and a notable fact is the absence of postoperative dislocations in this group. This fact contrasts with what happens in total hip arthroplasties when comparing fractures vs. degenerative pathology.
- The lower rate of complications in the fracture group could be related to highly selected indications (low comorbidity and absence of previous shoulder pathology), a fact that we must keep in mind in our daily practice.

5.6 Glenoid Bone Defects

This issue deserves a specific section because it affects both TSA and RSA, and it is undoubtedly the aspect that is currently under study to achieve better functional results and to reduce failure rates of the glenoid component. Treatment of glenoid bone defects is challenging. Fortunately, most cases of shoulder osteoarthritis and rotator cuff arthropathy are accompanied by small defects that do not require restoration for the arthroplasty to function properly. In cases of significant bone defect, if not treated properly, the glenoid component can loosen, triggering instability due to improper placement of the component or poor soft tissue balance. The first techniques described for its treatment were for the anatomical prostheses, both TSA and HA, with mixed results and ranging from 20 to 50% of failures [34].

Bone defects are usually classified according to the Walch classification. The original classification had 5 types: A1, A2, B1, B2, and C based on the preoperative image by two-dimensional CT [35], which was performed mainly to plan the type of shoulder prostheses to be implanted. The key to differentiate a type B glenoid from the other types is that the humeral head is posteriorly subluxated. However, this classification obtained a weak to moderate interobserver reproducibility using two-dimensional CT, even among experienced surgeons [36]. Thus, subsequent modifications have been made to improve this interobserver agreement, and three more types have been added: B3, C2, and D [37, 38]. This new classification has been developed with three-dimensional CT (Fig. 5.6). However, yet again, it did not achieve a greater interobserver reproducibility (kappa 0.37–0.43) although it did improve intraobserver reproducibility (kappa 0.51–0.63) [39]. The main problem that arises is the differentiation between types B3, C1, and C2, questioning if a defect was initially a type B1 that evolves to B2 and then to B3, or if it was a dysplasia (type C) from the very beginning. A summary that can help us to understand what type of glenoid defect

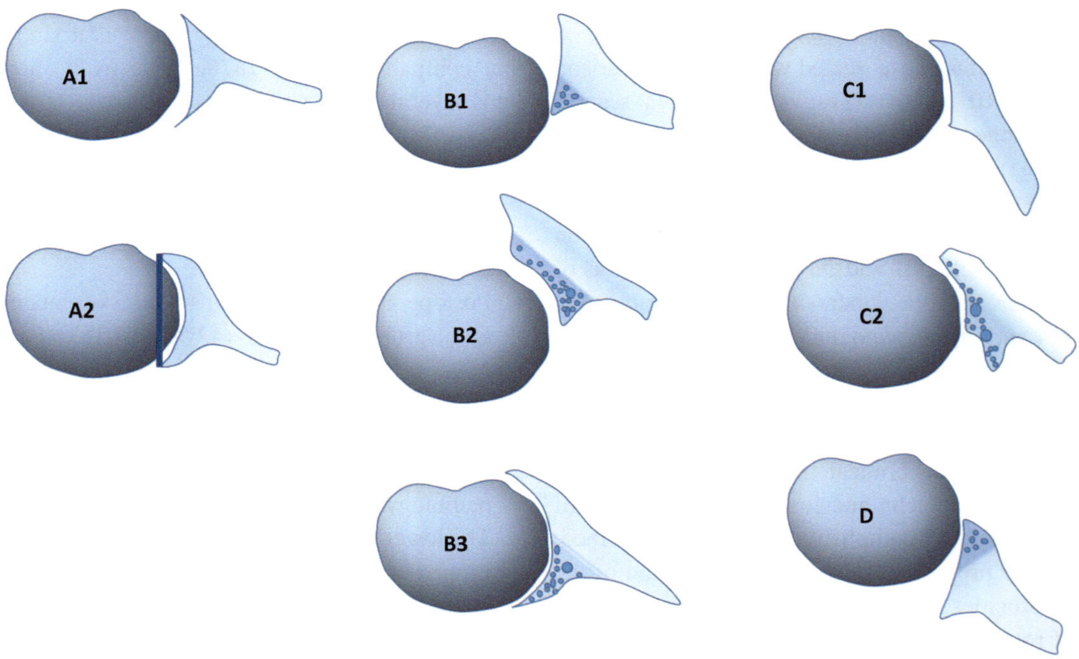

Fig. 5.6 The modified Walch classification. Bercik et al. published modification in 2016. The main modifications include the addition of B3 and D and clarification of the A2 glenoid. Ianotti et al. recently published an additional modification, in which they utilized the vault model theory to further define the B3 glenoid and introduced a new subtype, the C2 glenoid [35, 37, 38]

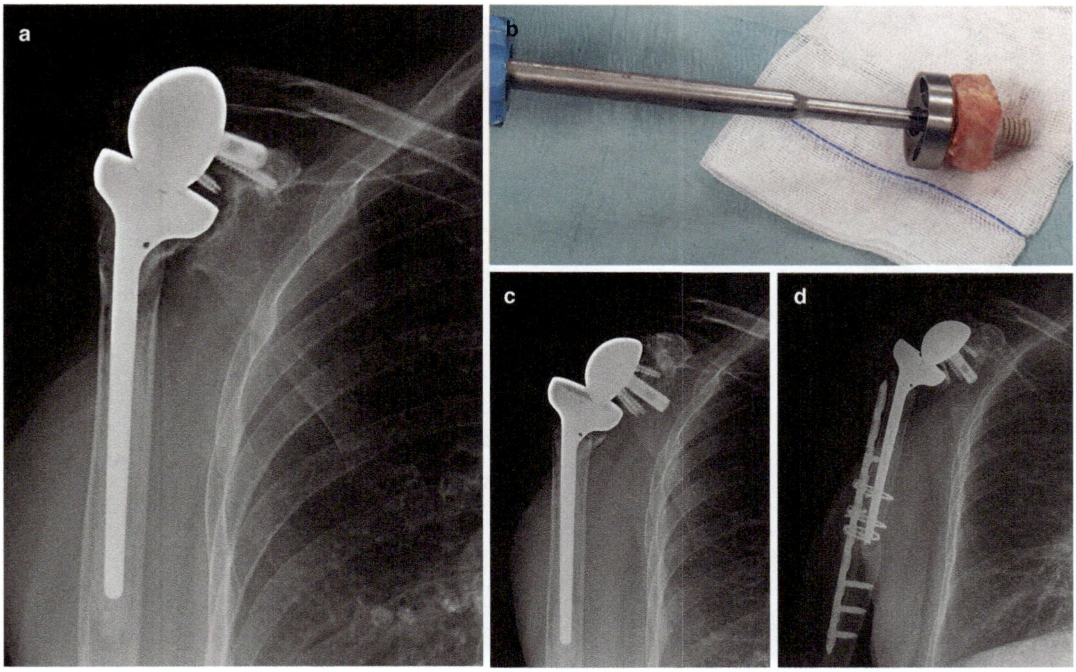

Fig. 5.7 A 75 year-old woman with rheumatoid arthritis. She underwent several surgeries because of shoulder arthritis. First surgery was a hemiarthroplasty 12 years ago then revised to TSA (adding the glenoid component) and finally a RSA. Suddenly, the patient started experiencing pain and loss of motion after continued overuse taking care of her sick mother. Anteroposterior radiograph shows aseptic loosening of the glenoid (**a**). Revision with allograft and a metaglene with longer central peg was implanted with great clinical success. However, anteroposterior radiograph shows the glenosphere slightly tilted upwards (**b** and **c**). Two years later the patient suffered a periprosthetic fracture after a fall that required open surgery with a locking plate. Fracture healing was obtained with good clinical results (**d**)

are we facing would be: a B2 type has a biconcave glenoid appearance; B3 has lost that biconcavity due to increased posterior erosion, with a version greater than 15° or at least 70% posterior humeral head subluxation (or both) and, most importantly, with no remnants of the native glenoid (or paleoglenoid) observed in the anterior area (therefore, it appears more concentric than a B2); type C has dysplastic glenoids, with an increase in retroversion above 25° and without signs of erosion; the C2 introduced by Ianotti et al. would have a biconcavity as an evolution of a C1. Another aspect that can help to define the glenoid defect is the etiology of the shoulder pathology that the patient presents. Thus, in glenohumeral osteoarthritis, it is common to observe either central (contained or not) or peripheral defects (mainly in the posterior aspect); in rotator cuff arthropathy, the main defect is found in the upper part; in patients with chronic anterior instability, the defect found will be anterior; and in revision cases, there will be global or combined defects (Fig. 5.7) [34]. The ideal approach to treat these defects is to use a structural bone graft, either from the native humeral head or from a humeral head allograft.

5.6.1 Reverse Shoulder Arthroplasty

Primary RSA is usually performed without providing structural graft (Fig. 5.8). However, there are authors who believe that it can be needed in up to 48% of primary cases. Other authors even state it would be required in up to 70% of cases [40]. In one study, better functional results were observed in reverse prostheses in which no graft was necessary compared to those that needed it [41].

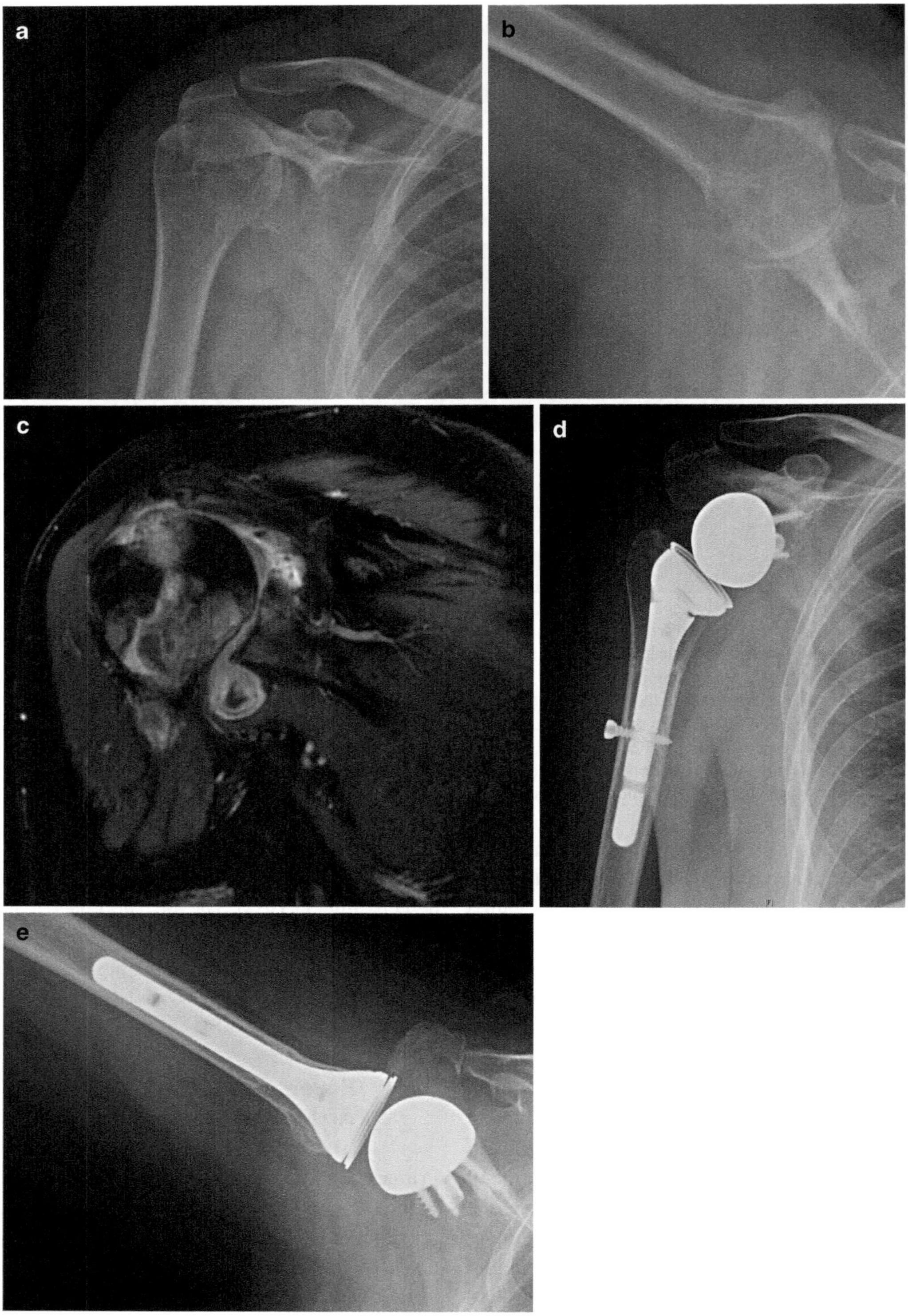

Fig. 5.8 Anteroposterior and axial X-rays of a 56-year-old female with rheumatoid arthritis. She underwent two unsuccessful rotator cuff repair surgeries (**a** and **b**). MRI images show important bone and cartilage lesions in both sides of the joint and an extensive synovial proliferation with some loose bodies (**c**). RSA was performed with good clinical and radiological results after a 4-year follow-up (**d** and **e**)

Undoubtedly, reverse prostheses allow better fixation of the glenoid component than total anatomical ones; and in cases with glenoid bone defects, a better graft incorporation has been described. There are studies that show good clinical results with the use of grafted RSA. Lorenzetti et al. observed a marked functional improvement with the incorporation of the graft in 98% of the cases, without any case of loosening (studied by postoperative CT). This work included patients with rotator cuff arthropathy and primary osteoarthritis. Another interesting data of the study is that the glenoid component was in contact with native bone in 0 to 50%, with an average of only 17% [42]. Boileau et al. used a trapezoidal-shaped autologous humeral head graft with the aim of correcting the version and inclination in patients with primary osteoarthritis and rotator cuff arthropathy and observed an integration of 94% of the grafts with good clinical and functional results [43]. In the work of Tashjan et al., they observed that the structural graft can achieve a good functional result with a low percentage of failure, observing a 93% glenoid implant survival and 100% short-term graft integration. They also believe that even a correction of as much as 35° could be resolved [34].

5.6.2 Total Shoulder Arthroplasty

In the case of a type B2 defect, the placement of a TSA is a challenge since the retroversion must be corrected, while at the same time re-centering the humeral that has subluxated is needed. To achieve this, different surgical techniques have been described, as we have mentioned previously: corrective eccentric glenoid reaming, posterior bone grafting, or augmented glenoid implants.

Corrective eccentric reaming, also referred to as high-side reaming, has the problem that it can lead to inadequate glenoid support, excessive medialization, and the risk of a fracture of the anterior glenoid rim. This type of surgery should be performed judiciously according to Mehta et al. in cases of excessive retroversion, over 15° [22].

The addition of structural bone graft has the purpose of correcting the glenoid version and at the same time recovering bone stock. The clinical results are mixed. Recent articles such as that by Nicholson et al. observed good clinical results with a mean follow-up of 4 years and with the incorporation of the graft in 100% of the cases [44]. On the other hand, Walch et al. reported a high frequency of complications. The goal for the correction of the version for these authors was less than 10°. Patients with bone graft were associated with poorer radiological and clinical results in terms of anterior flexion, Constant score, mobility, strength, and radiolucent lines. Graft resorption and even some cases of posterior dislocation were recorded as well [45]. In cases of TSA with retroversion of more than 27°, Walch et al. observed a 44% loosening of the glenoid component and, if the degree of posterior subluxation of the humeral head exceeded 80%, a risk of posterior instability of 11% [46]. In these instances, it is difficult to reproduce the glenoid anatomy, and frequently the implant pegs are not fully covered by bone. A reverse prosthesis can be considered in such cases, even with a functional rotator cuff, especially in the elderly patient.

Regarding the use of augmented glenoid implants, there are not many clinical studies, and most of the researched published is based on biomechanical studies or computer modeling. The preliminary results are promising, but studies with longer follow-up are required [22].

5.7 Short-Stem Shoulder Arthroplasty

It is the glenoid component which more frequently fails in TSA [47, 48]. The early uncemented components did not match the gold standard assumed by the cemented ones. However, modern uncemented components are achieving promising results [49], with advantages as less difficult revisions when compared to cemented ones. Current trends favor a metaphyseal rather than diaphyseal fixation, trying to recreate the proximal anatomy of the humerus while preserving the proximal bone stock. Short-stem humeral components avail these advantages, although they also have drawbacks such as the risk of misalignment and early loosening, especially in models without a proximal porous coating. Some studies have been published showing very good clinical results in terms of pain relief, mobility, and few complications [50]. However, it is noticeable that they observed medial resorption in the humeral calcar in 9.3% of cases on plain X-rays. This resorption is observed from the beginning, progressing slowly over time, and with only an average follow-up of as little as 3 years. The authors express their concern of possible resorption progression and associated complications.

Another study shows 2.6% loosening, 10.2% sinking, and a 15.4% risk of mobilization with a stem without proximal porous coating [51]. It has been advised for these stems to have a proximal porous or hydroxyapatite coating to obtain better results and to avoid the complications described. Further prospective studies are needed to compare standard-length humeral stems with short-stem components. Nowadays, short-stem humeral components can be useful in situations such as alteration of the normal anatomy due to a previous proximal diaphyseal fracture or prior elbow prostheses or in young patients seeking preservation of the humeral bone stock.

5.8 Complications of Shoulder Arthroplasties

5.8.1 Complications of RSA

The complications of RSA are numerous, the most frequent being scapular notching, already discussed; but others such as fractures of the acromion or the spine of the scapula and instability are also important.

5.8.1.1 Acromion and Scapula Spine Fractures

When facing a patient with good clinical progression after a RSA, the sudden onset of pain accompanied by loss of function should lead us to suspect a fracture in the insertion of the deltoid either in the acromion or in the spine of the scapula. The clinical suspicion can be confirmed either with simple radiology or with a CT scan. In the case of simple radiology, it should be suspected when typical changes are observed such as the tilt of the acromion or the decrease in acromiohumeral distance. There are two classifications that are used, that of Levy et al. and Crosby et al., to plan the adequate treatment [52, 53].

Undoubtedly, the biomechanics of the prosthesis, by producing greater tension on the deltoid, causes greater stress on its bone insertions, especially flexion forces upon the acromion. Added to this is the fact that these patients frequently associate reduced bone resistance, as observed in patients with rheumatoid arthritis or even in advanced cases of rotator cuff arthropathy [54, 55]. Other factors that can contribute to reduce bone resistance are previous acromioplasty, or acromioclavicular osteoarthritis, that implies greater stiffness at this level causing more stress on the acromion during movements [53–55].

In relation to the components of the prosthesis, the placement of the upper screw of the glenoid component has been associated with a higher rate of fractures. Thus, it may be advisable to take extreme care in its placement and when choosing the length. A lateralized humeral cut and a medialized glenoid have been suggested to provide greater protection against acromion fracture [54]. However, studies such as those by Marigi et al., after retrospectively reviewing 2000 reverse prostheses, only see a relationship with the occurrence of these fractures in women with osteopenia and a history of acromioplasty and not with other pathologies or with the type of prosthesis [55].

Treatment is conservative in most cases, although surgery is indicated in acute cases with displacement or in symptomatic chronic cases, either in terms of pain or loss of function (Fig. 5.9) [52, 53, 56].

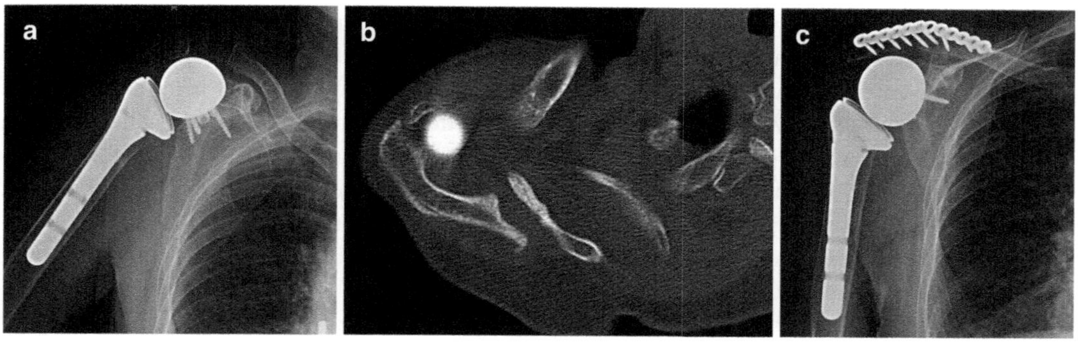

Fig. 5.9 A 70-year-old woman with rheumatoid arthritis is presented. RSA was performed to relieve her pain and loss of motion due to her disease. The patient underwent knee and spine surgeries as well due to her disease. She was performing well with the RSA, until suddenly she started experiencing loss of motion and pain in her right shoulder. In this scenario, an X-ray was performed where we can find increased distance between the acromion and the distal end of the clavicle (**a**). A CT scan confirmed a scapular spine fracture (**b**). The patient suffered some episodes of prosthesis dislocation that she could reduce by herself every time. Finally, the patient was recently operated using a reconstruction plate to fix the spine fracture (**c**)

5.8.1.2 Instability

Instability after RSA is one of the leading causes of revision, with devastating complications. Early instability can be related to inadequate soft-tissue tensioning and/or axillary nerve palsy or due to impingement or liner failure [57].

Cheung et al. found that postoperative instability was associated with male gender, history of prior open shoulder surgery, and preoperative diagnosis of fracture sequelae, including tuberosity nonunion. They identified a 9.2% incidence of early instability, and it is explained that nearly 50% of these patients had previous failed open surgeries. In their experience, addressing redislocation with only a thicker polyethylene insert was only effective in 5 of their 11 patients. Two underwent resection arthroplasty, and one had a conversion to a hemiarthroplasty [58].

Initial instability after RSA must be carefully managed and can be related to multiple causes, especially inadequate soft tissues management (either not tensioned or absent), mispositioned implants, or inadequate implant sizes [58, 59].

5.8.2 Complications of Total Anatomic Arthroplasty

In total anatomic arthroplasty, a change in the frequency of the complications originally described has been observed. Improvements in the composition of the components, in their design, and in the surgical technique have contributed to this [60].

In a review published in 2016, they observed that glenoid component loosening accounted for 37% of all complications, rotator cuff failure for 9%, and humeral component loosening for 1% [61]. However, these results were based on studies presented by groups that perform this surgery in large numbers, but we need to consider the complications experienced by surgeons who perform only few arthroplasties each year. Bearing this in mind and taking as a reference an organism as transparent as the FDA, it is observed that the loosening rate of the glenoid component is 20.4% [62]. A report from the Australian Orthopedic Society corroborates this, observing a glenoid loosening of 18% and confirming rotator cuff tear as a cause of revision in 26% of cases and instability in 22% [63]. Among the factors that have reduced glenoid loosening are a better surgical technique in treating glenoid defects, especially the posterior ones, with the use of grafts, and the decreasing popularity of the classic eccentric reaming, which places the fixation of the glenoid component at higher risk.

Matsen et al. recommend a minimum reaming but not with the intention of changing the version that the glenoid had. They report that out of 159 patients with osteoarthritis with type B1, B2, and B3 glenoid defects, at 2 years of follow-up, they did not need to carry out revisions of the glenoid component and only observed osteolysis around the central peg in 2 patients [64]. It is also noticeable that in a previous study by Somerson's group, they did not observe clinical or radiological differences between patients in whom the glenoid component was placed with a retroversion greater than 15° compared to those who were placed with a retroversion less than 15° at 2 years follow-up [65].

Grey et al., using a glenoid component with a posterior augmentation of 8° in 68 patients with a follow-up of 2 years, reported only the revision of 2 components, although radiolucent lines were observed in 37% (21 patients) [66]. Similar results were observed in the study by Priddy et al. using a full-wedge glenoid component in 37 patients. They reported only 2 revisions and only one of them because of the glenoid component itself [67]. They also found an important number of radiolucencies, 54% of patients. Further studies with longer follow-ups are still needed to evaluate the use of glenoid components with augmentations instead of bone graft, which had already shown good clinical results and high rates of integration.

Other developments proposed to reduce the failure of the glenoid component are the use of cross-linked cemented polyethylene instead of non-cross-linked polyethylene, metal-backed components, and uncemented components [68].

Regarding metal-backed components, a work by Boileau et al. draws attention to a greater failure of metal-backed glenoid components [69]. In another retrospective analysis of 21 studies that included 1571 arthroplasties, they showed a revision rate of 14% in the metal-backed components group versus 4% in the polyethylene components group. The authors believe that this is due to the thickness of the metal lateralizing the center of rotation and the differences in the stiffness of the three components: metal, polyethylene, and bone [70].

Regarding the fixation of the glenoid components either with keel or pegs, all published data before 2010 used components with keel. A randomized and controlled study in 2010 demonstrated better results of the components with pegs [71]; thus, the possibility of using them instead was introduced from then on. Along these lines, a more recent systematic work shows fewer revisions in the glenoid components with pegs, although this does not imply significant differences on the clinical level [72].

Undoubtedly, currently, the most frequent cause of failure of TSA is rotator cuff injury. A multicenter study found rotator cuff injury in 3.1% of patients, which in turn represented 28% of complications, thus being a factor to bear in mind when choosing which arthroplasty to be performed [73]. Nowadays, when facing a weakened rotator cuff, either thinned or partially torn, there is a tendency to use the RSA, especially in patients over 60 years of age. In order to determine the injury of the rotator cuff, we can use the parameters described by Young et al., like a rise of the humeral head greater than 25% in the true AP projection, and the factors that can predict a greater risk of rotator cuff tear like follow-up time, greater tilt of the glenoid component, and the degree of infraspinatus atrophy seen on CT [74]. Subscapularis muscle injury has been identified as the main cause of instability in TSA. Levy et al. reported that this involvement is due either to inadequate reinsertion of the tendon, poor rotation of the humeral component, larger components, injury of the capsule, or an inefficient deltoid [75].

The use of RSA in cases where TSA presented frequent complications like patients with rotator cuff arthropathy, large glenoid defects, or post-traumatic pathology has significantly reduced the complications reported in more recent series of TSA.

5.9 Conclusions

The shoulder has become the third most frequently replaced joint, after the hip and knee. Since Neer's early designs used for fractures, shoulder prostheses have evolved to accommodate the proximal humeral anatomy, but the most important step in the evolution of shoulder arthroplasty was undoubtedly the introduction of the reverse total shoulder prosthesis. These prostheses have undergone important changes since their first designs with the aim of minimizing the complications initially observed, especially scapular erosion. Nowadays, we are entering a new stage that has the objective of a better placement of the prostheses, especially of the glenoid component.

References

1. Boileau P, Watkinson DJ, Hatzidakis AM, Balg F. Grammont reverse prsothesis: design, rationale and biomechanics. J Shulder Elbow Surg. 2005;14: 148–61.
2. Levigne C, Boileau P, Favard L, Garaud P, Molé D, Sirveaux F, Walch G. Scapular notching in reverse shoulder arthroplasty. J Shoulder Elb Surg. 2008;17:925–35.
3. Werner CM, Steinmann PA, Gilbart M, Gerber C. Treatment of painful pseudoparesis due to irreparable rotator cuff dysfunction with the Delta III reverse-ball-and-socket total shoulder prosthesis. J Bone Joint Surg Am. 2005;87:1476–86.
4. Boileau P, Chuinard C, Roussanne Y, Bicknell RT, Rochet N, Trojani C. Reverse shoulder arthroplasty combined with a modified latissimus dorsi and Teres major tendon transfer for shoulder pseudoparalysis associated with dropping arm. Clin Orthop Relat Res. 2008;466:584–93.
5. Elhassan BT, Wagner ER, Werthel JD. Outcome of lower trapezius transfer to reconstruct massive irreparable posterior-superior rotator cuff tear. J Shoulder Elb Surg. 2016;25:1346–53.
6. Werner BS, Chaoui J, Walch G. The influence of humeral neck shaft angle and glenoid lateralization on range of motion in reverse shoulder arthroplasty. J Shoulder Elb Surg. 2017;26:1726–31.
7. Gutierrez S, Levy J, Frankle M, et al. Evaluation of abduction range of motion and avoidance of inferior scapular impingement in a reverse shoulder model. J Shoulder Elbw Surg. 2008;17:608–15.
8. Lädermann A, Geuorguiev B, Charbonnier C. Scapular notching on kinematic simulated range of motion after reverse shoulder arthroplasty is not the result of impingement in adduction. Medicini. 2015;94(38):e1615.
9. Collin P, Liu X, Denard PJ, Gain S, Nowak A, Lädermann A. Standard versus bony increased-offset reverse shoulder arthroplasty: a retrospective comparative cohort study. J Shoulder Elb Surg. 2018;27: 59–64.
10. Greiner S, Herrmann P, Perka. Clinical performance of lateralized versus non-lateralized reverse shoulder arthroplasty: a prospective randomized study. J Shoulder Elb Surg. 2015;24:1397–404.
11. Athwal GS, MacDermid JC, Reddy KM, Marsh JP, Faber KJ, Drosdowech D. Does bony increased–offset reverse shoulder arthroplasty decrease scapular notching? J Shoulder Elb Surg. 2015;24:468–73.
12. Lopiz Y, Rodriguez-Gonzalez A, Martín-Albarrán S, Marcel H, García-Fernández C, Marco F. Injury to the axillary and suprascapular nerves in rotator cuff arthropathy and after reverse shoulder arthroplasty: a prospective electromyographic analysis. J Shoulder Elb Surg. 2018;27:1275–82.
13. Tashjian RZ, Hillyard B, Childress V, Kawakami J, Presson AP, Zhang C, Chalmers PN. Outcomes after a Grammont-style reverse total shoulder arthroplasty? J Shoulder Elb Surg. 2021;30:e10–7.
14. Mollon B, Mahure SA, Roche CP, Zuckerman JD. Impact of glenosphere size on clinical outcomes after reverse total shoulder arthroplasty: an analysis of 297 shoulders. J Shoulder Elb Surg. 2016;25:763–71.
15. Torrens C, Guirro P, Miquel J, Santana F. Influence of glenosphere size on the development of scapular notching : a prospective randomized study. J Shoulder Elb Surg. 2016;25:1735–41.
16. Muller AM, Born M, Jung C, Flury M, Kolling C, Schwyzer HK, Audigé L. Glenosphere size in reverse shoulder arthroplasty: is larger better for external rotation and abduction strength? J Shoulder Elb Surg. 2018;27:44–52.
17. Dillon MT, Inacio MC, Burke MF, Navarro RA, Yian EH. Shoulder arthroplasty in patients 59 years of age and younger. J Shoulder Elb Surg. 2013;22: 1338–44.
18. Denard PJ, Raiss P, Sowa B, Walch G. Mid-to long-term follow-up of total shoulder arthroplasty using a keeled glenoid in young adults with primary glenohumeral arthritis. J Shoulder Elb Surg. 2013;22: 894–900.
19. Mitchell JJ, Warner BT, Horan MP, et al. Comprehesive arthroscopic management of glenohumeral osteoarthritis: preoperative factors predictive of treatment failure. Am J Sports Med. 2017;45:794–802.
20. Millett PJ, Horan MP, Pennock AT, et al. Comprehesive Arthroscopic Management (CAM) procedure: clinical results of a joint-preserving arthroscopic treatment for young, active patients with advanced shoulder osteoarthritis. Arthroscopy. 2013;29:440–8.
21. Bailie DS, Llinas PJ, Ellenbecker TS. Cementless humeral resurfacing arthroplasty in active patients less than fifty-five years of age. J Bone Joint Surg Am. 2008;90:110–7.
22. Mehta SK, Aleem AW. Management of the B2 glenoid in glenohumeral osteoarthritis. Orthop Clin N Am. 2019;50:509–20.
23. Domos P, Chechia CS, Walch G. Walch B0 glenoid: pre-osteoarthritic posterior subluxation of the humeral head. J Shoulder Elb Surg. 2018;27:181–8.
24. Melis B, Bonnevialle N, Neyton Walch G. Glenoid loosening and failure in anatomical total shoulder arthroplasty. J Shoulder Elb Surg. 2012;21:342–9.
25. Handoll HH, Brorson S. Interventions for treating proximal humeral fractures in adults. Cochrane

Database Syst Rev. 2015:CD000434. https://doi.org/10.1002/14651858.CD000434.pub4.
26. Anakwenze OA, Zoller S, Ahmad CS, Levine WN. Reverse shoulder arthroplasty for acute proximal humerus fractures: a syistematic review. J Shoulder Elb Surg. 2014;23:e73–80.
27. Favre P, Sussmann PS, Gerber C. The effect of component positioning on intrinsic stability of the reverse shoulder arthroplasty. J Shoulder Elb Surg. 2010;19:550–6.
28. Fraser AN, Bjordal J, Wagle TM, Karlberg AC, Lien OA, Eilertsen L, Mder K, Apold H, Larsen LB, Madsen JE, Fjalestad T. Reverse shoulder arthroplasty is superior to plate fixation at 2 years for displaced proximal humeral fractures in the elderly. J Bone Jt Surg Am. 2020;102:477–85.
29. Lopiz A-DG-O. Reverse shoulder arthroplasty versus nonoperative treatment for 3- or 4-part proximal humeral fractures in elderly patients: a prospective randomized controlled trial. J Shoulder Elb Surg. 2019:2259–71.
30. Sebastiá-Forcada CG, Cebrián-Gómez R, Lizaur-Utrilla A, Gil-Guillén V. Reverse shoulder arthroplasty versus hemiarthroplasty for acute proximal humeral fractures. A blinded, randomized, controlled, prospective study. J Shoulder Elbow Surg. 2014;23:1419–26.
31. Jonsson ES, Ekholm C, Salomonsson B, Demir Y, Olerud P, Collaborators in the SAPF Study Group. Reverse total shoulder arthroplasty provides better shoulder function than hemiarthroplasty for displaced 3- and 4-part proximal humeral fractures in patients over 70 years of age: a multicenter randomized controlled trial. J Shoulder Elbow Surg. 2021;30:994–1006.
32. NCT02075476 A. (2020). Effectiveness between two surgical techniques for reconstruction of humeral proximal extremity fractures. Recuperado el diciembre de 2020, de clinicaltrials.gov: https://clinicaltrials.gov/ct2/show/results/NCT02075476
33. Crespo AM, Luthringer TA, Frost A, Khabie L, Roche C, Zuckerman JD, Egol KA. Does reverse total shoulder arthroplasty for proximal humerus fracture portend poorer outcomes than for elective indications? J Shoulder Elb Surg. 2021;30:40–50.
34. Tashjian RZ, Granger E, Chalmers PN. Structural glenoid grafting during primary reverse total shoulder arthroplasty using humeral head autograft. J Shoulder Elb Surg. 2018;27:e1–8.
35. Walch G, Badet R, Boulahia A, Khoury A. Morphologic study of the glenoid in primary glenohumeral osteoarthritis. J Arthroplast. 1999;14:756–60.
36. Nowak DD, Gardner TR, Bigliani LU, Levine WN, Ahmad CS. Interobserver and intraobserver reliability of the Walch classification in primary glenohumeral arthritis. J Shoulder Elb Surg. 2010;19:180–3.
37. Bercik MJ, Kruse K 2nd, Yalizis M, Gauci MO, Chaoui J, Walch G. A modification to the Walch classification of the glenoid in primary glenohumeral osteoarthritis using three-dimensional imaging. J Shoulder Elb Surg. 2016;25:1601–6.
38. Iannotti JP, Jun BJ, Patterson TE, Ricchetti ET. Quantitative measurement of osseous pathology in advanced glenohumeral osteoarthritis. J Bone Joint Surg Am. 2017;99:1460–8.
39. Ricchetti ET, Khazzam S, Denard PJ, Dines DM. Reliability of the modified Walch classification for advanced glenohumeral osteoarthritis using 3-dimensional computed tomography analysis: a study of the ASES B2 Glenoid Multicenter Research Group. J Shoulder Elb Surg. 2021;30:736–46.
40. Kleim SM, Dunning P, Frankle MA. Effects of adquired glenoid bone. JBJS Am. 2010;92:1144–54.
41. McFarland EG, Huri G, Hyun YS, et al. Reverse total shoulder arthroplasty without bone-grafting for severe glenoid bone loss in patients with osteoartjritis and intact rotator cuff. J Bone Joint Surg Am. 2016;98:1801–7.
42. Lorenzetti A, Streit JJ, Cabezas AF, et al. Bone graft augmentation for severe bone glenoid loss in primary reverse total shoulder arthroplasty: outcomes and evaluation of host bone contact by 2D-3D image registration. JB JS Open Access. 2017;2(3):e0015.
43. Boileau P, Morin-Salvo N, Gauci MO, et al. Angled BIO-RSA (bony-increased offset-reverse shoulder arthroplasty): a solution for the management of glenoid bone loss and erosion. J Shoulder Elb Surg. 2017;26:2133–42.
44. Nicholson GP, Cvetanovich GL, Rao AJ, et al. Posterior glenoid bone grafting in total shoulder arthroplasty for osteoarthritis with severe posterior glenoid wear. J Shoulder Elb Surg. 2017;26:1844–53.
45. Walch G, Moraga C, Young A, et al. Results of anatomic nonconstrained prosthesis in primary osteoarthritis with biconcave glenoid. J Shoulder Elb Surg. 2012;21:1526–33.
46. Mizuno N, Denard PJ, Raiss P, et al. Reverse total shoulder arthroplasty for primary glenohumeral osteoarthritis in patients with a biconcave glenoid. J Bone Joint Surg Am. 2013;95:1297–304.
47. Walch G, Young AA, Boileau P, Loew M, Gazielly D, Molé D. Patterns of loosening of polyethylene keeled glenoid components after shoulder arthroplasty for primary osteoarthritis: results of a multicenter study with more than five years of follow-up. J Bone Joint Surg Am. 2012;94:145–50.
48. Young AA, Walch G, Bolieau P, Favard L, Gohlke F, Loew M, et al. A multicenter study of the long -term results of a flat—back polyethylene glenoid component in shoulder replacement for primary osteoarthritis. J Bone Joint Surg Br. 2011;93:210–6.
49. Sperling JW, Cofield RH, O'Driscoll SW, Torchia ME, Rowland CM. Radiographic assesment of ingrowth total shoulder arthroplasty. J Shoulder Elb Surg. 2000;9:507–13.
50. Szerlip BW, Morris BJ, Laughlin MS, Kilian CM, Edwards TB. Clinical and radiographic outcomes after total shoulder arthroplasty with an anatomic press-fit short stem. J Shoulder Elb Surg. 2018;27:10–6.
51. Morwood MP, Johnston PS, Garrigues GE. Proximal ingrowth coating decreases risk of loosening

following uncemented shoulder arthroplasty using mini-stem humeral components and lesser tuberosity osteotomy. J Shoulder Elb Surg. 2017;26:1246–52.
52. Levy JC, Anderson C, Samson A. Classification of postoperative acromial fractures following reverse shoulder arthroplasty. J Bone Joint Surg Am. 2013;95:e104.
53. Crosby LA, Hamilton A, Twiss T. Scapula fractures after reverse total shoulder arthroplasty: classification ant treatment. Clin Ortho Relat Res. 2011;469: 2544–9.
54. Cho CH, Rhee TG, Yoo JC, et al. Incidence and risk factors of acromial fracture following reverse total shoulder arthroplasty. J Shoulder Elb Surg. 2021;30:57–64.
55. Marigi E, Bartels D, Tangtiphaiboontana J, et al. Acromial and spine fracture after reverse arthroplasty: prevalence and risk factors. Semin Arthroplast. 2020;30:237–41.
56. Colliton EM, Jawa A. Acromion and scapular spine fractures following total shoulder arthroplasty. Orthop Clin N Am. 2021;52:257–68.
57. Kohan EM, Chalmers PN, Salazar D, Keener JD, Yamaguchi K, Chamberlain AM. Dislocation following reverse total shoulder arthroplasty. J Shoulder Elb Surg. 2017;26:1238–45.
58. Cheung EV, Sarkissian EJ, Sox-Harris A, Comer AC, Saleh JR, Diaz R, Costouros JG. Instabilitu after reverse total shoulder arthroplasty. J Shoulder Elb Surg. 2018;27:1946–52.
59. Gallo RA, Gamradt SC, Mattern CJ, Cordasco FA, Craig EV, Dines DM, Warren RF. On behalf of the sports medicine and shoulder Service at the Hospital for special surgery, New York. Instability after reverse total shoulder replacement. J Shoulder Elb Surg. 2011;20:584–90.
60. Weatherby PJ, Efejuku TA, Somerson JS. Complications after anatomic shoulder arthroplasty. Revisiting leading causes of failure. Orthop Clin N Am. 2021;52:269–77.
61. Bohsali KI, Bois AJ, Wirth MA. Complications of shoulder arthroplasty. J Bone Joint Surg. 2017;99:256–69.
62. Somerson JS, Hsu JE, Neradilek MB, et al. Analysis of 4063 complications of shoulder arthroplasty reported to the US Food and Drug Administration from 2012 to 2016. J Shoulder Elb Surg. 2018;27:1978–86.
63. Australian Orthopaedic Association National Joint Replacement Registry (AOAANJRR). Hip, Knee & Shoulder Arthroplasty Annual Report, AOA, Adelaide. Available at: https://aoanjrr.sahmri.com/annual-reports-2020.
64. Matsen FA, Whitson AJ, Somerson JS, et al. Anatomic total shoulder arthroplasty with all-polyethylene glenoid component for primary osteoarthritis with glenoid deficiencies. JBJS open Access. 2020;5(4):e20.00002.
65. Service BC, Hsu JE, Somerson JS, et al. Does postoperative glenoid retroversion affect the 2-year clinical and radiographic outcomes for total shoulder arthroplasty? Clin Orthop. 2017;475:2726–39.
66. Grey SG, Wright TW, Flurin P-H, et al. Clinical and radiographic outcomes with a posteriorly augmented glenoid for Walch B glenoids in anatomic total shoulder arthroplasty. J Shoulder Elb Surg. 2020;29: e185–95.
67. Priddy M, Zarezadeh A, Farmer KW, et al. Early results of augmented anatomic glenoid components. J Shoulder Elb Surg. 2019;28(Supplement):S138–45.
68. Page RS, Pai V, Eng K, et al. Cementless versus cemented glenoid components in conventional total shoulder joint arthroplasty: analysis from the Australian Orthopaedic Association National Joint Replacement Registry. J Shoulder Elb Surg. 2018;27: 1859–65.
69. Boileau P, Avidor C, Krishnan SG, et al. Cemented polyethylene versus uncemented metal-backed glenoid components in total shoulder arthroplasty: a prospective, double-blind randomized study. J Shoulder Elb Surg. 2002;11:351–9.
70. Papadonikolakis A, Matsen FA. Metal-backed glenoid components have a higher rate of failure and fail by different modes in comparison with all-polyethylene components. J Bone Joint Surg Am. 2014;96: 1041–7.
71. Edwards TB, Labriola JE, Stanley RJ, et al. Radiographic comparison of pegged and keeled glenoid components using modern cemented techniques: a prospective randomized study. J Shoulder Elb Surg. 2010;19:251–7.
72. Welsher A, Gohal C, Madden K, et al. A comparison of pegged vs keeled glenoid components regarding functional and radiographic outcomes in anatomic total shoulder arthroplasty: a systematic review and meta-analysis. JSES Open Access. 2019;3:136–44.e1.
73. Parada SA, Flurin P-H, Wright TW, et al. Comparison of complications types and rates associated with anatomic and reverse total shoulder arthroplasty. J Shoulder Elb Surg. 2020; https://doi.org/10.1016/j.jse.2020.07.028.
74. Young AA, Walch G, Pape G, et al. Secondary rotator cuff dysfunction following total shoulder arthroplasty for primary glenohumeral osteoarthritis: results of a multicenter study with more than five years of follow-up. J Bone Joint Surg Am. 2021;94:685–93.
75. Levy DM, Abrams GD, Harris JD, et al. Rotator cuff tears after total shoulder arthroplasty in primary osteoarthritis: a systematic review. Int J Shoulder Surg. 2016;10:78–84.

Clavicle Fractures: To Operate or Not?

6

Alonso Moreno-García
and E. Carlos Rodríguez-Merchán

6.1 Introduction

Clavicle fractures are common injuries, especially in young active individuals. A recent study on high school athletes reported an injury rate of 1.80 per 100,000 [1]. These fractures account for approximately 2.6–4% of all fractures in adults [2]. A study from the Swedish Fracture Register showed a male predominance, with 68% of the clavicle fractures occurring in males, the largest subgroup aged 15–24 years. However, over the age of 65, females sustained more clavicle fractures than males [3].

These fractures are usually related to sport injuries and road traffic accidents. A direct blow on the point of the shoulder is the commonest reported mechanism of injury. Most of these fractures occur in the midshaft of the clavicle, followed by the distal third. Fractures of the medial third are the most uncommon ones.

Clavicle fractures were originally divided by Allman into proximal (Group I), middle (Group II), and distal (Group III) third fractures. This classification was posteriorly enhanced by Neer and Rockwood in an attempt to take into account factors that influence treatment and outcome. Posteriorly, Robinson developed a classification scheme based on prognostic variables from a population-based study [2]. This classification keeps the division of the clavicle into thirds, adding variables that are of proven diagnostic value: intra-articular extension, displacement, and comminution. Robinson classification is based on an extensive database that helps to predict outcome and hence guide treatment.

Regarding the treatment of clavicle fractures, there is still controversy in the surgical indications. A comprehensive epidemiological study from Sweden revealed important changes in the rates of surgery over the time independently to the actual fracture rates [4]. Local traditions and surgeon preferences have been suggested as important factors for the choice of surgical treatment. In this chapter, we review the most updated evidence concerning treatment of clavicle fractures to help the reader to decide on the treatment approach based on the best clinical evidence available.

6.2 Fractures of the Middle Third of the Clavicle

Fractures of the middle third of the clavicle are the most common ones. Traditionally, these fractures have been treated conservatively with generally good results. Neer, in a classical study that dominated the clinical approach to clavicular fractures for decades, reported nonunion in only three of 2235 patients with middle-third fractures

A. Moreno-García · E. C. Rodríguez-Merchán (✉)
Department of Orthopedic Surgery, "La Paz" University Hospital-IdiPaz, Madrid, Spain

E. C. Rodríguez-Merchán, A. Moreno-Garcìa (eds.), *Controversies in Orthopedic Surgery of The Upper Limb*, https://doi.org/10.1007/978-3-031-04907-1_6

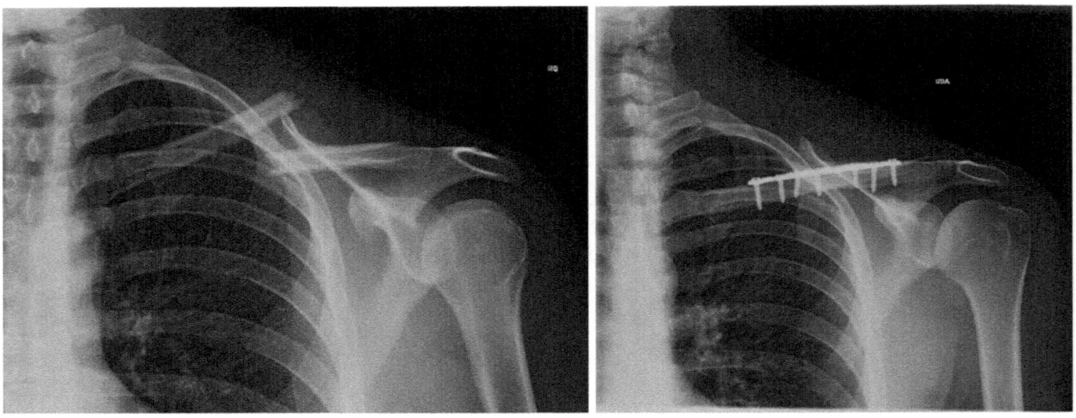

Fig. 6.1 Midshaft displaced fracture treated with open reduction and plate fixation (ORPF). Preoperative and postoperative X rays

treated by closed methods [5]. However, recent reports of large randomized control trials (RCT) have identified a subgroup of patients that may benefit from surgical treatment (Fig. 6.1). In a recent meta-analysis addressing this question, Qid et al. compared open reduction and plate fixation (ORPF) with nonsurgical treatment for displaced midshaft clavicle fractures. They conclude that ORPF yielded better results than conservative treatment in terms of fracture healing and appearance. However, the rate of complication was significantly lower in the nonsurgical treatment group, ranging from 3% to 7% when accounting for complications directly related to the surgery [6]. A multicenter randomized controlled trial comparing operative with nonoperative treatment of displaced midshaft clavicle fractures showed at 9 months a significantly lower proportion of nonunion ($p < 0.001$) in the operative group (0.8%) compared with the nonoperative group (11%). This study included 301 patients with an age of 18 to 65 years, with displaced midshaft fracture of the clavicle, Robinson classification 2B1 or 2B2, and being medically fit to undergo surgery. Fixation was performed using a precontoured titanium plate, while the conservative treatment consisted of a sling for up to 6 weeks or until there was clinical and/or radiographic evidence of union. The risk of complications in both treatment groups was low [7]. The DASH and Constant-Murley scores and patient satisfaction were all significantly better in the operative group than in the nonoperative group at 6 weeks and 3 months; however, they were equivalent at 9 months [7]. These findings of faster functional recovery in the surgical treated patients have been supported by Echalier et al. who reported a significant and clinically relevant difference in the functional scores favoring the surgical treatment in the first 6 weeks after the fracture event. Also, they showed that fracture fixation allows significantly faster return to work [8]. There is some discussion in relation to long-term clinical results, although the Canadian Orthopaedic Trauma Society reported in a large prospective clinical trial that Constant shoulder and DASH scores significantly improved in the operative fixation group at all time-points, with a total follow-up of 1 year [9]. Another interesting study evaluating the long-term results of nonsurgical treatment of midshaft clavicle fractures reported that patients with fractures with vertical displacement of ≥100% may eventually require surgical treatment due to unsatisfactory results secondary to residual deformities [10].

Under a societal perspective, and regarding cost-effectiveness, Sørensen et al. in a recent study concluded that operative treatment with locking plate fixation does not represent a cost-effective treatment option vs. nonoperative treatment in Denmark. However, the authors acknowledge that their results are subject to uncertainties and advise to interpret the results cautiously and take local context and patient profession into consideration [11]. Another study from the USA, however, found early operative fixation of displaced midshaft clavicle fractures more cost-effective than nonoperative treatment [12]. A systematic literature review on this matter have suggested that routine operative treatment seems to be more expensive, although cost-effective in some cases, recommending cost-effectiveness analysis in RCT studies in the future [13].

A recent meta-analysis including 11 high-quality trials has revealed a significantly lower relative risk of developing nonunion and symptomatic malunion in patients undergoing surgical treatment. A subgroup analysis of plate fixation versus intramedullary nailing was performed which suggested that the incidence of nonunion after plate fixation was lower as compared to intramedullary nailing [14]. Another reported complication of intramedullary nailing is axial instability resulting in telescoping and shortening of the clavicle length. To avoid this complication, a recent publication has proposed the use of S-shaped titanium endomedullary nails with good results [15]. For displaced midshaft fractures of the lateral diaphysis, and when using intramedullary nailing, a recent study advises the use of a lateral approach instead of the classical medial one. The authors report excellent functional results with this novel technique [16].

Currently, there is sufficient evidence to assume that surgical treatment of displaced midshaft fractures in adults produce better results when compared to the nonsurgical approach. In order to define displacement, it has been accepted, after the study of Hill et al., a distance >2 cm as the threshold for conservative management [17]. Regarding children and adolescents, surgical and conservative management may yield similar results, as presented by Swarup et al. in a recent study. Both operatively and nonoperatively treated patients had excellent functional and pain outcomes, similar refracture rates, and no nonunions [18]. Nonoperative management should be considered as first-line treatment for most pediatric displaced clavicle fractures, and operative management should potentially be reserved for atypical cases such as floating shoulder, multitrauma, open fractures, nonunions, and symptomatic malunions. Another study reporting long-term outcomes supports nonsurgical treatment as the treatment of choice for displaced midshaft clavicular fractures in adolescents [19].

Considering the surgical technique, ORPF is the most common procedure, but intramedullary nails can be also used. In a recent study comparing both techniques, no differences were found regarding clinical results or complications, leaving to the preference of the surgeon the choice of the implant used [20]. Skin erosion with the exposure of the synthesis material was the main complication in the group of ORPF reported in this study. Some authors have recommended incisions following the Langer's line to avoid skin complications; however, Anker et al. found in a recent study that an incision following Langer's lines does not reduce the rate of complications following fixation of displaced middle-third clavicle fractures [21].

Possible complications of ORPF were thoroughly reviewed by Wijdicks et al., finding the vast majority being implant related. Irritation or failure of the plate were consistently reported on average ranging from 9 to 64% [22]. The use of dual mini-fragment plating is an innovative approach to reduce complications. Compared to single plating, dual plating is biomechanically equivalent in axial loading and torsion yet offers better multi-planar bending stiffness despite the use of smaller plates. This technique may decrease the need for secondary surgery due to implant prominence and may aid in fracture reduction by buttressing butterfly fragments in two planes [23]. These good results have been substantiated by other authors [24, 25].When comparing local complications, a total of 8% of dual mini-fragment plating patients had symptomatic implant removal compared with 20% of single traditional plating patients [25]. A recent systematic review of the literature supports the aforementioned advantages of dual plating [26].

For midshaft clavicle fractures, the absence of cortical alignment in wedge and comminuted fractures directly influences the fixation stability of the synthesis, and complications like nonunion or malunion are more frequent [27]. The use of a lag screw in such instances have been recommended, and the AO/OTA advises a screw diameter of 3.5 mm. Wurm et al. have recently published a study comparing the use of lag screws of different diameter (3.5 mm vs. 2.0 mm), concluding that both groups showed comparable results with respect to fracture reduction, fixation, and stability as well as time to consolidation of the fracture, while the 2.0 mm screw diameter was associated with easier handling of small fracture fragments [28].

The floating shoulder, defined as combined clavicle and ipsilateral scapular neck fractures, is an entity that has recently been reviewed regarding its best therapeutic approach. An ample analysis of the literature found satisfactory outcomes following both surgical fixation and nonoperative management. However, floating shoulder injuries with significant displacement of the scapular neck may benefit from surgical fixation of both the clavicle and scapula fractures, while those with minimal or nondisplaced scapular neck fractures may achieve good outcomes when treated nonoperatively or with surgical fixation of the clavicle alone [29].

6.3 Fractures of the Distal Third of the Clavicle

In an ample review of the treatment of fractures of the distal clavicle, Oh et al. concluded that nonsurgical treatment resulted in a nonunion rate of 33.3% [30]. However, the same authors acknowledged no significant difference in the functional scores compared to the surgically treated group. There are up-to-date no high-quality studies to support either approach, and until then it seems prudent to treat these injuries nonoperatively initially and reserve surgery for severely displaced fractures and high-demand patients or for failures of nonoperative care (Fig. 6.2).

Regarding surgical treatment, several different techniques have been proposed, but none has been established as gold standard. Complications have been reviewed in the literature, finding for hook plate fixation a complication rate of 40.7% in one study [30] and 62.5% in another one [31]. Precontoured clavicle plate fixation showed a 16.2% complication rate in the same study, while no complications were found for coracoclavicular (CC) stabilization [31]. This low rate of complications for CC stabilization was reported as well by Oh et al. in a systematic review, reporting a complication rate of 4.8% [30].

A question that remains under discussion is the use of CC ligament augmentation when using

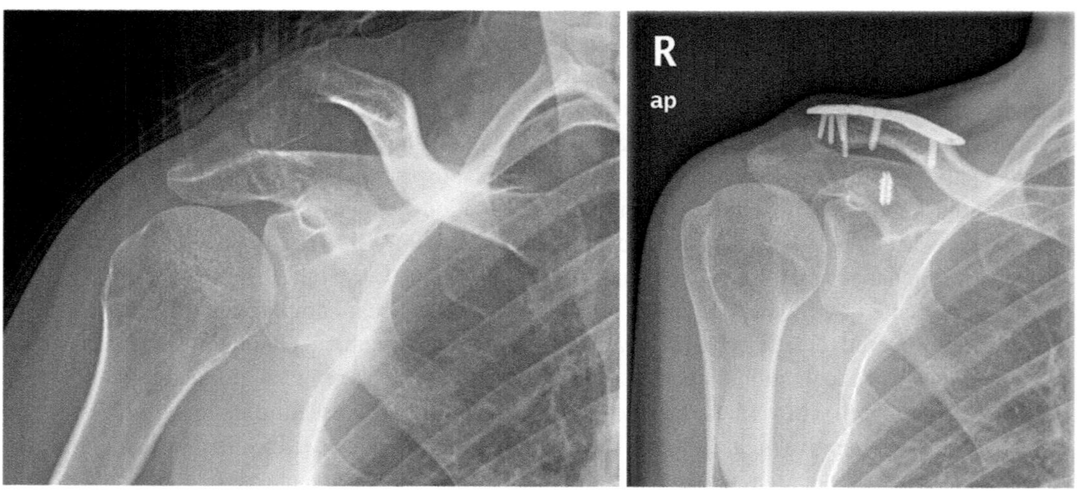

Fig. 6.2 Lateral displaced fracture treated with ORPF and CC augmentation. Preoperative and postoperative X rays

plate fixation of distal clavicle fractures. A recent study demonstrated comparable outcomes after locking plate fixation with and without CC ligament augmentation [32]. Other authors in contradistinction preconize the use of stand-alone coracoclavicular suture repair for the treatment of unstable distal clavicle fractures. In a case series study, the authors describe their technique of coracoclavicular stand-alone cow-hitch suture repair and report the results of 19 cases with a mean follow-up of 5 years [33].

In 2008, Kalamaras et al. described the use of locking T-plate for the treatment of distal clavicle displaced fractures. In an observational study of 9 cases, they reported good clinical results, achieving union in all the cases [34]. Posteriorly, precontoured-specific locking plates for distal clavicle fractures were developed. Vaishya et al., in a prospective study, reported the results of 32 patients treated with locking plates, showing good clinical and functional results with only one nonunion that did not require surgery. The authors consider this surgical treatment the best option available, awaiting for larger randomized studies [35]. A recent biomechanical study aimed to measure the screw angles and the number of screws that can be inserted in different fragment sizes and to elucidate the size limits for locking plate fixation. It concluded that other augmented fixation procedures should be considered for fractures with fragment sizes <25 mm that cannot be fixed with a sufficient number of screws [36].

The combination of locking plate fixation and CC ligament augmentations has been proposed recently based on the vertical and horizontal stress forces that intervene in these type of fractures and assuming that any technique counteracting both the forces should result in a better clinical outcome. Karuppaiah et al. published a prospective series of 19 patients treated with open reduction and internal fixation with lateral end locking plate augmented with a coracoid anchor. The authors reported good clinical and functional outcomes after a mean follow-up of 54 months, with a low rate of the need for implant removal (26%) and no difference in the functional outcome between intra-articular and extra-articular fractures [37]. Another case series of 22 patients treated surgically using precontoured locking plate and coracoclavicular reconstruction with Endobutton and FiberWire was reported by Vikas et al. In their study, clinical outcome was assessed using the University of California Los Angeles (UCLA) shoulder score and Constant-Murley score; the CC distance was also recorded. The CC distance did not vary significantly at a one-year interval when compared to the normal shoulder, there were no major complications in any of the patients, and all were able to return to their preinjury level of activity. Bony union was achieved in all the cases [38]. The use of a titanium alloy cable system-augmented reconstruction of the CC ligament, along with a precontoured locking compressive distal clavicular plate, has been recently proposed by Xie et al. In a case series study of 28 patients, the authors reported good restoration of function and high level of satisfaction. The mean CC distance was 9.61 ± 0.61 mm on the injured side vs. 9.62 ± 0.57 mm on the contralateral uninjured side. The reported complications were one delayed healing of the skin, one severe shoulder stiffness, three incidences of moderate shoulder stiffness, and five cases of symptomatic hardware [39]. With a similar technical approach, Zhang et al. published their results of a retrospective case series study of 21 patients, using a distal clavicle locking plate and a titanium cable. All patients achieved bony union within 6 months, with good clinical and functional results. They reported only one complication (wound infection), and two patients had the implant removed due to local irritation [40]. In a prospective cohort study, 36 patients with distal clavicle fracture were randomly allocated either to titanium cable group (fixed with a titanium cable in combination with a locking plate) and hook plate group (fixed with a clavicular hook plate only). The VAS score in the titanium cable group was significantly lower than that in the hook plate group 1 year after the operation, and the number of postoperative complications in the titanium cable group was significantly lower than that in the hook plate group. Both groups showed good clinical and functional outcomes [41].

6.4 Fractures of the Proximal Third of the Clavicle

Medial clavicle fractures are rare and traditionally acknowledged to account for only 2–3% of all clavicle fractures. However, a recent big data analysis elevated this figure to 11.6% [42]. They are more frequent in middle-aged males, and two-thirds of these fractures are undisplaced [43]. They are commonly associated with high-energy trauma, with a reported in-hospital mortality rates as high as 20% [44] and a 34% mortality rate at 5 years [45]. In a retrospective review study of this type of fractures, Salipas et al. found 68 cases over a 5-year period in a Level 1 Trauma Center. The majority of patients were males with a median age of 53.5 years. The fracture pattern was almost equally distributed between extra-articular and intra-articular, and 80.9% had minimal or no displacement. Operative fixation was performed for painful atrophic delayed union in only two patients (2.9%). Both patients were under 65 years of age and had a severely displaced fracture. Excellent functional results were reported in this study following conservative management [46].

Among patients with displaced fractures of the medial clavicle, surgical treatment has been advised although no randomized controlled study has been published to date. Sidhu et al. reported their results of 27 patients treated with plate and screws in 19 cases and with transosseous sutures in 8 cases. All patients had full shoulder range of motion at final follow-up and were able to return to preinjury occupational activities. There were no significant complications with a union rate of 100% at 12 months [47]. With the use of locking plates, Frima et al. published their results of a retrospective study including 15 patients. They concluded that operative treatment of displaced medial clavicle fractures with well-fitting "small fragment" locking plates provides an excellent long-term functional outcome. Regarding complications, one patient had an early revision operation and developed an infection after 1.5 years, no mal- or nonunions occurred, and eight patients had their implants removed [48]. Li et al. have recently proposed the use of a bridging plate technique across the sternum. For the one case presented, this technique maintained reduction and achieved union of a medial-end comminuted and displaced fracture. To the view of the authors, this approach is simple, safer, and promising [49]. Zúñiga et al. published a case report of a severely displaced proximal-third clavicle fracture managed with open reduction and double-plate internal fixation obtaining a good result [50].

Although uncommon, nonunions and/or failure of osteosynthesis of this type of fracture pose a difficult problem with scarce experience reported. In an innovative approach, Dion et al. proposed medial clavicle resection and stabilization to the sternum using a palmaris longus autograft as a salvage technique. Excellent functional outcomes at 3 years of follow-up were reported in the case presented [51].

6.5 Conclusions

Clavicle fractures are common injuries accounting for 2.6–4% of all fractures in adults. There are several classifications, but we advise the use of Robinson's which has proven diagnostic and prognostic value.

Fractures of the middle third are the commonest. They have been traditionally treated conservatively; however, in the cases of displacement, surgical treatment has inarguably reduced the rate of nonunions. When it comes to patient satisfaction and function, surgically treated patients showed a faster recovery although equivalent scores are reported on the long term. However, for pediatric and adolescent patients, nonoperative management should be considered as first-line treatment, and operative management should potentially be reserved for atypical cases such as floating shoulder, multitrauma, open fractures, nonunions, and symptomatic malunions.

Plate fixation (ORPF) is the most common procedure used for the treatment of middle-third clavicle fractures; however, intramedullary, nails can be also used with similar functional and clinical results, as well as complication rates. The vast majority of ORPF complications are implant related. Dual mini-fragment plating is an innovative approach which has shown to reduce these complications. The use of lag screws is advised in wedge and comminuted fractures to reduce complications, traditionally of 3.5 mm of diameter. A recent study using smaller diameter screws (2 mm) showed comparable results with easier handling of small fracture fragments. After a recent review, floating shoulder injuries with significant displacement of the scapular neck may benefit from surgical fixation of both the clavicle and scapula fractures. Cost-effectiveness of surgical treatment of middle-third clavicle fractures has been addressed recently with inconsistent results, for which it has been recommended to add economic studies in future RCT.

Fractures of the distal third of the clavicle treated conservatively are prone to nonunion with a reported rate of 33%. However, studies comparing surgical and conservative treatment have not shown differences regarding function and pain. There are up-to-date no high-quality studies to support either approach, and until then it seems prudent to treat these injuries nonoperatively initially and reserve surgery for severely displaced fractures, high-demand patients, or failures of nonoperative care. Hook plate fixation has a high reported rate of complications, for which locking plate fixation seems a wiser approach especially if using precontoured implants. The use of coracoclavicular (CC) ligament augmentation would add further stability to the construct facilitating faster recovery and better clinical outcomes. Encouraging case series in this respect have been published, but no RCTs are available to date.

Medial clavicle fractures account for 2–11% of all clavicle fractures and are usually associated with high-energy trauma. In displaced fractures, surgical treatment has been advised although no randomized controlled study has been published to date. Locking plates are the implants of choice in the published series. Recently, medial clavicle resection and stabilization to the sternum using a palmaris longus autograft as a salvage technique has been described.

References

1. McCarthy MM, Bihl JH, Frank RM, Salem HS, McCarty EC, Comstock RD. Epidemiology of clavicle fractures among US high school athletes, 2008-2009 through 2016-2017. Orthop J Sports Med. 2019;7:2325967119861812.
2. Robinson CM. Fractures of the clavicle in the adult: epidemiology and classification. J Bone Joint Surg. 1998;80:476–84.
3. Kihlström C, Möller M, Lönn K, Wolf O. Clavicle fractures: epidemiology, classification and treatment of 2 422 fractures in the Swedish Fracture Register; an observational study. BMC Musculoskelet Disord. 2017;18(1):82.
4. Huttunen TT, Launonen AP, Berg HE, Lepola V, Felländer-Tsai L, Mattila VM. Trends in the incidence of clavicle fractures and surgical repair in Sweden: 2001-2012. J Bone Joint Surg Am. 2016;98:1837–42.
5. Neer CS. Nonunion of the clavicle. J Am Med Assoc. 1960;172:1006–11.
6. Qin M, Zhao S, Guo W, Tang L, Li H, Wang X, et al. Open reduction and plate fixation compared with non-surgical treatment for displaced midshaft clavicle fracture: a meta-analysis of randomized clinical trials. Medicine (Baltimore). 2019;98(20):e15638.
7. Ahrens PM, Garlick NI, Barber J, Tims EM. The clavicle trial. J Bone Joint Surg Am. 2017;99:1345–54.
8. Echalier C, Sakek F, Soumagne T, el Rifaï S, Berthier F, Uhring J, et al. Prospective evaluation of early functional recovery of displaced fractures of the middle third of the clavicle whether operated or not. Orthop Traumatol Surg Res. 2021;107:102768.
9. Canadian Orthopaedic Trauma Society. Nonoperative treatment compared with plate fixation of displaced midshaft clavicular fractures. J Bone Joint Surg. 2007;89:1–10.
10. Lee GB, Kim H, Jeon I-H, Koh KH. Long-term outcomes of initially conservatively treated midshaft clavicle fractures. Clin Shoulder Elbow. 2021;24:9–14.
11. Sørensen A-KR, Hammeken LH, Qvist AH, Jensen SL, Ehlers LH. Operative treatment of displaced midshaft clavicular fractures is not cost-effective. J Shoulder Elb Surg. 2020;29:27–35.
12. Liu J, Srivastava K, Washington T, Hoegler J, Guthrie ST, Hakeos W, et al. Cost-effectiveness of operative versus nonoperative treatment of displaced midshaft clavicle fractures. J Bone Joint Surg. 2019;101:35–47.
13. Kask G, Raittio L, Mattila VM, Launonen AP. Cost-effectiveness of operative versus non-operative treatment for clavicle fracture: a systematic literature review. Curr Rev Musculoskeletal Med. 2020;13:391–9.
14. Amer K, Smith B, Thomson JE, Congiusta D, Reilly MC, Sirkin MS, et al. Operative versus nonoperative outcomes of middle-third clavicle fractures: a systematic review and meta-analysis. J Orthop Trauma. 2020;34:e6–e13.

15. Langenhan R, Bushuven S, Reimers N, Probst A. S-shaped titanium endomedullary nail reduces telescoping of comminuted midshaft clavicular fractures. Eur J Orthop Surg Traumatol. 2021;31:391–8.
16. Kabelitz N, Kabelitz M, Frima H, Rehm A, Sommer C, Michelitsch C. Lateral approach for intramedullary nailing of displaced midshaft clavicle fractures; a retrospective cohort study. Eur J Trauma Emerg Surg. 2021; https://doi.org/10.1007/s00068-021-01620-4. Online ahead of print.
17. Hill JM, McGuire MH, Crosby LA. Closed treatment of displaced middle-third fractures of the clavicle gives poor results. J Bone Joint Surg. 1997;79:537–9.
18. Swarup I, Maheshwer B, Orr S, Kehoe C, Zhang Y, Dodwell E. Intermediate-term outcomes following operative and nonoperative management of midshaft clavicle fractures in children and adolescents. JBJS Open Access. 2021;6:–e20.00036.
19. Riiser MO, Molund M. Long-term functional outcomes and complications in operative versus nonoperative treatment for displaced midshaft clavicle fractures in adolescents: a retrospective comparative study. J Pediatr Orthop. 2021;41:279–83.
20. Storti TM, Camilo MS, Silva RFA, Faria RSS, Simionatto CL, Paniago AF. Clinical evaluation of the treatment of clavicle fractures: intramedullary nail × plate. Acta Ortop Bras. 2021;29:34–8.
21. Ankers T, Sawalha S, Nixon M, Kenyon P, Webb M. Does a skin incision along Langer's lines reduce complications following fixation of displaced middle-third clavicle fractures? Arch Orthop Trauma Surg. 2021; https://doi.org/10.1007/s00402-021-03766-7. Online ahead of print.
22. Wijdicks F-JG, van der Meijden OAJ, Millett PJ, Verleisdonk EJMM, Houwert RM. Systematic review of the complications of plate fixation of clavicle fractures. Arch Orthop Trauma Surg. 2012;132:617–25.
23. Prasarn ML, Meyers KN, Wilkin G, Wellman DS, Chan DB, Ahn J, et al. Dual mini-fragment plating for midshaft clavicle fractures: a clinical and biomechanical investigation. Arch Orthop Trauma Surg. 2015;135:1655–62.
24. Chen MJ, DeBaun MR, Salazar BP, Lai C, Bishop JA, Gardner MJ. Safety and efficacy of using 2.4/2.4 mm and 2.0/2.4 mm dual mini-fragment plate combinations for fixation of displaced diaphyseal clavicle fractures. Injury. 2020;51:647–50.
25. DeBaun MR, Chen MJ, Campbell ST, Goodnough LH, Lai C, Salazar BP, et al. Dual mini-fragment plating is comparable with precontoured small fragment plating for operative diaphyseal clavicle fractures: a retrospective cohort study. J Orthop Trauma. 2020;34:e229–32.
26. Sheth U, Fernandez CE, Morgan AM, Henry P, Nam D. Are two plates better than one? A systematic review of dual plating for acute midshaft clavicle fractures. Shoulder Elbow. 2021; https://doi.org/10.1177/17585732211002495.
27. Hulsmans MH, van Heijl M, Houwert RM, Burger BJ, Verleisdonk E, Jan M, Veeger DJ, et al. Surgical fixation of midshaft clavicle fractures: a systematic review of biomechanical studies. Injury. 2018;49:753–65.
28. Wurm M, Zyskowski M, Greve F, Gersing A, Biberthaler P, Kirchhoff C. Comparable results using 2.0-mm vs. 3.5-mm screw augmentation in midshaft clavicle fractures: a 10-year experience. Eur J Med Res. 2021;26(1):122.
29. Dombrowsky AR, Boudreau S, Quade J, Brabston EW, Ponce BA, Momaya AM. Clinical outcomes following conservative and surgical management of floating shoulder injuries: a systematic review. J Shoulder Elb Surg. 2020;29:634–42.
30. Oh JH, Kim SH, Lee JH, Shin SH, Gong HS. Treatment of distal clavicle fracture: a systematic review of treatment modalities in 425 fractures. Arch Orthop Trauma Surg. 2011;131:525–33.
31. Singh A, Schultzel M, Fleming JF, Navarro RA. Complications after surgical treatment of distal clavicle fractures. Orthop Traumatol Surg Res. 2019;105:853–9.
32. Salazar BP, Chen MJ, Bishop JA, Gardner MJ. Outcomes after locking plate fixation of distal clavicle fractures with and without coracoclavicular ligament augmentation. Eur J Orthop Surg Traumatol. 2021;31:473–9.
33. Laux CJ, Villefort C, el Nashar R, Farei-Campagna JM, Grubhofer F, Bouaicha S, et al. Stand-alone coracoclavicular suture repair achieves very good results in unstable distal clavicle fractures at a minimum follow-up of 1 year. J Shoulder Elb Surg. 2021;30:2090–6.
34. Kalamaras M, Cutbush K, Robinson M. A method for internal fixation of unstable distal clavicle fractures: early observations using a new technique. J Shoulder Elb Surg. 2008;17:60–2.
35. Vaishya R, Vijay V, Khanna V. Outcome of distal end clavicle fractures treated with locking plates. Chin J Traumatol. 2017;20:45–8.
36. Abe S, Koizumi K, Murase T, Kuriyama K. Comparing the locking screw direction of three locking plates for lateral clavicle fractures: a simulation study. BMC Musculoskelet Disord. 2021;22(1):812.
37. Karuppaiah K, Bilal A, Colegate-Stone T, Sinha J, Tahmassebi R, Tavakkolizadeh A. Outcome following management of unstable lateral end clavicle fractures with locking plate and coracoid anchor augmentation. Shoulder Elbow. 2021; https://doi.org/10.1177/1758573220981708.
38. Vikas V, Bhatia N, Jalan D, Prakash J, Singh J, Khare S. Clinical outcome of Neer type II lateral end clavicle fractures with coracoclavicular ligament disruption treated with pre-contoured locking plate and endobutton. Cureus. 2021;13(1):e12585.
39. Xie Z, Song M, Zhou J, Yin G, Lin H. Precontoured locking compression plate with titanium alloy cable system: in treatment of Neer type IIb distal clavicle fracture. Orthop Surg. 2021;13:451–7.
40. Zhang F, Fu Q, Li Y, Lu N, Chen A, Zhao L. Locking plate combined with titanium cable for Neer type II

distal clavicle fractures. BMC Musculoskelet Disord. 2021;22(1):269.
41. Wang J, Guan J, Liu M, Cui Y, Zhang Y. Treatment of distal clavicle fracture of Neer type II with locking plate in combination with titanium cable under the guide. Sci Rep. 2021;11(1):4949.
42. Bakir MS, Unterkofler J, Haralambiev L, Kim S, Carbon R, Ekkernkamp A, et al. Medial injuries of the clavicle: more prevalent than expected? A big data analysis of incidence, age, and gender distribution based on nationwide routine data. Eur J Trauma Emerg Surg. 2021;47:1175–82.
43. Gumina S, Carbone S, Polizzotti G, Paglialunga C, Preziosi Standoli J, Candela V. The rare medial-end clavicle fractures: epidemiological study on inhabitants of a suburban area. Cureus. 2021;13(9):e18008.
44. Throckmorton T, Kuhn JE. Fractures of the medial end of the clavicle. J Shoulder Elb Surg. 2007;16:49–54.
45. Lindsey MH, Grisdela P, Lu L, Zhang D, Earp B. What are the functional outcomes and pain scores after medial clavicle fracture treatment? Clin Orthop Relat Res. 2021;479:2400–7.
46. Salipas A, Kimmel LA, Edwards ER, Rakhra S, Moaveni AK. Natural history of medial clavicle fractures. Injury. 2016;47:2235–9.
47. Sidhu VS, Hermans D, Duckworth DG. The operative outcomes of displaced medial-end clavicle fractures. J Shoulder Elb Surg. 2015;24:1728–34.
48. Frima H, Houwert RM, Sommer C. Displaced medial clavicle fractures: operative treatment with locking compression plate fixation. Eur J Trauma Emerg Surg. 2020;46:207–13.
49. Li Z, Liu H, Chen D, Chen C, Zhang Y, Xue E. A new technique for medial-end comminuted clavicle fractures. Injury. 2019;50:811–3.
50. Zúñiga DG, García LF, Leal JA. Biplanar osteosynthesis for severely displaced proximal-third clavicle fracture: a case report. JBJS case. Connect. 2021;11(2) https://doi.org/10.2106/JBJS.CC.20.00584.
51. Dion MO, Martel S, Pelet S. Surgical treatment of a medial clavicle fracture nonunion with medial clavicle resection and stabilization to the sternum with palmaris longus graft. Case Rep Orthop. 2019;2019:7123790.

Massive Rotator Cuff Tears: When and How to Repair

7

Diego de Godos-Martínez, Pablo Vadillo-Cardona, and Alfonso Vaquero-Picado

7.1 Introduction

Shoulder pain is one of the most frequent circumstances leading to consultation in orthopedic surgery. Rotator cuff disorders are among the most frequent causes of shoulder pain. In fact, they are considered to be the main cause of disability related to the shoulder [1]. Rotator cuff disorders include a wide range of pathologies, from simple subacromial bursitis and tendonitis to massive irreparable cuff tears and rotator cuff arthropathy. All are related to a common etiology and can be named as the "rotator cuff disease."

It is paramount to differentiate the terms "massive" and "irreparable." Rotator cuff tears are considered massive when two or more tendons are affected and/or retracted. A massive tear can be reparable or not. However, a cuff tear is irreparable when the possibilities of healing after repair are poor. An irreparable tear can be massive or not (i.e., a severe fatty infiltrated isolated supraspinatus tear is irreparable but not necessarily massive). Regarding massive rotator cuff tears, there is a controversy in what is the appropriate treatment for patients who suffer this pathology. It is of special interest to discuss the convenience or not of repairing this lesions and the best method to perform it. In this chapter, we will try to clarify these aspects according to the evidence that is available. We will mainly focus the content of our chapter on degenerative cuff tears.

7.2 Epidemiology

Prevalence of rotator cuff tears have been investigated in cadaver specimens and also in imaging studies performed in general population. Investigations in cadaver specimens have reported a prevalence of rotator cuff tendon defects ranging from 5% to almost 40% [2]. General population studies with ultrasonography have shown that rotator cuff tears are present in 20.7% of the explored shoulders, with a prevalence of 16.9% in asymptomatic subjects [3]. Overall, prevalence of rotator cuff abnormalities increases with age, from 9.2% in patients under 20 years to up to 62% in patients over 80 years of age [4]. Other risk factors for rotator cuff tears had been reported: dominant arm, history of trauma [3], smoking [5], genetics [6], and hypercholesterolemia [7].

7.3 Anatomy and Biomechanics

Rotator cuff is constituted of four muscles: supraspinatus, infraspinatus, teres minor, and subscapularis. Each one is prolonged by a tendon, inserting distally in a different point at the proxi-

D. de Godos-Martínez · P. Vadillo-Cardona
A. Vaquero-Picado (✉)
Upper Limb Unit, Department of Orthopedic Surgery, La Paz University Hospital, Madrid, Spain

E. C. Rodríguez-Merchán, A. Moreno-Garcìa (eds.), *Controversies in Orthopedic Surgery of The Upper Limb*, https://doi.org/10.1007/978-3-031-04907-1_7

mal humerus, keeping a consistent pattern [8, 9]. The primary function of cuff tendons is to balance forces in the glenohumeral joint, providing dynamic stability in two planes: vertical (coronal) and horizontal (axial). In addition, rotator cuff muscles contribute to humeral rotation and compress the humeral head against the glenoid fossa, centering the proximal humerus during all the range of motion [10].

In coronal plane, the supraspinatus counteracts the superior force produced by the deltoid muscle, centering the head. This is known as the vertical balance. In the horizontal plane, the anterior moment created by internal rotators (pectoralis major, subscapularis, teres major, and latissimus dorsi) is counteracted by the posterior moment created by external rotators (infraspinatus and teres minor). This subtle balance of forces may cease when rotator cuff disease appears, causing pain, disability, and joint degeneration. When shoulder is not balanced on vertical plane, the deltoid will pull the head superiorly without the opposition of the supraspinatus. The humeral head tends to scape superior (first) and anteriorly, leading to a pseudoparalytic shoulder. When the broken balance is on the horizontal plane, the bigger and stronger internal rotator muscles will not have the opposition of the external rotators, and the patient will lose the ability for external rotation. Cadaveric studies have shown the presence of a crescent-shaped structure that comprises supraspinatus and infraspinatus insertions from anterior to posterior: the rotator cable [11]. This structure may act as the cable of a suspension bridge, protecting function of the cuff when a tear occurs and aiding to maintain dynamic stability.

7.4 Natural History of Rotator Cuff Disease

When talking about rotator cuff disease, different types of lesions can be found, ranging from simple tendinosis to massive full thickness tears and rotator cuff arthropathy. These lesions are considered to be part of a continuous process of degeneration which starts with compression or impingement of the tendon against close structures (acromion, coracoid process, or coracoacromial ligament), causing at first acute tendinosis with edema and hemorrhage that progresses into chronic tendinitis with fibrosis and, finally, rotator cuff tears [12]. However, not all the cases fit into this sequence of progressive degenerative condition, and two subgroups of patients can be distinguished: young patients (usually under 40 years of age) with traumatic tears and older patients (over 50 years) with nontraumatic, degenerative tears [13].

There is a group of patients where rotator cuff tears are part of a degenerative process related with age. Several studies have shown that is frequent to find tears in asymptomatic subjects [3], with a 15% rate of full-thickness tears and a 20% rate of partial thickness tears [14]. Awareness of the natural evolution of these asymptomatic tears is useful in the understanding of rotator cuff disease. Yamaguchi et al. reported that 51% of asymptomatic patients with full-thickness tears became symptomatic over a period of 2.8 years [15]. Pain development is associated with tear enlargement. Larger tears are also more likely to develop symptoms and to progress [16]. Regarding symptomatic patients, it has been reported that larger tears have a chance of progression around 50% [17, 18]. On the other hand, smaller tears (under 1–1.5 cm) have shown lower risk of enlargement (25%) [19]. Natural history of rotator cuff disease and untreated tears must be taken into account when evaluating a patient presenting with this pathology.

7.5 Rotator Cuff Tears Classification: Definition of Massive Rotator Cuff Tear

Cofield subdivided tears in four groups according to the length of the greatest diameter of the tear: small (1 cm or less), medium (1–3 cm), large (3–5 cm), and massive (over 5 cm) [20]. Harryman et al. classified tears according to the number of tendons affected, without giving a specific definition for massive tears [21]. Gerber et al. also classified tears according to the number of tendons torn and defined massive tears as the detachment of at least two entire tendons [22]. Patte presented a complex classification that takes into account the extent of the tear and topography in the frontal and sagittal plane [23]. This system introduced the concept of tendon retraction: minimal retraction (stage 1), retraction to the level of the humeral head (stage 2), and retraction to the level of the glenoid (stage 3).

Davidson and Burkhart proposed a three-dimensional classification system in which tears are divided in four groups according to geometric patterns [24]: type 1 (crescent-shaped), type 2 (longitudinal U-shaped and L-shaped), type 3 (massive contracted, defined as too long for the tendon end to be pulled laterally directly to bone and too wide to be closed directly side to side), and type 4 (arthropathy, associated with glenohumeral osteoarthritis). The size established by Davidson and Burkhart to consider a tear as massive contracted was coronal length and sagittal width over 2–3 cm. As it can be inferred from this huge variety of classifications, there is not consensus about the definition of what a massive rotator cuff tear is. Probably, the most widely used is the one given by Gerber et al. [22]: detachment of two entire tendons, and that is the definition that will be employed in this chapter.

7.6 Massive Rotator Cuff Tears: When to Repair

When facing a massive rotator cuff tear, several issues must be taken into account: clinical factors (symptoms, function, age, activity of the patient, mechanism of tear), imaging, and intraoperative factors. All of them must be analyzed comprehensively to determine if a tear is amenable to be repaired or not.

7.6.1 Clinical Factors

Regarding clinical factors, an adequate physical examination must be performed. This should include inspection (signs of muscular atrophy), palpation (search for concomitant pathology around the shoulder), assessment of range of motion, and neurovascular examination (to assess the integrity of axillary and suprascapular nerve function).

Strength testing of all rotator cuff muscles is paramount [25]. Some patients with massive tears are able to maintain active overhead motion [26]. These are the patients with a "balanced shoulder" either vertical and/or horizontal. However, other patients present a pseudoparalytic shoulder, defined as the inability to raise the affected arm over 90° in association with preserved passive motion (unbalanced vertical shoulder) [27]. In a series published by Läderman et al., reversion of pseudoparalysis could be achieved in over 90% of patients with arthroscopic rotator cuff repair [28]. Functional results worsen when revision repair is tried in individuals with pseudoparalysis, with only 43% of subjects regaining forward flexion over 90° [29]. However, results of repair in massive tears with pseudoparalysis are not consistent through the literature, and indication for repair in these patients must be carefully addressed. It is now accepted (and the opinion of the authors), that pseudoparalysis is better addressed with a reverse shoulder arthroplasty, giving more consistent and reliable results.

7.6.2 Imaging Factors

Besides physical examination, imaging of the shoulder is necessary to evaluate treatment options for massive tears. Standard evaluation must include plain radiographs with different views (at least true anteroposterior and lateral views). Ultrasonography can be used in diagnosis, but it is highly technician dependent, so we prefer magnetic resonance in order to assess size and location of the tear, tendon retraction, or muscle degeneration.

Regarding plain radiographs, the presence of rotator cuff arthropathy must be assessed. Hamada et al. proposed a radiographic classification of arthritis in massive rotator cuff tears [30] that were subsequently complemented by Walch et al. [31]. It distinguishes 5 stages: stage 1 (acromiohumeral interval greater than 7 mm), stage 2 (acromiohumeral interval less than 7 mm), stage 3 (acromiohumeral interval less than 7 mm with acetabulization of the acromion), stage 4a (acromiohumeral interval less than 7 mm with glenohumeral arthritis without acetabulization of the acromion), stage 4b (acromiohumeral interval less than 7 mm with glenohumeral arthritis and acetabulization of the acromion), and stage 5 (acromiohumeral interval less than 7 mm with collapsed humeral head). Patients with decreased acromiohumeral interval (stage 2 or higher) have shown a higher rate of supraspinatus retear after repair when compared to subjects with preserved acromiohumeral distance (stage 1) [32], so a <7 mm acromiohumeral interval is usually considered a relative contraindication for repair. Recently, it has been proposed that acromiohumeral interval must be measured not only in standard radiographs but also in stress radiographs (with patient holding a 5 kg weight). This introduces the concept of "reducible" acromiohumeral distance: those patients with a differential value in acromiohumeral interval greater than 3.2 mm between standard and stress radiographs showed a lower failure rate and higher functional scores [33]. Supraspinatus tendon repair failure has been reported to be significantly more frequent in patients with osteoarthritis [34]. Therefore, the presence of degenerative changes in plain radiographs with reduced acromiohumeral distance is a factor that must be taken into account when deciding if a tear is amenable to repair or not. As we have mentioned before, ascended humeral head is considered a contraindication for repairing supraspinatus tears, as the risk of pseudoparalysis and re-tear is extremely high. In case of symptomatic ascended humeral head or glenohumeral osteoarthritis, palliative techniques should be considered.

Magnetic resonance (MRI) is the most accurate and widely used examination for studying rotator cuff tears (Fig. 7.1). One of the main aspects that can be (and should be) evaluated on MRI is the presence of fatty infiltration in rotator cuff muscles. Goutallier et al. proposed a classification system for fatty muscle degeneration that is widely used [35]. Although this system was initially described in CT scan images, it has been adapted for use on T1 imaging on MRI by Fuchs et al. [36]. It differentiates 5 grades: grade 1 (normal muscle), grade 2 (some fatty streaking), grade 3 (fatty infiltration present but less than muscle), grade 4 (equal amount of fatty infiltration than muscle), and grade 5 (more fat than muscle). Several authors have reported worse results in rotator cuff repair when muscles present a fatty degeneration index over grade 3 in the supraspinatus or over grade 2 in the infraspinatus, with higher rates of incomplete repair [37, 38]. Grade 2 fatty infiltration of the supraspinatus has been reported as a positive predictor for retears [39]. After repair, improvement of fatty degeneration has been observed in 25% of the cases [40].

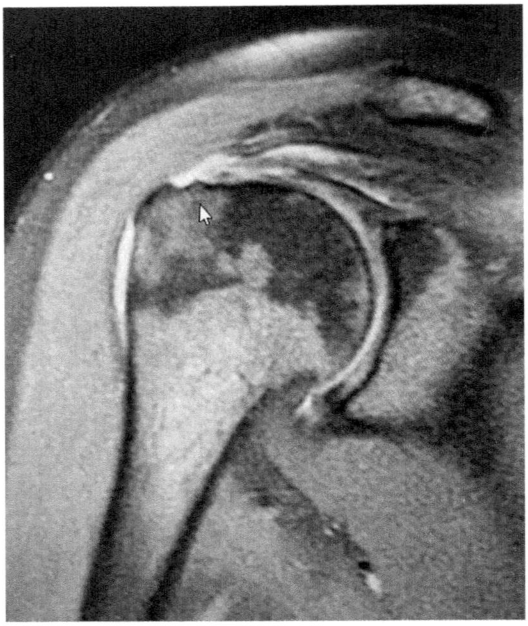

Fig. 7.1 Magnetic resonance imaging (MRI) showing a degenerative supraspinatus tear, Patte grade 1

Other aspects that should be assessed on MRI are tendon retraction and tear size. Preoperative musculotendinous junction position with respect to the glenoid has been reported to be a predictive factor of healing: tears that had a preoperative musculotendinous junction medial to glenoid level show lower healing rates when compared to those in which musculotendinous junction is lateral (56% vs. 94%) [41]. Patte classification equal or under stage 2 (tendon retraction that does not reach glenoid level) has been associated with good results after repair [42]. Anteroposterior and mediolateral tear size have also shown correlation with reparability in large to massive rotator cuff tears [38].

Age has also been reported as a critical factor in tendon healing, with patients under 65 years presenting significantly higher rates of healing (86% vs. 43%) [43]. Traumatic tears have shown significantly better postoperative results as well [13]. Taking into account the risk of progression in symptomatic tears [17, 18] and the good healing rates, the indication of repair is clear in young patients, and it should be attempted in almost all cases. However, in old patients with degenerative tears, repair is not always indicated. Conservative treatment provides good results in older patients [44] and allows to avoid surgery in near half of the subjects, with some series reporting intervention rates of only 26% after appropriate physical therapy [45]. Moreover, delaying surgery for 3 months does not seem to influence the outcome negatively [46]. For thus, conservative management before considering surgery seems an adequate practice in many patients sustaining degenerative tears.

7.6.3 Intraoperative Factors

Rotator cuff tears are not only defined as irreparable according to preoperative factors: a tear in which we cannot reduce the tendon to its footprint or in which the tendon is reduced but we foresee that the repair is going to fail is also an irreparable tear. It has been reported that the possibility of re-tear increases when tension over 35 N is required to reach the articular margin of the footprint [47].

In brief, a comprehensive evaluation of the patient and imaging is necessary when pondering the treatment of a massive cuff tear. However, we must be aware that these are not the only factors involved and that intraoperative findings are important too. Rotator cuff arthropathy, high-grade fatty infiltration, and tendon retraction are relative contraindications for repair, and risks and benefits must be taken into account before indicating surgery, especially in older patients with lower healing potential.

7.7 Massive Rotator Cuff Tears: How to Repair

Once the decision of repairing a rotator cuff tear has been made, the surgeon has to choose what is the best method to perform it. A huge variety of techniques have been described, not only for primary repair but also for helping in tendon reduction and for reinforcement or augmentation of the construct. A good choice between this myriad of surgical options can maximize the chances for obtaining a complete and functional tendon healing.

Open repair in massive tears has shown good long-term clinical outcomes with adequate functional scores and subjective patient satisfaction, although re-tear rates as high as 57% in 10 years have been reported [48]. One advantage of this technique is the shorter learning curve. Classically, the possibility of performing fixation through transosseous tunnels was mentioned as another advantage of open repair. However, with improved suture-anchors designs, it has been reported that bone fixation by suture-anchors is significantly less prone to failure than fixation through bone tunnels [49]. Regarding disadvantages of the open technique, some authors have reported higher infection rates when compared with arthroscopic repair [50].

Arthroscopic treatment has risen as a reliable alternative to open repair of rotator cuff tears in the last two decades. Faster recovery, better cosmetic results, and decreased postoperative pain have been cited as possible advantages of this technique. However, there is no evidence on the superiority of arthroscopic versus open repair concerning the postoperative pain relief [51]. Although initial comparative studies reported worse outcomes in massive tears when compared to the open treatment (82% vs. 77% of satisfactory results) [52], more recent meta-analyses have shown no differences in pain, functional scores, range of motion, or complications between both techniques [53, 54]. Considering this, we think that both techniques are still valid options, and the choice must be taken according to the surgeon's experience and preference.

When choosing the technique of repair, a key aspect that must be taken into account is the geometric pattern of the tear. As previously mentioned, Davidson and Burkhart classified rotator cuff tears according to a three-dimensional pattern and proposed a repair method for each one [24]: crescent-shaped tears (type 1) are proposed to be operated with a direct tendon to-bone repair; U-shaped and L-shaped longitudinal tears (type 2) are better repaired with a side-to-side/margin convergence technique along with lateral suture anchors; massive contracted tears (type 3) are considered too long for the tendon end to be pulled laterally directly to bone and too wide to be closed directly side to side, so release and interval slides are often required. In some cases, partial repair may be the best choice. Arthropathy tears (type 4) are considered irreparable.

There is controversy on what is the best treatment option for massive contracted tears (type 3). Single and double interval slide techniques have demonstrated improvement in active motion, strength, and function [55]. However, long-term studies have shown a high re-tear rate (88%) in those tears treated with aggressive release and complete repair. This re-tear rate is similar to the one of those patients treated with partial repair (85%). When comparing both techniques, there are not significant differences in clinical outcomes [56]. Therefore, in this kind of lesions, it may be preferable to perform a partial repair.

Another concern regarding tear repair is if it is a necessary anatomic complete repair, with full coverage of the footprint. Several studies have shown that partial repair yields comparable outcomes to complete repair [57], with similar re-tear rates and functional scores [58]. However, the percentage of head coverage achieved has been directly correlated with more favorable outcomes [58]. A recent systematic review reported that complete repair is associated with at least equal or better functional outcomes compared to partial repair [59]. We think that complete repair should be the aim of treatment, accepting partial repair for those cases in which full coverage of the footprint is not possible.

Other technical aspect that remains controversial is the convenience of performing a double-row repair versus a simpler single-row repair. Meta-analyses have shown that double-row repair provides a significantly higher rate of tendon healing than single-row repair, especially in large or massive tears. However, this does not reflect on clinical results, and differences on functional outcomes have not been demonstrated [60]. In addition, it has been reported that double-row repair is not cost-effective for any size of tear when compared to single-row repair [61]. Consequently, some authors recommend using double-row repair only in selected cases. Probably those with larger and more contracted tears would be good candidates, aiming to improve the lower rate of healing of these cases.

Another issue under debate is the convenience of performing additional surgical gestures when repairing a rotator cuff tear, like tenotomy of the long head of the biceps, acromioplasty, or suprascapular nerve decompression.

Regarding tenotomy of the long head of the biceps, there are few studies comparing repair alone with repair plus tenotomy. The long head of the biceps has been reported as a possible source of pain in rotator cuff tears [62]. However, patients treated with rotator cuff repair plus tenotomy showed no benefit with respect to those treated with repair alone [63]. For that reason, our recommendation is not to perform tenotomy in all patients, reserving it for those cases in which the long head of the biceps tendon presents advanced degeneration or as an adjuvant treatment for pain in patients with irreparable tears but with good shoulder function, in which partial repair plus biceps tenotomy is frequently performed [64].

With respect to acromioplasty, several studies have reported that there are no differences in functional outcomes or re-tear rates between patients in which acromioplasty was performed in addition to the repair and those in which simple repair was done [63, 65]. We do not recommend to perform acromioplasty unless there is an objective compression between acromion and supraspinatus after the repair.

Regarding suprascapular nerve decompression, no differences between groups with or without decompression have been reported [66]. Accordingly, and due to the risk of suprascapular nerve palsy, we do not perform this routinely.

With respect to augmentation of the repair, there is a huge variety of methods described to reinforce the repair: grafts (autograft, allograft, or xenograft), extracellular matrix, and synthetic or biologic patches. This wide range of options yields a lack of homogeneity in the bibliography, which makes difficult to conclude what is the real advantage provided by these techniques. Nevertheless, some authors have tried to analyze the information available, and several systematic reviews have been published shedding some light on this question [67]. It has been reported that allograft augmentation is functionally and structurally superior to primary repair, with a significantly higher rate of intact repairs. In contrast, xenograft augmentation has failed to demonstrate superiority to primary repair and presents a worse healing rate. Polypropylene patches showed improved outcomes with respect to primary repair and collagen patches [68], although there is a lack of randomized data. Grafts can be used to reinforce the repair or as a "bridge" between the tendon and its footprint when complete repair is not possible. Bridging grafts have not shown significant difference in healing or clinical outcomes when compared to grafts used for augmentation [69]. Other augmentation systems, like extracellular matrix grafts, seem to reduce the incidence of re-tears and improve patient outcomes when compared to simple repair [70].

Surgical techniques in which the biceps tendon is used for augmentation have been described (either tenotomizing the tendon or just incorporating it to the repair without detachment). Several authors have reported reduced failure rates using this technique, with similar clinical outcomes and better strength improvement than repair alone [71, 72].

In summary, there are many options described to augment rotator cuff repair, some of them with promising results. As these techniques may imply longer surgical time, complexity, and higher costs, author's advice is to limit augmentation use to those cases in which repair failure, even when repair is an accurate indication, is highly predictable or when a revision of a previously failed repair is done.

Another point that is frequently discussed regarding massive rotator cuff repair is the convenience of using platelet-rich plasma (PRP) as adjuvant treatment. Some meta-analyses have reported that the use of PRP reduces the failure risk after repair, regardless of tear size [73]. However, systematic reviews of meta-analyses failed to demonstrate this point [74]. All the studies agree to indicate the great heterogeneity of PRP preparations as an obstacle to generalize outcomes. We consider that at this moment, it is not possible to make a specific recommendation with respect to PRP use.

7.8 Conclusions

Rotator cuff tears are very common and can cause important disability, especially massive tears. When facing patients with this pathology, knowledge of natural history, adequate physical examination, comprehensive analysis of imaging studies, and awareness of risk factors for repair failure are essential for the selection of the best treatment. If repair is performed, a deep understanding of anatomy, tear geometry, and surgical techniques available is necessary. Our recommendation is to choose between open or arthroscopic repair according to the surgeon's preference and experience. Complete single-row repair must be attempted, and geometric pattern of the tear must be taken into account. Double-row repair and augmentation techniques must be considered in specific cases. No additional surgical gestures are recommended as a routine.

References

1. Chakravarty K, Webley M. Shoulder joint movement and its relationship to disability in the elderly. J Reum. 1993;20:1359–61.
2. Tashjian RZ. Epidemiology, natural history, and indications for treatment of rotator cuff tears. Clin Sports Med. 2012;31:589–604.
3. Yamamoto A, Takagishi K, Osawa T, Yanagawa T, Nakajima D, Shitara H, et al. Prevalence and risk factors of a rotator cuff tear in the general population. J Shoulder Elb Surg. 2010;19:116–20.
4. Teunis T, Lubberts B, Reilly BT, Ring D. A systematic review and pooled analysis of the prevalence of rotator cuff disease with increasing age. J Shoulder Elb Surg. 2014;23:1913–21.
5. Baumgarten KM, Gerlach D, Galatz LM, Teefey SA, Middleton WD, Ditsios K, et al. Cigarette smoking increases the risk for rotator cuff tears. Clin Orthop Relat Res. 2010;468:1534–41.
6. Harvie P, Ostlere SJ, Teh J, McNally EG, Clipsham K, Burston BJ, et al. Genetic influences in the aetiology of tears of the rotator cuff. Sibling risk of a full-thickness tear. J Bone Jt Surg Ser B. 2004;86:696–700.
7. Abboud JA, Kim JS. The effect of hypercholesterolemia on rotator cuff disease. Clin Orthop Relat Res. 2010;468:1493–7.
8. Curtis AS, Burbank KM, Tierney JJ, Scheller AD, Curran AR. The insertional footprint of the rotator cuff: an anatomic study. Arthroscopy. 2006;22:603–609.e1.
9. Huegel J, Williams AA, Soslowsky LJ. Rotator cuff biology andbBiomechanics: a review of normal and pathological conditions. Curr Rheumatol Rep. 2015;17:1–9.
10. Hsu JE, Gee AO, Lippitt SB, Iii FAM. Chapter 14—The rotator cuff [Internet]. In: Rockwood and Matsen's the shoulder. 5th ed. Elsevier Inc.; 2020, pp. 651–719.e7.
11. Burkhart SS, Esch JC, Jolson RS. The rotator crescent and rotator cable: an anatomic description of the shoulder's "suspension bridge.". Arthroscopy. 1993;9:611–6.
12. Neer CS. Impingement lesions. Clin Orthop Relat Res. 1983;173:70–7.
13. Braune C, von Eisenhart-Rothe R, Welsch F, Teufel M, Jaeger A. Mid-term results and quantitative comparison of postoperative shoulder function in traumatic and non-traumatic rotator cuff tears. Arch Orthop Trauma Surg. 2003;123:419–24.
14. Sher JS, Uribe JW, Posada A, Murphy BJ, Zlatkin MB. Abnormal findings on magnetic resonance images of asymptomatic shoulders. J Bone Jt Surg Ser A. 1995;77:10–5.
15. Yamaguchi K, Tetro AM, Blam O, Evanoff BA, Teefey SA, Middleton WD. Natural history of asymptomatic rotator cuff tears: a longitudinal analysis of asymptomatic tears detected sonographically. J Shoulder Elb Surg. 2001;10:199–203.
16. Mall NA, Kim HM, Keener JD, Steger-May K, Teefey SA, Middleton WD, et al. Symptomatic progression of asymptomatic rotator cuff tears a prospective study of clinical and sonographic variables. J Bone Joint Surg Am. 2010;92:2623–33.
17. Maman E, Harris C, White L, Tomlinson G, Shashank M, Boynton E. Outcome of nonoperative treatment of symptomatic rotator cuff tears monitored by magnetic resonance imaging. J Bone Jointt Surg Am. 2009;91:1898–906.
18. Safran O, Schroeder J, Bloom R, Weil Y, Milgrom C. Natural history of nonoperatively treated symptomatic rotator cuff tears in patients 60 years old or younger. Am J Sports Med. 2011;39:710–4.
19. Fucentese SF, Von Roll AL, Pfirrmann CWA, Gerber C, Jost B. Evolution of nonoperatively treated symptomatic isolated full-thickness supraspinatus tears. J Bone Joint Surg Am. 2012;94:801–8.
20. DeOrio JK, Cofield RH. Results of a second attempt at surgical repair of a failed initial rotator-cuff repair. J Bone Joint Surg Am. 1984;66:563–7.
21. Harryman D, Mack L, Wang K, Jackins S, Richardson M, Matsen F, et al. Repairs of the rotator cuff. Correlation of functional results with integrity of the cuff. J Bone Joint Surg Am. 1991:982–9.
22. Gerber C, Fuchs B, Hodler J. The results of repair of massive tears of the rotator cuff. J Bone Joint Surg Am. 2000;82:505–15.
23. Patte D. Classification of rotator cuff lesions. Clin Orthop Relat Res. 1990;254:81–6.
24. Davidson J, Burkhart SS. The geometric classification of rotator cuff tears: a system linking tear pattern to treatment and prognosis. Arthroscopy. 2010;26:417–24.
25. Mancuso F, Di Benedetto P, Tosolini L, Buttironi MM, Beltrame A, Causero A. Treatment options for massive rotator cuff tears: a narrative review. Acta Biomed. 2021;92
26. Burkhart SS. Fluoroscopic comparison of kinematic patterns in massive rotator cuff tears: a suspension bridge model. Clin Orthop Relat Res. 1992;284:144–52.
27. Collin P, Matsumura N, Lädermann A, Denard PJ, Walch G. Relationship between massive chronic rotator cuff tear pattern and loss of active shoulder range of motion. J Shoulder Elb Surg. 2014;23:1195–202.
28. Denard PJ, Lädermann A, Brady PC, Narbona P, Adams CR, Arrigoni P, et al. Pseudoparalysis from a massive rotator cuff tear is reliably reversed with an arthroscopic rotator cuff repair in patients without preoperative glenohumeral arthritis. Am J Sports Med. 2015;43:2373–8.
29. Denard PJ, Lädermann A, Jiwani AZ, Burkhart SS. Functional outcome after arthroscopic repair of massive rotator cuff tears in individuals with pseudoparalysis. Arthroscopy. 2012;28:1214–9.
30. Hamada K, Fukuda H, Mikasa M, Kobayashi Y. Roentgenographic findings in massive rotator cuff tears. A long-term observation. Clin Orthop Relat Res. 1990;254:92–6.

31. Walch G, Edwards TB, Boulahia A, Nové-Josserand L, Neyton L, Szabo I. Arthroscopic tenotomy of the long head of the biceps in the treatment of rotator cuff tears: clinical and radiographic results of 307 cases. J Shoulder Elb Surg. 2005;14:238–46.
32. Hamada K, Yamanaka K, Uchiyama Y, Mikasa T, Mikasa M. A radiographic classification of massive rotator cuff tear arthritis. Clin Orthop Relat Res. 2011;469:2452–60.
33. Jeon YD, Yoon JY, Jeong HJ, Nam GW, Heo K, Kim JU, et al. Significance of the acromiohumeral distance on stress radiography for predicting healing and function after arthroscopic repair of massive rotator cuff tears. J Shoulder Elb Surg. 2021;30:e471–81.
34. Herve A, Thomazeau H, Favard L, Colmar M, Mansat P, Walch G, et al. Clinical and radiological outcomes of osteoarthritis twenty years after rotator cuff repair. Orthop Traumatol Surg Res. 2019;105:813–8.
35. Goutallier D, Postel JM, Bernageau J, Lavau L, Voisin MC. Fatty muscle degeneration in cuff ruptures: pre- and postoperative evaluation by CT scan. Clin Orthop Relat Res. 1994;304:78–83.
36. Fuchs B, Weishaupt D, Gerber C, Hodler J. Fatty degeneration of the musclesof the rotator cuff: assessment by computed tomography versus magnetic resonance imaging. J Shoulder Elb Surg. 1999;8:599–605.
37. Yoo JC, Ahn JH, Yang JH, Koh KH, Choi SH, Yoon YC. Correlation of arthroscopic repairability of large to massive rotator cuff tears with preoperative magnetic resonance imaging scans. Arthroscopy. 2009;25:573–82.
38. Kuptniratsaikul V, Laohathaimongkol T, Umprai V, Yeekian C, Prasathaporn N. Pre-operative factors correlated with arthroscopic reparability of large-to-massive rotator cuff tears. BMC Musculoskelet Disord. 2019;20:1–9.
39. Liem D, Lichtenberg S, Magosch P, Habermeyer P. Magnetic resonance imaging of arthroscopic supraspinatus tendon repair. J Bone Joint Surg Am. 2007;89:1770–6.
40. Yamaguchi H, Suenaga N, Oizumi N, Hosokawa Y, Kanaya F. Will preoperative atrophy and fatty degeneration of the shoulder muscles improve after rotator cuff repair in patients with massive rotator cuff tears? Adv Orthop. 2012;2012:1–7.
41. Tashjian RZ, Erickson GA, Robins RJ, Zhang Y, Burks RT, Greis PE. Influence of preoperative musculotendinous junction position on rotator cuff healing after double-row repair. Arthroscopy. 2017;33:1159–66.
42. Kim JY, Park JS, Rhee YG. Can preoperative magnetic resonance imaging predict the reparability of massive rotator cuff tears? Am J Sports Med. 2017;45:1654–63.
43. Boileau P, Brassart N, Watkinson DJ, Carles M, Hatzidakis AM, Krishnan SG. Arthroscopic repair of full-thickness tears of the supraspinatus: does the tendon really heal? J Bone Joint Surg Am. 2005;87:1229–40.
44. Merolla G, Paladini P, Saporito M, Porcellini G. Conservative management of rotator cuff tears: literature review and proposal for a prognostic. Prediction Score. Muscles Ligaments Tendons J. 2011;1:12–9.
45. Kuhn JE, Dunn WR, Sanders R, An Q, Baumgarten KM, Bishop JY, et al. Effectiveness of physical therapy in treating atraumatic full-thickness rotator cuff tears: a multicenter prospective cohort study. J Shoulder Elb Surg. 2013;22:1371–9.
46. Mirzoyan H, Handelberg F, Pouliart N. Outcome at 3 to 5 years of a treatment algorithm for rotator cuff tears in an elderly population. Acta Orthop Belg. 2018;84:509–15.
47. Park SG, Shim BJ, Seok HG. How much will high tension adversely affect rotator cuff repair integrity? Arthroscopy. 2019;35:2992–3000.
48. Zumstein MA, Jost B, Hempel J, Hodler J, Gerber C. The clinical and structural long-term results of open repair of massive tears of the rotator cuff. J Bone Joint Surg Am. 2008;90:2423–31.
49. Burkhart SS, Diaz Pagàn JL, Wirth MA, Athanasiou KA. Cyclic loading of anchor-based rotator cuff repairs: confirmation of the tension overload phenomenon and comparison of suture anchor fixation with transosseous fixation. Arthroscopy. 1997;13:720–4.
50. Hughes JD, Hughes JL, Bartley JH, Hamilton WP, Brennan KL. Infection rates in arthroscopic versus open rotator cuff repair. Orthop J Sport Med. 2017;5:8–10.
51. Pham TT, Bayle Iniguez X, Mansat P, Maubisson L, Bonnevialle N. Postoperative pain after arthroscopic versus open rotator cuff repair. A prospective study. Orthop Traumatol Surg Res. 2016;102:13–7.
52. Ide J, Maeda S, Takagi K. A comparison of arthroscopic and open rotator cuff repair. Arthroscopy. 2005;21:1090–8.
53. Morse K, Davis AD, Afra R, Krall Kaye E, Schepsis A, Voloshin I. Arthroscopic versus mini-open rotator cuff repair: a comprehensive review and meta-analysis. Am J Sports Med. 2008;36:1824–8.
54. Ji X, Bi C, Wang F, Wang Q. Arthroscopic versus mini-open rotator cuff repair: An up-to-date meta-analysis of randomized controlled trials. Arthrosc J Arthrosc Relat Surg. 2015;31:118–24.
55. Lo IKY, Burkhart SS. Arthroscopic repair of massive, contracted, immobile rotator cuff tears using single and double interval slides: technique and preliminary results. Arthroscopy. 2004;20:22–33.
56. Jeong JY, Kim S-J, Yoon T-H, Eum K-S, Chun Y-M. Arthroscopic repair of large and massive rotator cuff tears. J Bone Joint Surg. 2020;102:1248–54.
57. Iagulli ND, Field LD, Hobgood ER, Ramsey JR, Savoie FH. Comparison of partial versus complete arthroscopic repair of massive rotator cuff tears. Am J Sports Med. 2012;40:1022–6.
58. Farazdaghi A, Paschos NK, Kelly JD. Comparison between partial and full coverage repair in massive rotator cuff tears. A minimum five year follow-up. Orthop Traumatol Surg Res. 2021;107:102911.
59. Malahias MA, Chytas D, Kostretzis L, Gkiatas I, Kokkineli S, Antonogiannakis E. Arthroscopic ana-

tomic complete versus non-anatomic repair of massive rotator cuff tears: a systematic review of comparative trials. Musculoskelet Surg. 2020;104:145–54.
60. Chen M, Xu W, Dong Q, Huang Q, Xie Z, Mao Y. Outcomes of single-row versus double-row arthroscopic rotator cuff repair: a systematic review and meta-analysis of current evidence. Arthroscopy. 2013;29:1437–49.
61. Genuario JW, Donegan RP, Hamman D, Bell JE, Boublik M, Schlegel T, et al. The cost-effectiveness of single-row compared with double-row arthroscopic rotator cuff repair. J Bone Joint Surg Am. 2012;94:1369–77.
62. Kempf JF, Gleyze P, Bonnomet F, Walch G, Mole D, Frank A, et al. A multicenter study of 210 rotator cuff tears treated by arthroscopic acromioplasty. Arthrosc J Arthrosc Relat Surg. 1999;15:56–66.
63. Ríos-Fak J, Olivos-Meza A, Sierra-Suárez L, Almazán-Díaz A, Pérez-Jiménez F, Cruz-López F. Comparación de los resultados funcionales de los pacientes con reparación artroscópica de rupturas masivas del manguito rotador sola o combinada con acromioplastía y/o tenotomía del bíceps TT—comparison of the functional outcomes of patients with arthr. Acta Ortopédica Mex. 2018;32:17–21.
64. Boileau P, McClelland WB, Rumian AP. Massive irreparable rotator cuff tears: how to rebalance the cuff-deficient shoulder. Instr Course Lect. 2014;63:71–83.
65. Waterman BR, Newgren J, Gowd AK, Cabarcas B, Lansdown D, Bach BR, et al. Randomized trial of arthroscopic rotator cuff with or without acromioplasty: no difference in patient-reported outcomes at long-term follow-up. Arthroscopy. 2021;37:3072–8.
66. Yamakado K. Arthroscopic rotator cuff repair with or without suprascapular nerve decompression in posterosuperior massive rotator cuff tears. Int Orthop. 2019;43:2367–73.
67. Ferguson DP, Lewington MR, Smith TD, Wong IH. Graft utilization in the augmentation of large-to-massive rotator cuff repairs. Am J Sports Med. 2016;44:2984–92.
68. Ciampi P, Scotti C, Nonis A, Vitali M, Di Serio C, Peretti GM, et al. The benefit of synthetic versus biological patch augmentation in the repair of posterosuperior massive rotator cuff tears: a 3-year follow-up study. Am J Sports Med. 2014;42:1169–75.
69. Ono Y, Dávalos Herrera DA, Woodmass JM, Boorman RS, Thornton GM, Lo IKY. Graft augmentation versus bridging for large to massive rotator cuff tears: a systematic review. Arthroscopy. 2017;33:673–80.
70. Gilot GJ, Alvarez-Pinzon AM, Barcksdale L, Westerdahl D, Krill M, Peck E. Outcome of large to massive rotator cuff tears repaired with and without extracellular matrix augmentation: a prospective comparative study. Arthroscopy. 2015;31:1459–65.
71. Cho NS, Yi JW, Rhee YG. Arthroscopic biceps augmentation for avoiding undue tension in repair of massive rotator cuff tears. Arthroscopy. 2009;25:183–91.
72. Ji JH, Shafi M, Jeong JJ, Park SE. Arthroscopic repair of large and massive rotator cuff tears using the biceps-incorporating technique: mid-term clinical and anatomical results. Eur J Orthop Surg Traumatol. 2014;24:1367–74.
73. Cavendish PA, Everhart JS, DiBartola AC, Eikenberry AD, Cvetanovich GL, Flanigan DC. The effect of perioperative platelet-rich plasma injections on postoperative failure rates following rotator cuff repair: a systematic review with meta-analysis. J Shoulder Elb Surg. 2020;29:1059–70.
74. Saltzman BM, Jain A, Campbell KA, Mascarenhas R, Romeo AA, Verma NN, et al. Does the use of platelet-rich plasma at the time of surgery improve clinical outcomes in arthroscopic rotator cuff repair when compared with control cohorts? A systematic review of meta-analyses. Arthroscopy. 2016;32:906–18.

8 Humeral Shaft Fixation in Adults: Plate Fixation, Intramedullary Nail, or Nonoperative?

Elena Gálvez-Sirvent, Aitor Ibarzabal-Gil, and E. Carlos Rodríguez-Merchán

8.1 Introduction

Fractures of the proximal humerus account for 1%–5% of all fractures [1], with an incidence of 13–14 cases per 100,000 population and a bimodal distribution, with a peak in young adults aged 20–30 years related to high-energy trauma and another in the elderly due to falls from their own height and lower-energy trauma associated with osteoporosis [1, 2].

There are several treatment options for this type of fracture, with controversy in the current literature and much variability in surgeon preferences [3].

8.2 Anatomy

To understand how these fractures behave and to establish the basis for their treatment, it is important to know certain anatomy details of the humeral diaphysis and its vasculonervous relationships.

The humeral diaphysis extends from the surgical neck of the proximal humerus [4] or superior border of the pectoralis major insertion [5] to the epicondyles or supracondylar crest [4, 5]. This is cylindrical in its proximal half and then becomes triangular, with three surfaces—anterolateral, anteromedial, and posterior [4, 5]—and a narrower diameter, which is important to take into account in the case of intramedullary fixations. Most of the vascularization of the humeral diaphysis arrives via a nutritional artery along the anteromedial border between the insertion of the coracobrachialis and anterior brachial muscles [4].

There are important and close vasculonervous relationships and structures to be considered, which can be injured by both the fracture itself and iatrogenically either by manipulations or in its surgical management. The humeral diaphysis has certain areas that the surgeon must know how to recognize because they are key points in these vasculonervous relationships. The deltoid tuberosity is a slight V-shaped bony outgrowth on the anterolateral surface where, as its name indicates, the deltoid muscle inserts [4]. This fact is important because, in diaphyseal fractures of the proximal third of the humerus below the deltoid V, the deltoid tends to pull on the proximal end and displaces it. Another important landmark is the radial groove that develops posteriorly at the insertion of the lateral belly of the triceps and extends distally and laterally and houses the radial nerve along with the brachial artery [4].

The vasculonervous structures in relation to the humeral diaphysis are the brachial artery and

E. Gálvez-Sirvent
Department of Orthopaedic Surgery, "Infanta Elena" University Hospital, Valdemoro, Madrid, Spain

A. Ibarzabal-Gil · E. C. Rodríguez-Merchán (✉)
Department of Orthopaedic Surgery, "La Paz" University Hospital-IdiPaz, Madrid, Spain

E. C. Rodríguez-Merchán, A. Moreno-Garcìa (eds.), *Controversies in Orthopedic Surgery of The Upper Limb*, https://doi.org/10.1007/978-3-031-04907-1_8

axillary nerve in the most proximal part and the radial, ulnar, median, and lateral antebrachial cutaneous nerves, sensory branches of the musculocutaneous nerve, in the most distal part. Special mention should be made of the radial nerve, the most commonly injured structure in this type of fractures, and the lateral antebrachial cutaneous nerve, present in the anterior mid-distal third approach.

The radial nerve is the main structure that can be affected in diaphyseal fractures of the humerus, with a reported rate of injury of 7–17% [6], which can be primary or iatrogenic. Iatrogenic injury rates in the literature range around 7%, but rates of up to 32% have been reported in some series [7, 8]. It is therefore important to have a good knowledge of the pathway and relationships of this nerve. It comes from the posterior fascicle of the brachial plexus, from nerve fibers coming from the spinal roots C5, C6, C7, and C8. It passes through the anterior aspect of the subscapularis muscle, descends medially along with the brachial artery, then separates from it, passes posteriorly between 18.1 and 20.7 cm proximal to the medial epicondyle, and enters the torsion canal [9, 10]. It leaves the latter between 10.1 and 14.8 cm proximal to the lateral epicondyle and crosses the lateral intermuscular septum of the arm to pass into the anterior compartment between 7.5 and 10 cm proximal to the elbow joint [11], an important anatomical relationship due to the possible injury of this nerve in Holstein Lewis fractures [12].

The lateral antebrachial cutaneous nerve is a terminal branch of the musculocutaneous nerve, which, after innervating the biceps and anterior brachial muscles, becomes superficial crossing the bicipital aponeurosis innervating the cutaneous region of the radial border of the forearm.

It is important to know the anatomy and relationships of these structures to avoid injury during surgical approaches. As we have said, the structure with the highest rate of injury in these fractures, both primary and iatrogenic, is the radial nerve, which we will make special mention of throughout this chapter.

8.3 Classification of Diaphyseal Humeral Fractures

Fractures of the humeral diaphysis can be defined according to location (proximal to the pectoralis major insertion, between the pectoralis major and deltoid insertions, or below the deltoid insertion) [5], fracture morphology (transverse, oblique, spiroid), angulation, displacement, and comminution or whether the fracture is open or closed. The most commonly used classification for open fractures is the Gustilo classification [13].

According to the fracture pattern, the most commonly used classification is that of the AO/OTA (Arbeitsgemeinschaft für Osteosynthesefragen (AO)/Orthopaedic Trauma Association (OTA) [14], which classifies fractures into 3 types—type A (simple fractures 63.3%), type B (wedge or butterfly wing fractures), and type C (complex comminuted fractures)—and then subdivides them into three distinct patterns according to the magnitude of comminution. Interobserver agreement for the 3 fracture types and for the 9 fracture groups was moderate ($\kappa = 0.46$ and $\kappa = 0.48$, respectively) [14].

There are also eponyms to describe certain fracture patterns, such as the Holstein-Lewis fracture, described in 1963 [15], an extra-articular spiroid displaced fracture of the distal third of humerus, where the proximal peak of the distal fragment deviates laterally, thus resulting in a high rate of radial involvement, since at that level this nerve crosses the lateral intermuscular septum to pass into the anterior compartment. It constitutes 7.5% of all humeral diaphyseal fractures [8, 12] (Fig. 8.1).

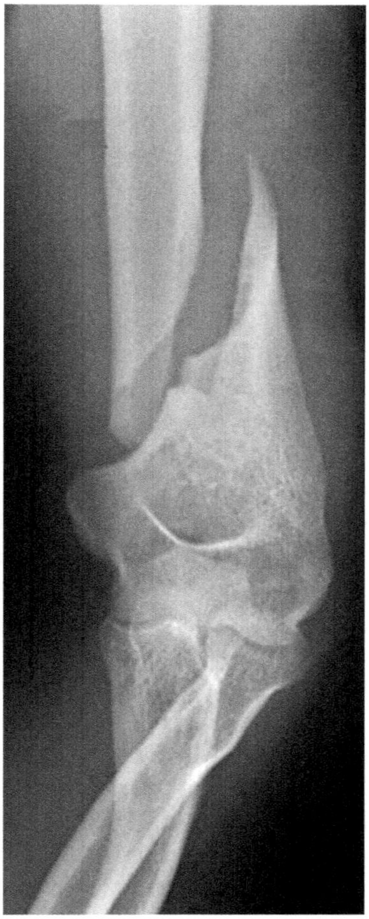

Fig. 8.1 Holstein-Lewis fracture

8.4 Initial Patient Assessment

During the anamnesis, the mechanism of injury should be ascertained; a fall from its own height with low-energy trauma indicates possible bone fragility, whether previously diagnosed or not. A high-energy trauma should warn us about possible associated injuries, both vasculonervous lesions at the fracture level and possible associated injuries.

In the physical examination, we will find pain, functional impairment, swelling, and frequent deformity at arm level. It will be necessary to verify a correct state of soft tissues and to rule out wounds that turn the injury into an open fracture.

It is essential to perform and record in the clinical history an initial neurovascular evaluation before any manipulation or surgical intervention and, again after them, paying special attention to the radial nerve, the most frequently injured, by checking the ability to extend the wrist and fingers. We will also check the ulnar nerve by means of Froment's sign and the median nerve by means of the extension of the first finger. The axillary nerve should be examined by means of the sensitivity in the deltoid area since the functional impotence due to the same fracture prevents us from abducting the arm. Finally, it is important to check the radial and ulnar pulses to rule out the involvement of the brachial artery.

A simple radiography in two projections will generally be sufficient for a correct diagnosis and characterization of the injury, including the adjacent joints, elbow, and shoulder. Other tests such as magnetic resonance imaging (MRI) or CT scan are reserved for a second time to evaluate possible lesions of the rotator cuff or other associated shoulder structures or consolidation delays, respectively.

The initial treatment will be immobilization by means of a hanging cast or U-splint. We would opt for an external fixator in open fractures with significant exposure (Gustilo III) where we consider that primary closure and definitive treatment is not possible or in the case of polytraumatized patients with injuries at other levels for damage control.

8.5 Treatment

The treatment of these fractures can be classified as conservative or surgical, the latter being an open reduction and internal fixation by means of a plate or a closed reduction and internal fixation by means of an intramedullary nail. In recent years, percutaneously placed plates have also been increasingly used.

As early as 1977, Sarmiento described good results with conservative treatment [15], which have been corroborated by numerous studies by the same author and others [16, 17]. For many surgeons, it is still considered the gold standard treatment. However, there has been a growing trend toward surgical management of these fractures, despite the lack of evidence in the literature on its superiority over orthopedic treatment. A study analyzing the Finland National Hospital Discharge Registry showed an increase in surgical treatment in the last two decades, doubling in men and almost tripling in women [18].

8.5.1 Conservative Treatment

As we have said, this is a treatment option with good results described decades ago [15–17, 19]. Before Sarmiento's description of functional immobilization, rigid immobilizations involving the shoulder and elbow (brachial splints, U-splints, hanging casts, Velpeau bandages) were used, which caused joint stiffness of the shoulder and elbow. In addition, it was also observed that functional rather than rigid immobilization created a larger and stronger callus [20].

Conservative treatment is performed sequentially. Initially, the fracture is immobilized in a hanging cast or U-splint for one to 2 weeks [15]. After this period, the immobilization is replaced by a prefabricated functional brace that can be adapted to the patient's arm by means of straps and can be tightened over the weeks as the swelling goes down. This system is based on external compression of the fracture through the musculature and other soft tissues, achieving good control of angulation and rotation, although not so much of the shortening, which depends more on the initial pattern of the fracture. Thanks to this system, the patient will be able to mobilize the elbow and shoulder according to tolerance to avoid stiffness [21]. To control the possible secondary displacement of the fracture, a control X-ray should be taken at 1 week of evolution and then serial X-rays every 2 weeks until the treatment is completed, which will last between 10 and 12 weeks on average [1].

Consolidation rates of between 77.4 and 100% have been described. Sarmiento published in 2000 a large series of 620 patients treated in this way with a nonunion rate of less than 2% in closed fractures and 6% in open fractures. Furthermore, this consolidation was achieved in 87% with less than 16 degrees of varus angulation and less than 16 degrees of anterior angulation [17]. Since then, numerous studies have been published confirming these good results.

In addition, in some studies, certain fracture patterns were observed to have worse healing rates with conservative treatment. Koch published a series of 67 fractures in 2002, with 87% healing in an average period of 10 weeks. Of the 9 cases of nonunions that required surgery, 6 were single-trait transverse fractures [16]. Rutgers published in 2006 a series of 49 patients with 44 of them (90%) consolidating. Of the five that did not consolidate, four were proximal third [19]. Ekholm published in 2006 a series of 78 patients with 90% consolidation after conservative treatment. The majority of nonunions, with a nonunion rate of 20%, were single-stroke fractures (type A of the AO classification) in the proximal third. He also reflected that functional outcomes were good in patients in whom the fracture consolidated with conservative treatment from the beginning but worse in those who required surgery for nonunion, even if consolidation was finally achieved, so this author recommended assessing a surgical treatment from the beginning for simple fractures of the proximal third, due to a higher risk of nonunion [22]. Ali published in 2015 a series of 138 fractures, with a consolidation rate of 83%, observing worse rates also in proximal third fractures and better rates in comminuted fractures than in simpler traces, being more specifically oblique proximal third fractures the ones with the lowest union rate [23]. These results are reflected in Table 8.1 [16, 17, 19, 22, 23].

Table 8.1 Published healing rates of conservative treatment of diaphyseal humerus fractures

Author	Year	*N*	Healing rate
Sarmiento [17]	2000	620	97.4
Koch [16]	2002	67	86.6
Rutgers [19]	2006	49	89.8
Ekholm [22]	2006	78	89.7
Ali [23]	2015	138	83

N Number of cases

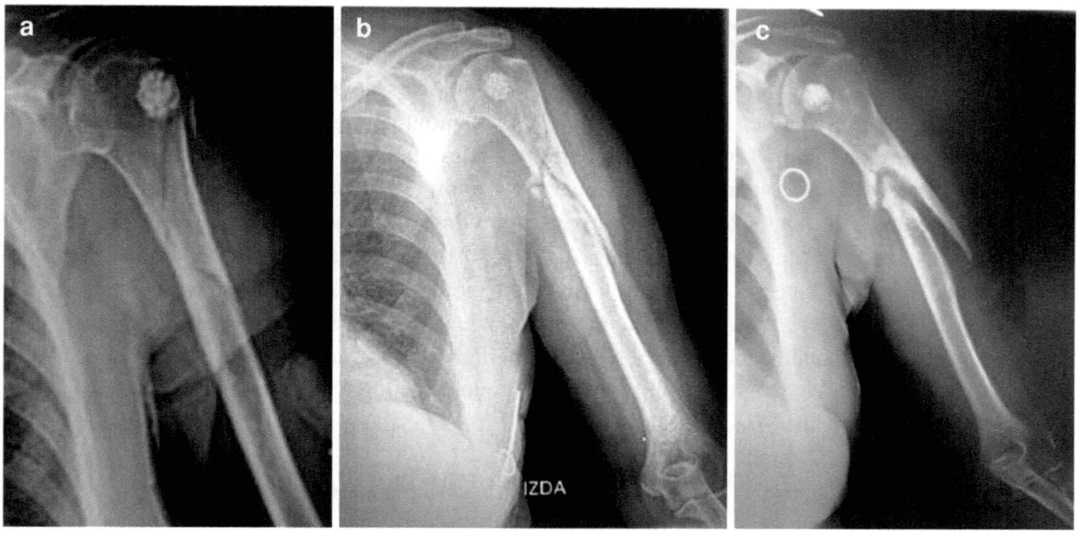

Fig. 8.2 (**a–b**) Diaphyseal fracture of the proximal third of the humerus with oblique trace, treated conservatively (**a**). Six months later, the fracture showed no signs of healing (**b**). Eighteen months later the fracture was in nonunion status (**c**)

Papsoulis conducted a literature review in 2021 with 16 case series and two comparative studies and observed a 94.5% healing rate in a mean time of 10.7 weeks, also observing a higher rate of nonunion in single-trace fractures (type A) in the proximal third [24]. It is suggested that the cause of this fact may rely on the action of the deltoid and pectoralis major displacing the proximal fragment and producing a muscular interposition in the fracture line. The same conclusion was reached by Ring et al. in their 2007 study [25]. They studied 32 patients with nonunions after orthopedic treatment of diaphyseal fractures of the humerus, 17 of which were in the proximal humerus, 14 in the middle third, and 1 in the distal third. Twenty-seven fractures had an oblique or simple spiral trace.

Regarding residual angulation, Klenerman described a sagittal angulation of 20° and a varus angulation of 30° as tolerable for good function as early as 1966 [26]. Since then, these parameters have been accepted. A valgus of 30°, a malrotation of 15°, and a maximum shortening of 3 cm have also been established as tolerable [27].

Therefore, conservative treatment of humerus diaphyseal fractures is a good option, with high healing rates and good functional results even with significant angulations. However, we know that certain fracture patterns, mainly single and proximal third traces, specifically a long oblique proximal third trace, probably due to muscle traction, have a higher risk of nonunion, and we could consider surgical treatment from the beginning (Fig. 8.2).

However, there are still absolute indications for surgery [13], which can be classified into several causes, summarized in Table 8.2:

Table 8.2 Indications for surgery in diaphyseal fractures of the humerus

- No tolerance to conservative treatment
- Fracture pattern
  - Inadequate reduction
  - Intra-articular extension
  - Floating elbow
  - Metastasis
  - Polytraumatized (relative)
  - Bilateral (relative)
- Soft tissue involvement (Gustilo III, burns, extensive abrasions)
- Brachial plexus injury
- Vascular injury in need of repair

– Because of non-tolerance to conservative treatment: obese patients, with poor pain control with immobilization or who simply refuse this type of treatment, since there is evidence that, for optimal conservative treatment, the patient must be satisfied with this method [22].

- By fracture pattern: whether adequate angulation cannot be obtained by functional immobilization or whether secondary displacement occurs after this treatment. Close follow-up by serial radiographs is therefore important. As mentioned above, the accepted angulation values are 30° of varus or valgus, 20° of anterior angulation, 15° of malrotation, and 3 cm of shortening [26, 27]. We would also opt for surgical treatment if the fracture has intra-articular extension, which would bring us closer to the plate option. Finally, if it is a floating elbow or in case of a pathological fracture due to metastasis, we would consider pin fixation. A polytraumatized patient or bilateral fractures would be a relative indication for surgery.
- Due to poor condition of soft tissues: open Gustilo type III fractures, burns, or extensive abrasions requiring frequent dressing.
- Associated vascular lesions that need to be surgically repaired, since fracture fixation, preferably rigid fixation with a plate, would be indicated to protect the anastomosis [1].
- Brachial plexus injuries: in these cases, high rates of nonunion have been observed in conservative treatment with functional plaster, due to poor muscle tone, not achieving adequate compression. In addition, this situation delays rehabilitation [28].

Regarding primary radial nerve involvement, it is not currently considered by itself a criterion for surgery. The literature has described high (73–95%) and similar rates of nerve recovery with both expectant management and early surgical revision, so it has been advised to avoid surgical indication from the outset [29–32]. However, other authors disagree and have created decision algorithms when facing radial palsy. The recommendation is to perform an electromyogram between week 3 and 4 and week 6 and week 12. Progressive reinnervation should be observed, although full recovery may take 6–12 months. If at week 12 there is no recovery, some authors suggest surgical revision of the nerve. For other authors, this date may be extended to the 4th–sixth month [33]. In the case of fractures with radial symptoms that require surgical treatment for another reason (described in Table 8.1), it is recommended that a revision of the radial nerve be performed at the same time. The osteosynthesis method of choice in these cases would be the plate, since there is a possibility of the nerve being in the fracture site and getting injured during intramedullary nail insertion [33].

8.5.2 Intramedullary Nailing

In comparison with open fixation with a plate, intramedullary fixation provides greater respect for the soft tissues and periosteal circulation, thus improving the biological environment for the repair of the fracture [1, 4]. In addition, being an intramedullary implant, it is aligned with the loading axis of the humerus, contributing to a better load distribution and more resistance to bending. It would be the implant of choice in cases of pathological fractures or bifocal fractures [1, 4].

Its main drawback would be residual pain and functional impairment of the shoulder in anterograde nails, the most commonly used, due to damage to the cuff in the hypovascular area near its insertion or subacromial occupation by protrusion of the material [34, 35]. For this reason, modifications in the entry point have been considered to try to minimize damage to the cuff insertion, making it more medial, more lateral, through the Neviaser portal or through the rotator interval [36–39]. It is also important to perform a good reduction, even if it is not direct as in plate placement. In oblique proximal traces, which are displaced by the action of the deltoid and pectoralis, a mini-open may be necessary to start introducing the nail with the fracture already reduced by a clamp or cerclage, in order to avoid possible nonunion of these traces, which is also greater in conservative treatment (Figs. 8.3 and 8.4).

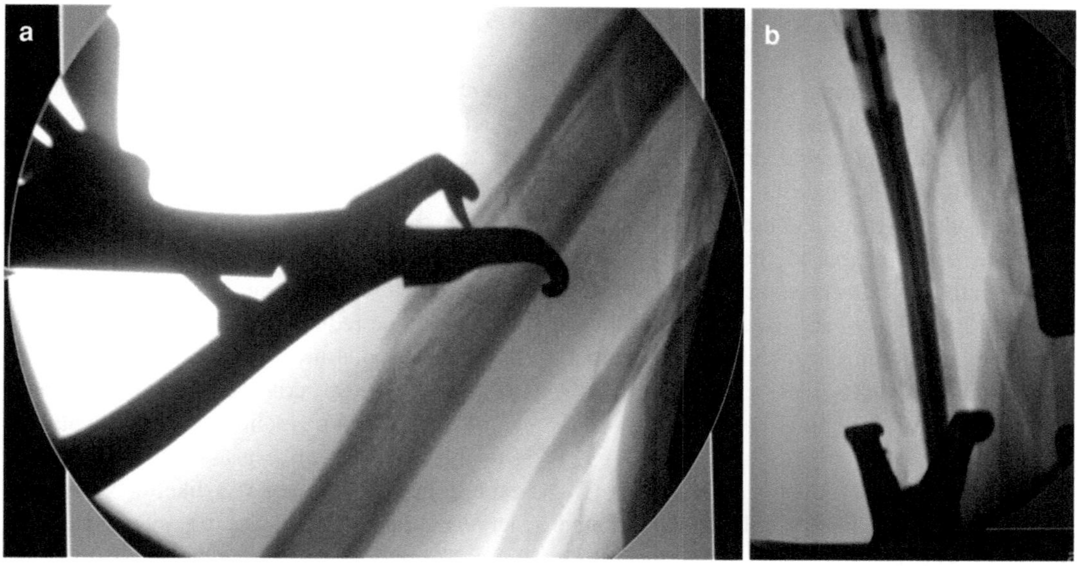

Fig. 8.3 (**a**–**b**) Reduction of diaphyseal fracture of the proximal third of the humerus with long oblique line by mini-open prior to intramedullary nailing (**a**). Nail insertion while maintaining the reduction (**b**)

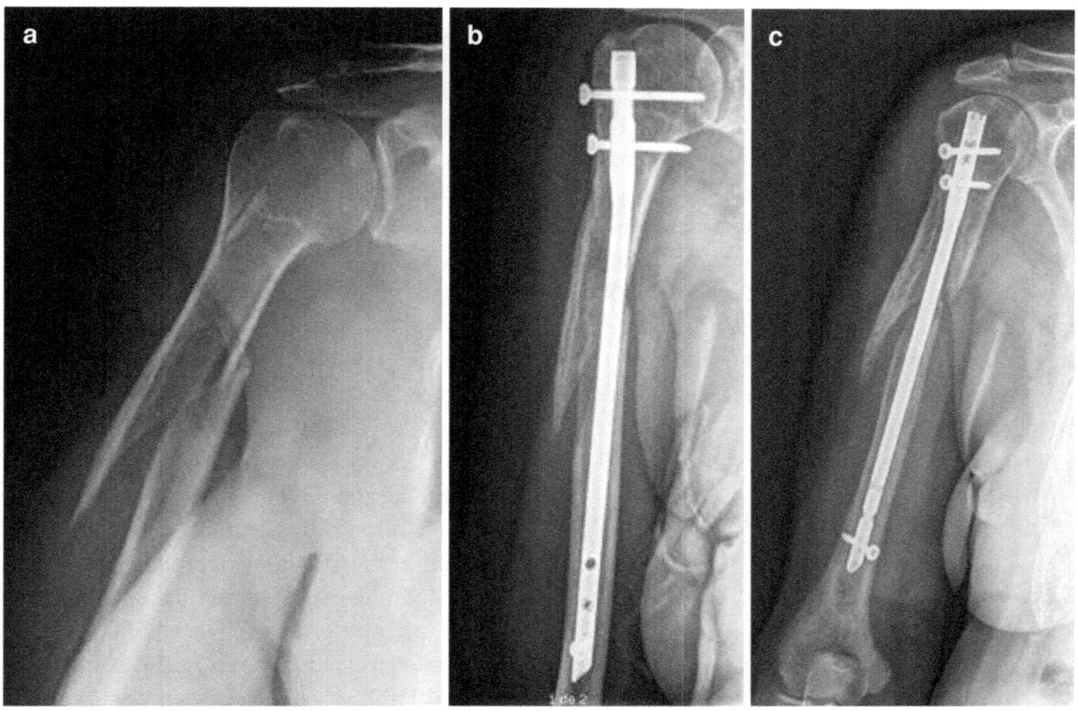

Fig. 8.4 (**a**–**c**) Diaphyseal fracture of the proximal third of the humerus with oblique trace treated by intramedullary nailing (**a**). Five months later showed no signs of healing (**b**). At 21 months after the fracture, the fracture was in nonunion (**c**)

As for retrograde nails, which are less commonly used, there is a risk of supracondylar humerus fracture during placement, as well as elbow joint stiffness and heterotopic calcifications, although they would prevent rotator cuff damage [40, 41]. In addition, they have shown similar results in terms of consolidation and complications with respect to the antegrade ones. However, they are less used probably due to their technical difficulty at the insertion point, requiring an oval entry area of several centimeters to avoid producing iatrogenic fracture of the anterior cortex of the humerus.

8.5.2.1 Results

The union rates are high, similar to conservative treatment, between 85% and 100%; the results are reflected in Table 8.3 [34, 42–47]. In contrast, high rates of residual pain and functional impairment of the shoulder have been reported, ranging from 6% to 100% in some series [48]. The longest published series [34] retrospectively reviewed 99 patients treated with intramedullary nailing, 54 antegrade, and 45 retrograde. A 97% consolidation rate was observed, 3 cases of radial paresis after surgery, which recovered spontaneously. Regarding shoulder function, measured by the Constant scale, 91.3% showed excellent function and 5.4% good. Elbow function, using the Mayo Elbow Score, was excellent in 81.5% and good in 14.1%. All patients with shoulder function deficits corresponded to antegrade nails, and all those with elbow function deficits corresponded to retrograde nails.

Table 8.3 Healing rates of humerus diaphyseal fractures treated with intramedullary nailing

Author	Year	*N*	Healing rate
McCormark[a] [46]	2000	19	89%
Chapman[a] [47]	2000	38	95%
Changulani[a] [44]	2007	21	85.7%
Rommens [34]	2008	99	97%
Putti[a] [42]	2009	16	100%
Singisetti[a] [43]	2010	20	95%
Benegas[a] [45]	2014	19	94.7%

[a]Comparative studies with plate; *N* Number of cases

8.5.3 Internal Fixation with Plate

In the case of opting for surgical treatment, the indications for a plate instead of a nail would be the need for an arterial repair taking advantage of the same approach and thus achieving a rigid fixation that protects the anastomosis [49] and the articular extension, either distal or proximal, of the fracture, since an anatomical reduction would then be required (Fig. 8.5). As previously mentioned, radial involvement in a fracture with surgical treatment criteria for another reason would make us more inclined to opt for a plate as a method of osteosynthesis associated with radial exploration, since there is a likelihood that the nerve is trapped in the fracture site and can be injured during the intramedullary nail insertion [33].

8.5.3.1 Surgical Approaches

For the proximal and middle third, the anterolateral approach is commonly used, a prolongation of the shoulder deltopectoral approach that goes down the lateral area of the biceps, displaces it medially, and goes deeper through the brachialis muscle, between its middle and lateral thirds, taking advantage of the double innervation of this muscle. In fact, some authors have proposed a new division of this muscle into two independent fascicles [50]. The only vasculonervous structure to be taken into account at this level is the lateral antebrachial cutaneous nerve, a sensory branch of the musculocutaneous nerve, which is located between the biceps and the brachialis. This approach allows a large exposure of the diaphysis in the middle and proximal thirds.

For the distal third, the most commonly used approach is the posterior approach, which can expose both the diaphysis and the elbow in case of intra-articular extension. In addition, a good exposure of the radial nerve is also achieved at proximal level, when it is located posteriorly, in the torsion canal, being able to place a plate under it if the fracture extends more proximally. Deep planes are accessed through the triceps fibers by separating them longitudinally or through lateral

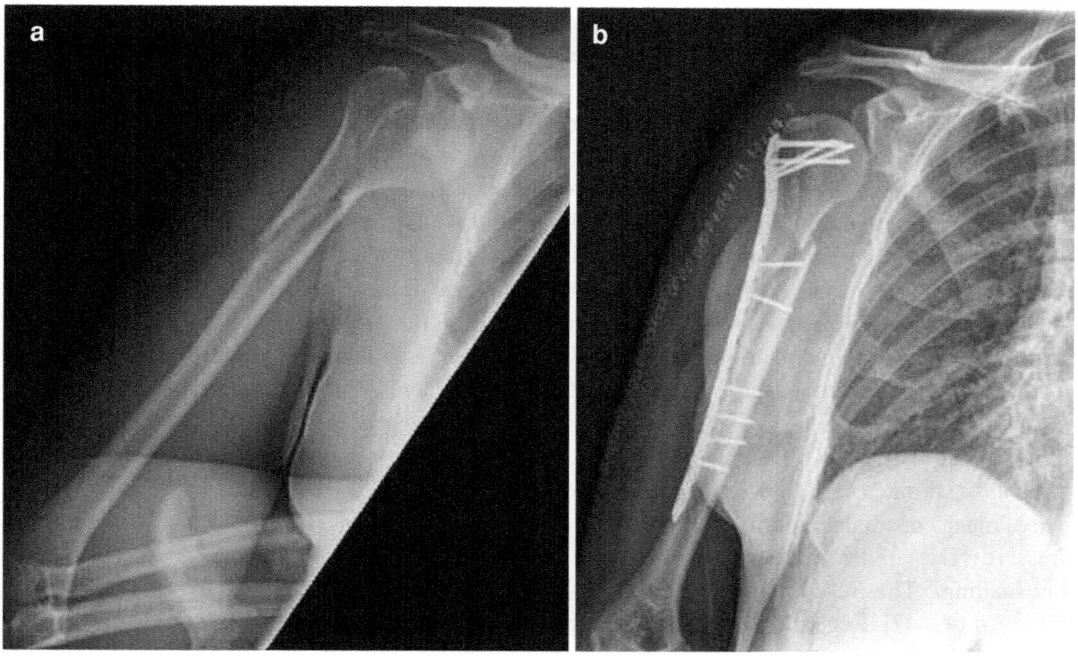

Fig. 8.5 (**a–b**) Diaphyseal fracture of the proximal humerus with intra-articular extension (**a**). Treatment by open reduction and internal fixation with plate (**b**)

and medial paratricipital windows, thus avoiding injury to the muscle belly. Gerwin published an anatomical study on 10 specimens where three types of posterior approach were performed [51]. Through triceps-splitting, 15.4 +/− 0.8 cm of humerus was exposed, from the epicondyle proximally, where the radial nerve crosses the posterior part of the humerus, seeing a total of 55% of the humerus. A second modification also mobilizes the radial nerve toward proximal and visualizes 6 cm more of the humerus toward proximal, 76% of the humerus. Finally, the third variant is the modified posterior approach, where the radial nerve was located in the distal and lateral area of the humerus and the triceps was retracted medially, being able to expose 26.2 ± 0.4 cm of the humeral diaphysis from the epicondyle to the proximal, 94% of the humerus. Clinical studies have also shown good results with the latter approach, emphasizing the large exposure achieved [52].

Other authors have proposed less used approaches such as the medial approach, although reserved only for the middle third, neither proximal nor distal, demonstrating the same results as with the anterolateral approach and proposing it as a more aesthetic alternative to the latter [53]. There are also groups that have used neurostimulators in their approaches to avoid radial injury [3].

8.5.3.2 Type and Placement of Plates

Following the principles of AO, the plates, generally of large fragments, can be arranged to give compression to the fracture, as neutralization plates of an interfragmentary compression with one or more screws or as bridging plates. This arrangement will depend on the fracture trace. In a simple trace, direct reduction and interfragmentary compression can be applied by plate in short transverse or oblique traces and by interferential screws plus neutralization plate in longer spiroid or oblique traces. In a comminuted fracture, a bridging plate assembly would be best option [54]. Regarding locked or unlocked screws, no significant differences in bending or torsional strength have been reported in cases with good bone quality [55], unlike in osteoporotic models [56], where locked plates would be beneficial. In cases of bone defects due to severe comminution, a shortening of the humerus, acceptable up to 3–4 cm, can be considered, despite the possible residual muscle weakness.

As for the use of double plates, there are several biomechanical and more recently clinical studies that support their use because they provide greater stability [57–61], so they could be useful for fractures where intraoperatively satisfactory stability is not achieved. It is also possible to associate a small fragment, reconstruction, or third shank plate as initial fixation to maintain the reduction and then place the large fragment plate.

8.5.3.3 Results

Consolidation rates vary between 87% and 96% with a mean consolidation time of 12 weeks; figures are very similar to conservative treatment and nailing. The results are summarized in Table 8.4 [42–47]. Regarding radial nerve injury, a study of 261 fractures treated by open reduction and internal fixation showed an injury rate of 12.2%, finding no differences in fracture location or type of approach [62]. In one study, these were significantly related to surgeon experience and not to fracture location or fracture pattern [63]. Most of these palsies recover spontaneously [64].

Regarding the attitude to radial paresis after surgical treatment, i.e., considered iatrogenic, there has classically been controversy between maintaining a wait-and-see attitude as in primary paresis or performing an early surgical revision. In a study of 707 surgically treated diaphyseal fractures of the humerus, 46 radial palsies were observed, in no case having been recorded during the operation of obvious radial lesions. Thirty-nine had been treated with plate, three with intramedullary nail, and four with Ender nails. Five cases were surgically revised, in none of which a macroscopic radial lesion was found. All cases recovered spontaneously in an average of 15 weeks. Therefore, these authors advocate a wait-and-see attitude unless there is any suspicion of injury, for example, by a loss of reduction or mobilization of the material in the post-surgical radiological control [65]. In a 2019 review, the authors observed a similar radial recovery pattern in primary and secondary paresis and observed no advantage to early surgical exploration [66]. In another recent review, they also recommend a wait-and-see approach unless there is an obvious suspicion of injury at surgery [67].

Table 8.4 Healing rates of diaphyseal humerus fractures treated with plates

Author	Year	*N*	Healing rate
McCormark[a] [46]	2000	22	95%
Chapman[a] [47]	2000	46	93%
Changulani[a] [44]	2007	24	87.5%
Putti[a] [42]	2009	18	94%
Singisetti[a] [43]	2010	16	94%
Benegas[a] [45]	2014	21	100%

[a]Comparative studies with plate; *N* Number of cases

8.5.3.4 MIPO (Minimally Invasive Plate Osteosynthesis) Technique

Minimally invasive plating has grown in recent years. In 2002, Fernandez Dell'Oca introduced the idea of helical implants for several types of fractures, including humerus diaphyseal fractures, presenting two cases with good results [68]. A helical conformation placed the proximal part of the plate in the lateral zone, while the distal zone remained in the anterior zone, avoiding the radial nerve. Livani published in 2004 his series of 15 patients with diaphyseal fractures treated by this technique where he described the percutaneous placement of a large fragment plate in the anterior zone of the humerus, a safe area in terms of vasculonervous structures and also flat, so it was not necessary to conform the plate, as proposed by Fernandez Dell'Oca, whose placement in the lateral zone of the humerus of his preconformed plate put the axillary nerve at risk [69]. The proximal approach involved a 3–5 cm anterolateral mini-approach between the biceps on one side and the deltoid and cephalic vein on the other. The distal approach was also made about 3–5 cm along the lateral aspect of the biceps, more deeply crossing the brachialis muscle and leaving the musculocutaneous nerve medially and the radial nerve laterally, which are the two nerves that supply this muscle, thus going through an interneural plane. A submuscular and extraperiosteal tunneling was then performed connecting the two approaches. The plate was introduced from proximal to distal, taking special care to place the plate medial to the long portion of the biceps and not trapping it. The plate was then fixed to the proximal fragment with 3 screws, followed by an indirect reduction of the distal fragment on the plate. Once verified by radioscopy, the distal fixation is performed with three more screws. In the case of very distal fractures, he opted to curve the end zone of the plate anteriorly and place it in the anterior zone of the lateral column, in this case performing the Kocher approach in this distal area [69]. From this point on, increasing series with similar surgical technique and good results continued to be published [70–82], and since then dozens of comparative studies, reviews, and several recent meta-analyses have been published showing excellent results compared to conventional open reduction, with less radial nerve injury rate, less bleeding, less surgical time, and even less nonunions. When compared to intramedullary nail fixation, better functional shoulder scales have been reported [83–86] (Table 8.5). The MIPO seem to correspond to the current trend as opposed to the wide approaches previously described (Fig. 8.6).

A cadaveric study in 2005 already described this method as very safe regarding the radial nerve. When sliding the plate through the anterior zone, it remained in the distal zone between 2 and 4.9 mm from the radial nerve in full supination and between 0 and 3 in pronation, so it is recommended to keep the arm in supination during percutaneous sliding of the plate [71]. Caution should also be taken to avoid tensioning the lateral area of the distal approach with Hohman-type spreaders to avoid radial paresis. The surgical technique and the confirmation of the safety of vasculonervous structures are maintained to this day. There are authors who consider radial paresis as a contraindication to perform a percutaneous technique, but others such as Livani already in 2005 published a small series of six patients with distal humerus fractures and radial paresis where he performed a percutaneous technique but through a distal Kocher approach, locating the radial nerve and introducing the plate from distal to proximal. All patients recovered from paresis [72].

More recently, the idea of helical implants for diaphyseal fractures with metaphyseal or proximal articular extension has been taken up again, either because there is insufficient space for an anterior plate placement proximally or because an associated articular reduction is needed. García-Virto et al. have recently published a series of 15 patients with fractures of this type where osteosynthesis was performed using the MIPO technique with preconformed helical plates. In the proximal area, a lateral transdeltoid mini-approach of 3–5 cm is performed, and in the distal area the anterior approach is similar to the anterior placement of straight plates. The helical

Table 8.5 Comparative studies between different surgical treatments of humerus diaphyseal fractures

Author	Year	Type of study	Comparative treatments	Results
Hohmann [84]	2016	Systematic review and meta-analysis of 8 prospective randomized controlled trial (**n = 376**)	ORIF vs. MIPO vs. IMN	MIPO: – Lower risk radial palsy – Shorter operation time – Better clinical outcomes
Tesworth [83]	2018	Review of 24 clinical case series, 5 comparatives trials, 6 RCTs and 4 meta-analysis	ORIF vs. MIPO	MIPO: – Lower risk for non-union – Lower risk radial palsy
Keshav [85]	2021	Meta-analysis and systematic review of 5 RCTs and 6 nonrandomized comparative studies (**n = 582**)	ORIF vs. MIPO	MIPO: – Lower risk radial palsy – Lesser blood loss – Shorter operation time
Beeres [86]	2021	Meta-analysis and systematic review of 2 RCT's (98 patients) and 7 observational studies (263 patients) (**n = 361**)	ORIF vs. MIPO	MIPO: – Lower risk of non-union – Lower secondary radial palsy

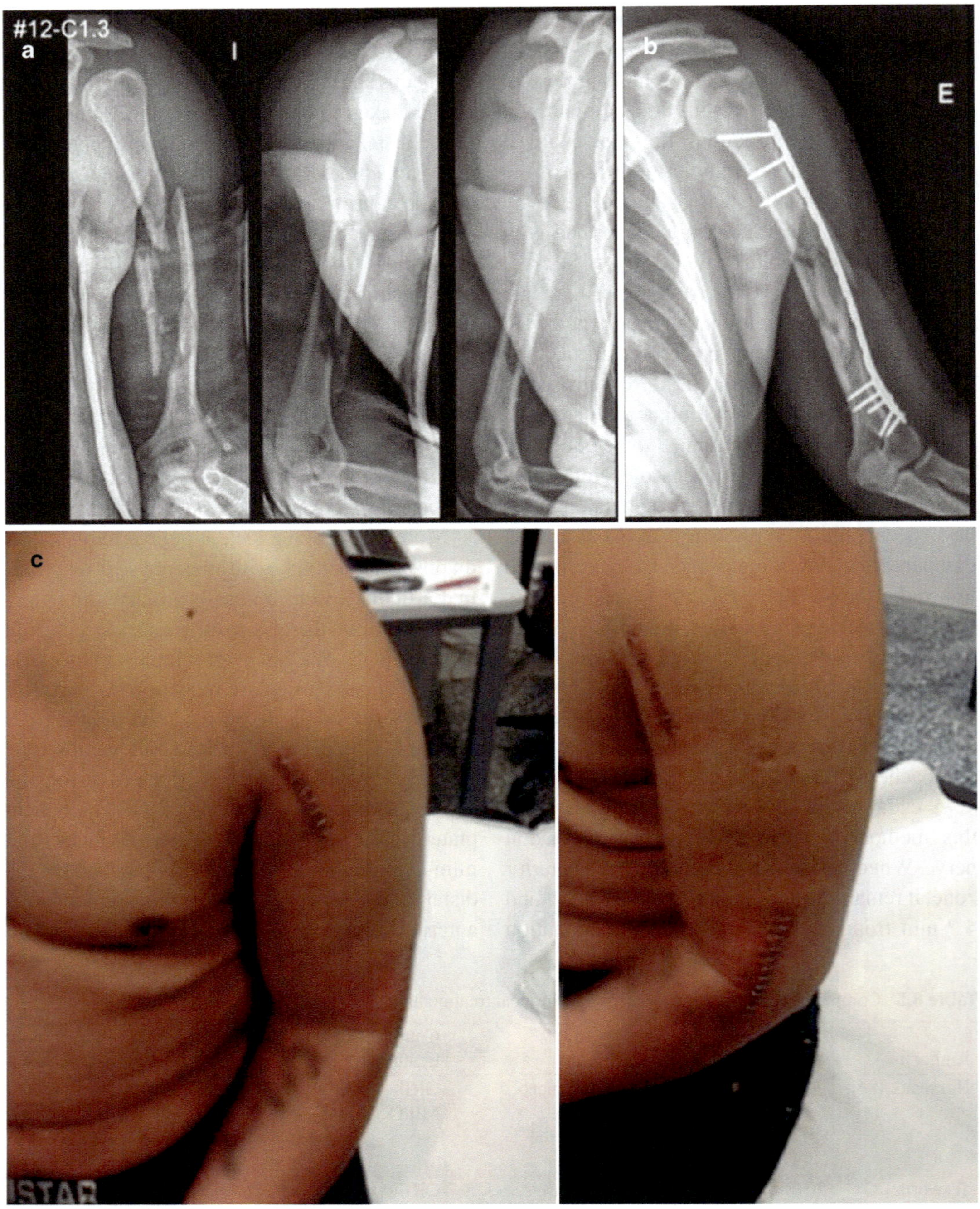

Fig. 8.6 (**a**–**c**) Comminuted diaphyseal humerus fracture (**a**). Closed reduction and fixation with straight plate using MIPO (minimally invasive plate osteosynthesis) technique (**b**). Surgical mini-approaches: proximal anterolateral and distal Kocher (**c**). Images provided by Dr. Miquel Videla, Traumatology and Orthogeriatrics Unit, Hospital Moisés Broggi

plate is introduced from proximal to distal taking special care with the axillary nerve. They had one case of nonunion, with no radial paresis and good to excellent functional results [87] (Fig. 8.7).

This technique offers a middle ground between ORIF and intramedullary nailing, incorporating benefits of both. From the nail, minimally invasive surgery provides greater respect for the soft

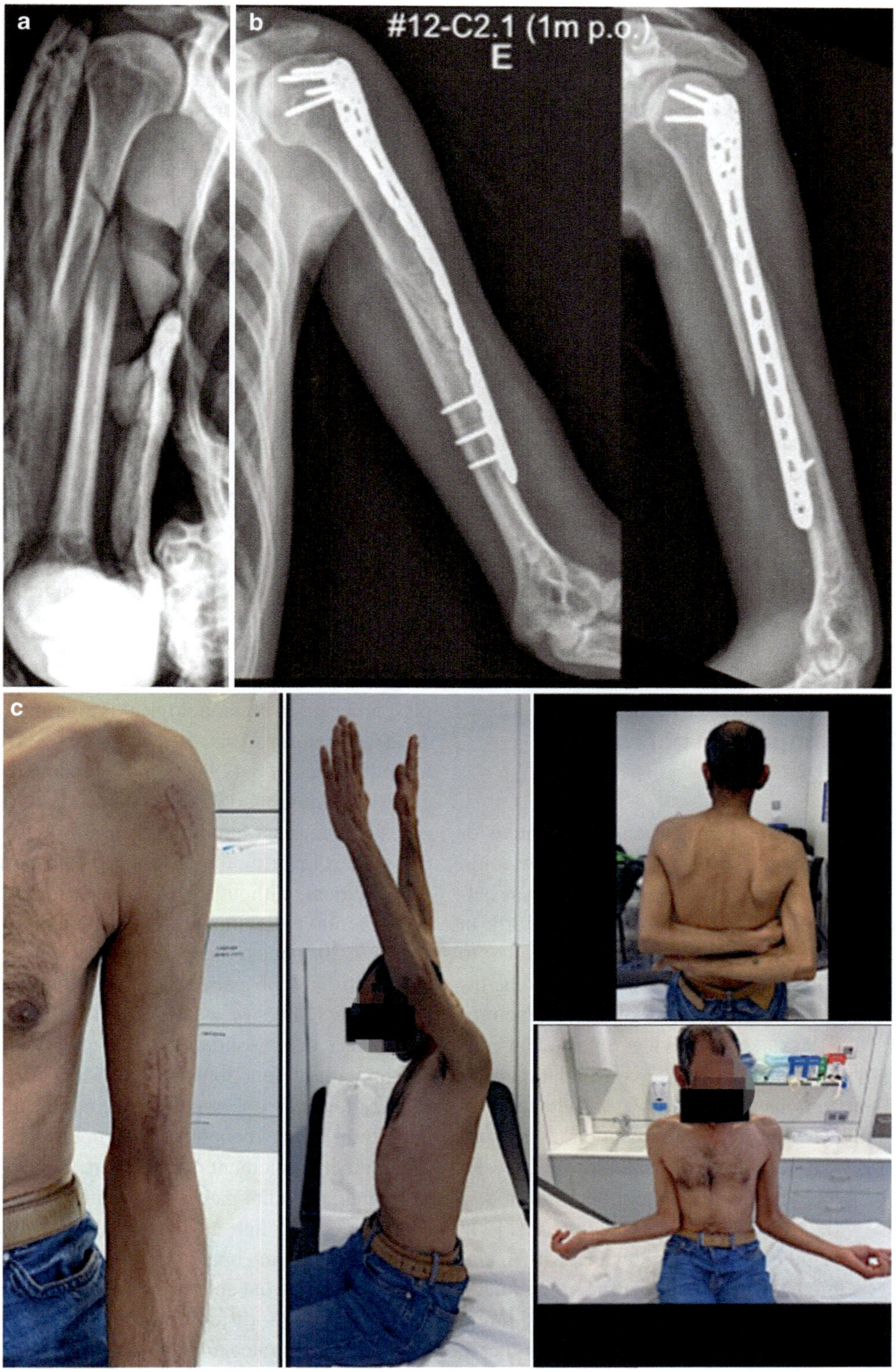

Fig. 8.7 (**a**–**c**) Diaphyseal fracture of the proximal humerus with insufficient space in the proximal fragment for placement of an anterior plate (**a**). Closed reduction and fixation with precontoured helical plate using MIPO (minimally invasive plate osteosynthesis) technique (**b**). Excellent functional result (**c**). Images provided by Dr. Miquel Videla, Traumatology and Orthogeriatrics Unit, Hospital Moisés Broggi

tissues and relative stability, thus obtaining a more biological fixation but avoiding damage to the cuff at its entry point, such as the plate. It also reduces radial nerve injuries, more frequently observed in open reductions and internal fixations with plate.

8.5.4 External Fixator

Generally, treatment with an external fixator is reserved for damage control in polytraumatized patients and for open fractures with a large defect (Gustilo III). In cases where definitive surgical treatment cannot be carried out after placement, either because of the general condition of the patient or because of the poor condition of the soft tissues, there are studies that describe good results using this method as definitive treatment [88]. It is important to be familiar with the anatomy and the changing situation of the radial nerve along the humerus to avoid injuring it with the pins [89].

8.6 Comparison of Treatment Options

Regarding the choice between conservative or surgical treatment, a 2012 Cochrane review could not conclude whether surgical treatment was better or worse than conservative treatment [90]. In 2015, another systematic review continued to state that there was no level 1 evidence in the literature on the management of these fractures [91]. A 2019 systematic review reflects that conservative treatment has better consolidation rates (6.3% nonunions versus 17.6%), with lower rates of complications such as iatrogenic radial injury or infection. Radiological malunion rates were higher in conservative treatment but did not correlate with worse functional outcomes [2]. In contrast, another systematic review with meta-analysis in 2020 showed a lower rate of nonunion in surgical treatment but a higher rate of infection, with no differences in malunion or nerve injury. Therefore, it does not seem to be a superiority of surgical treatment over conservative management, as long as there are no absolute indications for the latter (no tolerance to conservative treatment, inadequate reduction, intra-articular extension, floating elbow, metastasis, open Gustilo III fractures, brachial plexus lesions, vascular lesion).

As for the option of plate or nail if surgical treatment is chosen, this has been a matter of debate for decades, even when non-locked intramedullary implants were used. A 1995 study by Rodríguez-Merchán compared the use of plates with Hackethal nails in 40 patients with diaphyseal humerus fractures, finding no differences in healing and complication rates. He also proposed a classification for functional outcomes after treatment of these fractures [92].

In more recent literature and after many comparative studies, a 2010 meta-analysis of four randomized studies (n = 203 patients) reflected that there were no significant differences between both treatments in the rates of complications, nonunions, infection, radial palsy, or need for reintervention, although authors acknowledged there was heterogeneity in the studies, small samples, and certain methodological limitations [93]. A 2013 meta-analysis of 10 randomized controlled studies (n = 429 patients) found no differences in nonunion, delayed consolidation, radial paresis, or implant failure. In contrast, there were differences favoring the plate use in subacromial impingement, although the increased need for reinterventions for this reason was unclear [94]. A recent 2021 meta-analysis of 18 observational studies (n = 4906 patients) and 10 randomized controlled studies (n = 525 patients) showed no differences in consolidation rates, quality of life, and upper limb functional scales. A higher rate of reoperation was observed in the intramedullary nail group, most frequently for symptoms of subacromial impingement. There were lower rates of temporary radial paresis in the intramedullary nail group, although all but one case recovered spontaneously in both groups. Consolidation time was somewhat shorter in the intramedullary nail group (slight difference of 1.9 weeks), with lower infection rates and shorter operative time. All these differences, although significant, were small and advocate that both treatments achieve good results [48].

As for minimally invasive plating, developing in recent years, studies seem to point to it as the best option not only superior to ORIF but also to intramedullary nailing. A dozen of meta-analyses in the last 5 years report a statistically significant difference in favor of the MIPO technique in terms of consolidation rate, radial paresis, bleeding, operative time, and shoulder pain (Table 8.5).

8.7 Conclusions

After several decades of controversy in the literature on the treatment of diaphyseal fractures of the humerus, it can now be stated that whenever there are no contraindications, conservative treatment should be chosen, paying special attention to the need for close clinical and radiological follow-up and the patient's compliance and tolerance of this treatment. This mode of treatment is carried out sequentially, first with a hanging cast or U-splint immobilization, to be replaced in 1 or 2 weeks by a custom-made prefabricated brace, achieving a functional immobilization with early mobilization of the shoulder and elbow. Special attention should be paid to a fracture pattern: proximal third oblique line, in which higher rates of nonunion have been demonstrated, and surgical treatment can then be chosen at the outset.

In the case of deciding for surgical treatment, in fractures with metaphyseal or articular extension or in the case of vascular lesions in need of repair, we would opt for a plate, and, in bifocal or pathological fractures, we would opt for a nail. In all other cases, both treatments seem equally effective, with residual shoulder pain being the major disadvantage of the intramedullary nail, so special care should be taken to ensure that the material does not protrude into the subacromial space and try to minimize damage to the cuff at the point of entry. A more recent and superior treatment option to the previous ones are the plates placed in a minimally invasive way, its main limitation being the need for a learning curve, which once overcome seems to make this treatment the one of choice in case of deciding for a surgical treatment.

Regarding the most frequent complication, radial paresis, whether primary or iatrogenic, there seems to be general agreement that most of them have a spontaneous recovery, and therefore we should maintain an expectant attitude and not consider an early surgical revision unless there is a high suspicion of a clear lesion.

References

1. Gallusser N, Barimani B, Vauclair F. Humeral shaft fractures. EFORT Open Rev. 2021;6:24–34.
2. Sargeant HW, Farrow L, Barker S, Kumar K. Operative versus non-operative treatment of humeral shaft fractures: a systematic review. Shoulder Elbow. 2020;12:229–42.
3. Gulcek M, Gamli M. Anterior humeral approach with nerve stimulator. J Orthop Surg (Hong Kong). 2018;26:2309499018803002.
4. Updegrove GF, Mourad W, Abboud JA. Humeral shaft fractures. J Shoulder Elb Surg. 2018;27:e87–97.
5. Browner BD, Jupiter JB, Levine AM, Trafton PG, Krettek C, editors. Skeletal trauma basic science, management, and reconstruction, vol. 1 & 2. 4th ed. Philadelphia: Saunders Elsevier; 2009. ISBN: 978-1416022206.
6. Bishop J, Ring D. Management of radial nerve palsy associated with humeral shaft fracture: a decision analysis model. J Hand Surg Am. 2009;34(6):991–6.e1. https://doi.org/10.1016/j.jhsa.2008.12.029. Epub 2009 Apr 10.
7. Claessen FM, Peters RM, Verbeek DO, Helfet DL, Ring D. Factors associated with radial nerve palsy after operative treatment of diaphyseal humeral shaft fractures. J Shoulder Elb Surg. 2015;24(11):e307–11. https://doi.org/10.1016/j.jse.2015.07.012. Epub 2015 Sep 2.
8. Hak DJ. Radial nerve palsy associated with humeral shaft fractures. Orthopedics. 2009;32(2):111.
9. Guse TR, Ostrum RF. The surgical anatomy of the radial nerve around the humerus. Clin Orthop Relat Res. 1995;320:149–53.
10. Zlotolow DA, Catalano LW, Barron OA, Glickel SZ. Surgical exposures of the humerus. J Am Acad Orthop Surg. 2006;14:754–65.
11. McCann PA, Smith GC, Clark D, Amirfeyz R. The tricipital aponeurosis—a reliable soft tissue landmark for humeral plating. Hand Surg. 2015;20(1):53–8. https://doi.org/10.1142/S0218810415500070.
12. Holstein A, Lewis GM. Fractures of the humerus with radial-nerve paralysis. J Bone Joint Surg Am. 1963;45:1382–8.
13. Gustilo RB, Mendoza RM, Williams DN. Problems in the management of type III (severe) open fractures: a new classification of type III open fractures. J Trauma.

1984;24(8):742–6. https://doi.org/10.1097/00005373-198408000-00009.
14. Mahabier KC, Van Lieshout EM, Van Der Schaaf BC, Roukema GR, Punt BJ, Verhofstad MH, et al. Reliability and reproducibility of the OTA/AO classification for humeral shaft fractures. J Orthop Trauma. 2017;31:e75–80.
15. Sarmiento A, Kinman PB, Galvin EG, Schmitt RH, Phillips JG. Functional bracing of fractures of the shaft of the humerus. J Bone Joint Surg Am. 1977;59(5):596–601.
16. Koch PP, Gross DF, Gerber C. The results of functional (Sarmiento) bracing of humeral shaft fractures. J Shoulder Elb Surg. 2002;11(2):143–50. https://doi.org/10.1067/mse.2002.121634.
17. Sarmiento A, Zagorski JB, Zych GA, Latta LL, Capps CA. Functional bracing for the treatment of fractures of the humeral diaphysis. J Bone Joint Surg Am. 2000;82(4):478–86. https://doi.org/10.2106/00004623-200004000-00003.
18. Huttunen TT, Kannus P, Lepola V, Pihlajamäki H, Mattila VM. Surgical treatment of humeral-shaft fractures: a register-based study in Finland between 1987 and 2009. Injury. 2012;43(10):1704–8. https://doi.org/10.1016/j.injury.2012.06.011. Epub 2012 Jul 6.
19. Rutgers M, Ring D. Treatment of diaphyseal fractures of the humerus using a functional brace. J Orthop Trauma. 2006;20(9):597–601. https://doi.org/10.1097/01.bot.0000249423.48074.82.
20. Rüedi T, Moshfegh A, Pfeiffer KM, Allgöwer M. Fresh fractures of the shaft of the humerus—conservative or operative treatment? Reconstr Surg Traumatol 1974;14:65–74
21. Sarmiento A, Horowitch A, Aboulafia A, Vangsness CT Jr. Functional bracing for comminuted extra-articular fractures of the distal third of the humerus. J Bone Joint Surg Br. 1990;72(2):283–7. https://doi.org/10.1302/0301-620X.72B2.2312570. Erratum in: J Bone Joint Surg Br 1990 Jul;72(4):752.
22. Ekholm R, Tidermark J, Törnkvist H, Adami J, Ponzer S. Outcome after closed functional treatment of humeral shaft fractures. J Orthop Trauma. 2006;20(9):591–6. https://doi.org/10.1097/01.bot.0000246466.01287.04.
23. Ali E, Griffiths D, Obi N, Tytherleigh-Strong G, Van Rensburg L. Nonoperative treatment of humeral shaft fractures revisited. J Shoulder Elb Surg. 2015;24(2):210–4. https://doi.org/10.1016/j.jse.2014.05.009. Epub 2014 Aug 1.
24. Papasoulis E, Drosos GI, Ververidis AN, Verettas DA. Functional bracing of humeral shaft fractures. A review of clinical studies. Injury. 2010;41(7):e21–7. https://doi.org/10.1016/j.injury.2009.05.004. Epub 2009 Jun 11.
25. Ring D, Chin K, Taghinia AH, Jupiter JB. Nonunion after functional brace treatment of diaphyseal humerus fractures. J Trauma. 2007;62(5):1157–8. https://doi.org/10.1097/01.ta.0000222719.52619.2c.
26. Klenerman L. Fractures of the shaft of the humerus. J Bone Joint Surg Br. 1966;48(1):105–11.
27. Shields E, Sundem L, Childs S, Maceroli M, Humphrey C, Ketz JP, Soles G, Gorczyca JT. The impact of residual angulation on patient reported functional outcome scores after non-operative treatment for humeral shaft fractures. Injury. 2016;47(4):914–8. https://doi.org/10.1016/j.injury.2015.12.014. Epub 2015 Dec 23.
28. Brien WW, Gellman H, Becker V, Garland DE, Waters RL, Wiss DA. Management of fractures of the humerus in patients who have an injury of the ipsilateral brachial plexus. J Bone Joint Surg Am. 1990;72(8):1208–10.
29. Ekholm R, Ponzer S, Törnkvist H, Adami J, Tidermark J. The Holstein-Lewis humeral shaft fracture: aspects of radial nerve injury, primary treatment, and outcome. J Orthop Trauma. 2008;22(10):693–7. https://doi.org/10.1097/BOT.0b013e31818915bf.
30. Shao YC, Harwood P, Grotz MR, Limb D, Giannoudis PV. Radial nerve palsy associated with fractures of the shaft of the humerus: a systematic review. J Bone Joint Surg Br. 2005;87(12):1647–52. https://doi.org/10.1302/0301-620X.87B12.16132.
31. Pollock FH, Drake D, Bovill EG, Day L, Trafton PG. Treatment of radial neuropathy associated with fractures of the humerus. J Bone Joint Surg Am. 1981;63(2):239–43.
32. Bumbasirević M, Lesić A, Bumbasirević V, Cobeljić G, Milosević I, Atkinson HD. The management of humeral shaft fractures with associated radial nerve palsy: a review of 117 cases. Arch Orthop Trauma Surg. 2010;130(4):519–22. https://doi.org/10.1007/s00402-009-0951-4. Epub 2009 Aug 11.
33. Rocchi M, Tarallo L, Mugnai R, Adani R. Humerus shaft fracture complicated by radial nerve palsy: is surgical exploration necessary? Musculoskelet Surg. 2016;100(Suppl 1):53–60. https://doi.org/10.1007/s12306-016-0414-3. Epub 2016 Nov 30.
34. Rommens PM, Kuechle R, Bord T, Lewens T, Engelmann R, Blum J. Humeral nailing revisited. Injury. 2008;39(12):1319–28. https://doi.org/10.1016/j.injury.2008.01.014. Epub 2008 Apr 15.
35. Jang Y, Kempton LB, Mckinley TO, Sorkin AT. Insertion-related pain with intramedullary nailing. Injury. 2017;48(Suppl 1):S18–21. https://doi.org/10.1016/j.injury.2017.04.029. Epub 2017 May 5.
36. Christ AB, Gausden EB, Warner SJ, Nellestein AM, Thacher RR, Lorich DG. Rotator cuff-sparing approach for antegrade humeral nailing with biceps tenodesis: a technical trick with clinical implications. J Orthop Trauma. 2017;31(2):e60–5. https://doi.org/10.1097/BOT.0000000000000684.
37. Park JY, Pandher DS, Chun JY, Md ST. Antegrade humeral nailing through the rotator cuff interval: a new entry portal. J Orthop Trauma. 2008;22(6):419–25. https://doi.org/10.1097/BOT.0b013e318173f751.
38. Dimakopoulos P, Papadopoulos AX, Papas M, Panagopoulos A, Lambiris E. Modified extra rotator-cuff entry point in antegrade humeral nailing. Arch Orthop Trauma Surg. 2005;125(1):27–32. https://doi.org/10.1007/s00402-004-0757-3. Epub 2004 Nov 3.

39. Tanaka Y, Gotani H, Sasaki K, Yoshimura T, Yagi H. Evaluation of intramedullary nail fixation via the Neviaser portal for proximal humerus fracture. J Clin Orthop Trauma. 2019;10(3):474–9. https://doi.org/10.1016/j.jcot.2019.02.007. Epub 2019 Feb 8.
40. Rommens PM, Blum J, Runkel M. Retrograde nailing of humeral shaft fractures. Clin Orthop Relat Res. 1998;350:26–39.
41. Rommens PM, Verbruggen J, Broos PL. Retrograde locked nailing of humeral shaft fractures. A review of 39 patients. J Bone Joint Surg Br. 1995;77(1):84–9.
42. Putti AB, Uppin RB, Putti BB. Locked intramedullary nailing versus dynamic compression plating for humeral shaft fractures. J Orthop Surg (Hong Kong). 2009;17(2):139–41. https://doi.org/10.1177/230949900901700202.
43. Singisetti K, Ambedkar M. Nailing versus plating in humerus shaft fractures: a prospective comparative study. Int Orthop. 2010;34(4):571–6. https://doi.org/10.1007/s00264-009-0813-2. Epub 2009 Jun 9.
44. Changulani M, Jain UK, Keswani T. Comparison of the use of the humerus intramedullary nail and dynamic compression plate for the management of diaphyseal fractures of the humerus. A randomised controlled study. Int Orthop. 2007;31(3):391–5. https://doi.org/10.1007/s00264-006-0200-1. Epub 2006 Aug 10.
45. Benegas E, Ferreira Neto AA, Gracitelli ME, Malavolta EA, Assunção JH, Prada Fde S, Bolliger Neto R, Mattar R Jr. Shoulder function after surgical treatment of displaced fractures of the humeral shaft: a randomized trial comparing antegrade intramedullary nailing with minimally invasive plate osteosynthesis. J Shoulder Elb Surg. 2014;23(6):767–74. https://doi.org/10.1016/j.jse.2014.02.010. Epub 2014 Apr 24.
46. McCormack RG, Brien D, Buckley RE, McKee MD, Powell J, Schemitsch EH. Fixation of fractures of the shaft of the humerus by dynamic compression plate or intramedullary nail. A prospective, randomised trial. J Bone Joint Surg Br. 2000;82(3):336–9. https://doi.org/10.1302/0301-620x.82b3.9675.
47. Chapman JR, Henley MB, Agel J, Benca PJ. Randomized prospective study of humeral shaft fracture fixation: intramedullary nails versus plates. J Orthop Trauma. 2000;14(3):162–6. https://doi.org/10.1097/00005131-200003000-00002.
48. Beeres FJP, van Veelen N, Houwert RM, Link BC, Heng M, Knobe M, Groenwold RHH, Babst R, van de Wall BJM. Open plate fixation versus nailing for humeral shaft fractures: a meta-analysis and systematic review of randomised clinical trials and observational studies. Eur J Trauma Emerg Surg. 2021; https://doi.org/10.1007/s00068-021-01728-7. Epub ahead of print.
49. Paryavi E, Pensy RA, Higgins TF, Chia B, Eglseder WA. Salvage of upper extremities with humeral fracture and associated brachial artery injury. Injury. 2014;45(12):1870–5. https://doi.org/10.1016/j.injury.2014.08.038.
50. Chang AC, Ha NB, Sagar C, Bain GI, Leonello DT. The modified anterolateral approach to the humerus. J Orthop Surg (Hong Kong). 2019;27(3):2309499019865954. https://doi.org/10.1177/2309499019865954.
51. Gerwin M, Hotchkiss RN, Weiland AJ. Alternative operative exposures of the posterior aspect of the humeral diaphysis with reference to the radial nerve. J Bone Joint Surg Am. 1996;78(11):1690–5. https://doi.org/10.2106/00004623-199611000-00008.
52. Páramo-Díaz P, Arroyo-Hernández M, Rodríguez Vega V, Aroca-Peinado M, León-Baltasar JL, Caba-Doussoux P. Surgical treatment of extra-articular distal-third diaphyseal fractures of the humerus using a modified posterior approach and an extra-articular plate. Rev Esp Cir Ortop Traumatol. 2017;61(6):404–11. https://doi.org/10.1016/j.recot.2017.07.001. English, Spanish. Epub 2017 Sep 7.
53. Lu S, Wu J, Xu S, Fu B, Dong J, Yang Y, Wang G, Xin M, Li Q, He TC, Wang F, Zhou D. Medial approach to treat humeral mid-shaft fractures: a retrospective study. J Orthop Surg Res. 2016;11:32. https://doi.org/10.1186/s13018-016-0366-1.
54. Rellán I, Gallucci GL, Donndorff AG, De Carli P, Zaidenberg EE, Richard MJ, Boretto JG. Time until union in absolute vs. relative stability MIPO plating in simple humeral shaft fractures. Eur J Orthop Surg Traumatol. 2021; https://doi.org/10.1007/s00590-021-02920-6. Epub ahead of print.
55. O'Toole RV, Andersen RC, Vesnovsky O, Alexander M, Topoleski LD, Nascone JW, Sciadini MF, Turen C, Eglseder WA Jr. Are locking screws advantageous with plate fixation of humeral shaft fractures? A biomechanical analysis of synthetic and cadaveric bone. J Orthop Trauma. 2008;22(10):709–15. https://doi.org/10.1097/BOT.0b013e31818df8cb.
56. Gardner MJ, Griffith MH, Demetrakopoulos D, Brophy RH, Grose A, Helfet DL, Lorich DG. Hybrid locked plating of osteoporotic fractures of the humerus. J Bone Joint Surg Am. 2006;88(9):1962–7. https://doi.org/10.2106/JBJS.E.00893.
57. Karakasli A, Basci O, Ertem F, Sekik E, Havitcioglu H. Dual plating for fixation of humeral shaft fractures: a mechanical comparison of various combinations of plate lengths. Acta Orthop Traumatol Turc. 2016;50(4):432–6. https://doi.org/10.1016/j.aott.2016.07.002. Epub 2016 Jul 29.
58. Kosmopoulos V, Nana AD. Dual plating of humeral shaft fractures: orthogonal plates biomechanically outperform side-by-side plates. Clin Orthop Relat Res. 2014;472(4):1310–7. https://doi.org/10.1007/s11999-013-3379-7. Epub 2013 Nov 12.
59. Seo JB, Heo K, Yang JH, Yoo JS. Clinical outcomes of dual 3.5-mm locking compression plate fixation for humeral shaft fractures: comparison with single 4.5-mm locking compression plate fixation. J Orthop Surg (Hong Kong). 2019;27(2):2309499019839608. https://doi.org/10.1177/2309499019839608.

60. Sharaby M, Elhawary A. A simple technique for double plating of extraarticular distal humeral shaft fractures. Acta Orthop Belg. 2012;78(6):708–13.
61. Lee JK, Choi YS, Sim YS, Choi DS, Han SH. Dual plate fixation on distal third diaphyseal fracture of the humerus. Int Orthop. 2017;41(8):1655–61. https://doi.org/10.1007/s00264-016-3355-4. Epub 2016 Dec 1.
62. Streufert BD, Eaford I, Sellers TR, Christensen JT, Maxson B, Infante A, Shah AR, Watson DT, Sanders RW, Mir HR. Iatrogenic nerve palsy occurs with anterior and posterior approaches for humeral shaft fixation. J Orthop Trauma. 2020;34(3):163–8. https://doi.org/10.1097/BOT.0000000000001658.
63. Lee WY, Shin HD, Kim KC, Cha SM, Jeon YS. Relationship between incidence of postoperative radial nerve palsy and surgical experience in the treatment of humeral shaft fractures through a posterior triceps splitting approach: a retrospective study. Acta Orthop Traumatol Turc. 2021;55(4):338–43. https://doi.org/10.5152/j.aott.2021.20415.
64. Chang G, Ilyas AM. Radial nerve palsy after humeral shaft fractures: the case for early exploration and a new classification to guide treatment and prognosis. Hand Clin. 2018;34(1):105–12. https://doi.org/10.1016/j.hcl.2017.09.011.
65. Wang JP, Shen WJ, Chen WM, Huang CK, Shen YS, Chen TH. Iatrogenic radial nerve palsy after operative management of humeral shaft fractures. J Trauma. 2009;66(3):800–3. https://doi.org/10.1097/TA.0b013e31816142cf.
66. Vaishya R, Kandel IS, Agarwal AK, Vijay V, Vaish A, Acharya K. Is early exploration of secondary radial nerve injury in patients with humerus shaft fracture justified? J Clin Orthop Trauma. 2019;10(3):535–40. https://doi.org/10.1016/j.jcot.2018.11.002. Epub 2018 Nov 9.
67. Hegeman EM, Polmear M, Scanaliato JP, Nesti L, Dunn JC. Incidence and management of radial nerve palsies in humeral shaft fractures: a systematic review. Cureus. 2020;12(11):e11490. https://doi.org/10.7759/cureus.11490.
68. Fernández Dell'Oca AA. The principle of helical implants. Unusual ideas worth considering. Injury. 2002;33(Suppl 1):SA1–27. https://doi.org/10.1016/s0020-1383(02)00064-5.
69. Livani B, Belangero WD. Bridging plate osteosynthesis of humeral shaft fractures. Injury. 2004;35(6):587–95. https://doi.org/10.1016/j.injury.2003.12.003.
70. van de Wall BJM, Baumgärtner R, Houwert RM, Link BC, Heng M, Knobe M, Groenwold RHH, Babst R, Beeres FJP. MIPO versus nailing for humeral shaft fractures: a meta-analysis and systematic review of randomised clinical trials and observational studies. Eur J Trauma Emerg Surg. 2021; https://doi.org/10.1007/s00068-020-01585-w. Epub ahead of print.
71. Apivatthakakul T, Arpornchayanon O, Bavornratanavech S. Minimally invasive plate osteosynthesis (MIPO) of the humeral shaft fracture. Is it possible? A cadaveric study and preliminary report. Injury. 2005;36(4):530–8. https://doi.org/10.1016/j.injury.2004.05.036.
72. Livani B, Belangero WD, Castro de Medeiros R. Fractures of the distal third of the humerus with palsy of the radial nerve: management using minimally-invasive percutaneous plate osteosynthesis. J Bone Joint Surg Br. 2006;88(12):1625–8. https://doi.org/10.1302/0301-620X.88B12.17924.
73. Zhiquan A, Bingfang Z, Yeming W, Chi Z, Peiyan H. Minimally invasive plating osteosynthesis (MIPO) of middle and distal third humeral shaft fractures. J Orthop Trauma. 2007;21(9):628–33. https://doi.org/10.1097/BOT.0b013e31815928c2.
74. Apivatthakakul T, Phornphutkul C, Laohapoonrungsee A, Sirirungruangsarn Y. Less invasive plate osteosynthesis in humeral shaft fractures. Oper Orthop Traumatol. 2009;21(6):602–13. https://doi.org/10.1007/s00064-009-2008-9.
75. Kobayashi M, Watanabe Y, Matsushita T. Early full range of shoulder and elbow motion is possible after minimally invasive plate osteosynthesis for humeral shaft fractures. J Orthop Trauma. 2010;24(4):212–6. https://doi.org/10.1097/BOT.0b013e3181c2fe49.
76. Concha JM, Sandoval A, Streubel PN. Minimally invasive plate osteosynthesis for humeral shaft fractures: are results reproducible? Int Orthop. 2010;34(8):1297–305. https://doi.org/10.1007/s00264-009-0893-z. Epub 2009 Oct 21.
77. Lee HJ, Oh CW, Oh JK, Apivatthakakul T, Kim JW, Yoon JP, Lee DJ, Jung JW. Minimally invasive plate osteosynthesis for humeral shaft fracture: a reproducible technique with the assistance of an external fixator. Arch Orthop Trauma Surg 2013;133(5):649–657. doi: https://doi.org/10.1007/s00402-013-1708-7. Epub 2013 Mar 5.
78. Giordano M, Giordano V, Gameiro VS, Belangero W, Livani B, Giannoudis PV, Krettek C. Anterior minimally invasive plating osteosynthesis technique (MIPO) for humeral shaft fractures: an anatomical study of neuromuscular structures at risk. Eur J Orthop Surg Traumatol. 2021;31(3):449–58. https://doi.org/10.1007/s00590-020-02792-2. Epub 2020 Sep 14.
79. Shin SJ, Sohn HS, Do NH. Minimally invasive plate osteosynthesis of humeral shaft fractures: a technique to aid fracture reduction and minimize complications. J Orthop Trauma. 2012;26(10):585–9. https://doi.org/10.1097/BOT.0b013e318254895f.
80. López-Arévalo R, de Llano-Temboury AQ, Serrano-Montilla J, de Llano-Giménez EQ, Fernández-Medina JM. Treatment of diaphyseal humeral fractures with the minimally invasive percutaneous plate (MIPPO) technique: a cadaveric study and clinical results. J Orthop Trauma. 2011;25(5):294–9. https://doi.org/10.1097/BOT.0b013e3181f98421.
81. Ziran BH, Kinney RC, Smith WR, Peacher G. Submuscular plating of the humerus: an emerging technique. Injury. 2010;41(10):1047–52. https://doi.org/10.1016/j.injury.2010.04.021.

82. Ziran BH, Belangero W, Livani B, Pesantez R. Percutaneous plating of the humerus with locked plating: technique and case report. J Trauma. 2007;63(1):205–10. https://doi.org/10.1097/01.ta.0000231870.11908.3e.
83. Tetsworth K, Hohmann E, Glatt V. Minimally invasive plate osteosynthesis of humeral shaft fractures: current state of the art. J Am Acad Orthop Surg. 2018;26(18):652–61. https://doi.org/10.5435/JAAOS-D-17-00238.
84. Hohmann E, Glatt V, Tetsworth K. Minimally invasive plating versus either open reduction and plate fixation or intramedullary nailing of humeral shaft fractures: a systematic review and meta-analysis of randomized controlled trials. J Shoulder Elb Surg. 2016;25(10):1634–42. https://doi.org/10.1016/j.jse.2016.05.014. Epub 2016 Aug 10.
85. Keshav K, Baghel A, Kumar V, Neradi D, Kaustubh K, Mishra P. Is minimally invasive plating osteosynthesis better than conventional open plating for humeral shaft fractures? A systematic review and meta-analysis of comparative studies. Indian J Orthop. 2021;55(Suppl 2):283–303. https://doi.org/10.1007/s43465-021-00413-6.
86. Beeres FJ, Diwersi N, Houwert MR, Link BC, Heng M, Knobe M, Groenwold RH, Frima H, Babst R, van de Wall BJ. ORIF versus MIPO for humeral shaft fractures: a meta-analysis and systematic review of randomized clinical trials and observational studies. Injury. 2021;52(4):653–63. https://doi.org/10.1016/j.injury.2020.11.016. Epub 2020 Nov 6.
87. García-Virto V, Santiago-Maniega S, Llorente-Peris A, Simón-Pérez C, Álvarez-Ramos BA, García-Florez L, Aguado HJ. MIPO helical pre-contoured plates in diaphyseal humeral fractures with proximal extension. Surgical technique and results. Injury. 2021;52(Suppl 4):S125–30. https://doi.org/10.1016/j.injury.2021.01.049. Epub 2021 Feb 13.
88. Kurup H, Hossain M, Andrew JG. Dynamic compression plating versus locked intramedullary nailing for humeral shaft fractures in adults. Cochrane Database Syst Rev. 2011;6:CD005959. https://doi.org/10.1002/14651858.CD005959.pub2.
89. Gausepohl T, Koebke J, Pennig D, Hobrecker S, Mader K. The anatomical base of unilateral external fixation in the upper limb. Injury. 2000;31(Suppl 1):11–20. https://doi.org/10.1016/s0020-1383(99)00258-2.
90. Gosler MW, Testroote M, Morrenhof JW, Janzing HM. Surgical versus non-surgical interventions for treating humeral shaft fractures in adults. Cochrane Database Syst Rev. 2012;1:CD008832. https://doi.org/10.1002/14651858.CD008832.pub2.
91. Clement ND. Management of humeral shaft fractures; non-operative versus operative. Arch Trauma Res. 2015;4(2):e28013. https://doi.org/10.5812/atr.28013v2.
92. Rodríguez-Merchán EC. Compression plating versus hackethal nailing in closed humeral shaft fractures failing nonoperative reduction. J Orthop Trauma. 1995;9(3):194–7. https://doi.org/10.1097/00005131-199506000-00003.
93. Heineman DJ, Poolman RW, Nork SE, Ponsen KJ, Bhandari M. Plate fixation or intramedullary fixation of humeral shaft fractures. Acta Orthop. 2010;81(2):216–23. https://doi.org/10.3109/17453671003635884. Erratum in: Acta Orthop 2010;81(5):647.
94. Ouyang H, Xiong J, Xiang P, Cui Z, Chen L, Yu B. Plate versus intramedullary nail fixation in the treatment of humeral shaft fractures: an updated meta-analysis. J Shoulder Elb Surg. 2013;22(3):387–95. https://doi.org/10.1016/j.jse.2012.06.007. Epub 2012 Sep 1.

9 Controversies in the Management of Intra-Articular Distal Humerus Fractures in Adults

César García-Mauriño, Pablo Vadillo-Cardona, and Alfonso Vaquero-Picado

9.1 Introduction

Distal humerus fractures in adults are challenging injuries for trauma surgeons. These fractures comprise complex regional anatomy, poor outcomes, and common complications, even when recent advances in surgical technique and implants have improved clinical outcomes [1]. These fractures have an estimated incidence of 5.7 per 100,000 persons per year in adults and represent between 0.5 and 7% of all fractures in adults and 30% of all humerus fractures [2, 3]. As in other fractures in adults, it is noted a bimodal distribution of these injuries regarding age and sex, with an early peak of incidence in young males due to high-energy trauma (traffic and sport accidents), and a late peak of incidence in elderly females as a result of low-energy trauma, such as falling from standing height [4, 5].

It is expected a raise in the incidence of these injuries as the older population increases and the motorization of the developing world continues. Working up strategies such as osteoporosis treatment and fall prevention that may reduce the incidence of these injuries should be taken into account [5].

Until the development of the AO principles of fracture management, treatment of distal humerus fractures was predominantly nonsurgical, carrying on a high probability of functional disability. Nowadays, open reduction and internal fixation (ORIF) is the gold standard of treatment. Elderly patients, with insufficient bone stock and high degree of comminution, pose a true challenge to suitable fixation [2, 6, 7]. In spite of significant advances in the treatment of distal humerus fractures, controversy remains regarding the most adequate surgical approach, fixation method, and handling of ulnar nerve [8].

9.2 Clinical Assessment

When facing a distal humerus fracture, physical examination should always include the evaluation of ipsilateral shoulder and wrist, not to overlook associated fractures in adjacent joints, which may be present in up to 16% of patients [4, 9]. In patients sustaining high-energy trauma, associated injuries must be ruled out as well [10].

A circumferential inspection of the limb should be conducted in order to assess open fractures, which are relatively common. When open fracture occurs, they are often posterior as the injury usually results in hyperextension on an extended elbow [1, 2]. Open elbow fractures should be managed following standard open fracture protocols which include early antibiotics and tetanus prophylaxis administration, extremity stabilization and dressing, timely irrigation and

C. García-Mauriño · P. Vadillo-Cardona
A. Vaquero-Picado (✉)
Upper Limb Unit, Department of Orthopedic Surgery, La Paz University Hospital, Madrid, Spain

E. C. Rodríguez-Merchán, A. Moreno-Garcìa (eds.), *Controversies in Orthopedic Surgery of The Upper Limb*, https://doi.org/10.1007/978-3-031-04907-1_9

debridement, and soft tissue coverage. Vascular injury should always be assessed by inspecting distal extremity color, capillary filling, and peripheral pulses. It is important to remember that due to great collateral blood supply around the elbow, it is possible to have distal pulse presence even in the setting of a brachial artery injury [1]. Sometimes, correcting the deformity by gentle traction could be needed in order to improve the vascular status on emergency setting. If it is not normalized after traction, a computed tomography (CT) angiography or surgical exploration is necessary [2]. Neurological examination must include radial, median, and ulnar nerves. Motor and sensitive status should be documented preoperatively and postoperatively. Up to 26% of incomplete ulnar neuropathy is observed in type C distal humerus fractures [4, 9].

Special attention should be paid to the development of compartment syndrome. Unrelenting pain and the inability to bear finger extension indicate the possibility of that complication. The clinical evaluation must also include data on the patient's functional status, hand dominance, comorbidities, and living situation, which may help with the therapeutic decision-making process and preoperative risk assessment [4, 10].

9.3 Anatomy and Classification

A precise knowledge of elbow anatomy is fundamental for understanding these injuries.

In the coronal plane, distal humerus has a triangular shape, which is formed by two diverging columns (the medial and lateral columns) and the articular block. Distally, the medial column consists of the medial epicondyle (origin of the flexor-pronator mass) and the most medial side of the trochlea; meanwhile, the lateral column distally comprises the capitellum and, more proximally, the lateral epicondyle (origin of the extensor muscle mass). The bone between both columns, which include the coronoid fossa and olecranon fossa, is very thin or absent. The condylar mass is in 4–8 degrees of valgus relative to the shaft [5, 6]. In the sagittal plane, the articular segment is flexed 40° relative to the longitudinal axis of the humerus shaft, so, in the lateral side, the center of the capitellum aligns with the anterior humeral shaft line [1, 5].

There are several classification systems, but internationally the most commonly used is the Orthopedic Trauma Association (OTA/AO) classification. It distinguishes three main fracture patterns with increased complexity (A, B, and C) with further subdivision (1, 2, and 3) based on fracture pattern, location, and degree of comminution [7–9]:

- Type A fractures. Extra-articular fractures, which may involve the epicondyles (extracapsular fractures) or the metaphyseal region (intracapsular fractures).
- Type B fractures. Partial articular fractures. The fracture involves a segment of the articular mass, but the remaining is still connected to the metaphysis and diaphysis. It includes unicondylar fractures and coronal fractures of the capitellum, trochlea, or both.
- Type C fractures. Complete articular fractures. The fracture establishes a total lack of continuity between the condylar mass and the humeral shaft.

Up to 96% of distal humerus fractures in adults are intra-articular fractures, either affecting both columns or partial articular fractures [1, 9].

9.4 Imaging

Standard high-quality anteroposterior, lateral, and oblique radiographs should be obtained in all patients. Proximal and distal joints (ipsilateral shoulder and wrist) should be included in X-ray studies, in order to be sure concomitant fractures are not overlooked [2, 4, 6, 9, 10].

The Mckee's double arc sign can be observed in coronal fractures of the articular surface, one arc representing the capitellum and the other arc representing the lateral part of the trochlea. Characterization of intra-articular fractures of distal humerus, especially those with multiplanar fracture patterns or coronal plane injuries, can be challenging only with plain radiographs. In these situations, performing a CT scan is of great help for assessing articular involvement, comminution, and surgical planning [11].

9.5 Treatment

In the treatment decision-making process, one must take the age of the patient, medical comorbidities, job occupation, functional status and expectations, degree of comminution, inadequate bone stock, bone quality, or underlying arthritis [2, 4, 12].

9.5.1 Nonoperative Management

Conservative management has been associated with poor functional outcomes, decreased elbow range of motion, and high rate of delayed union and nonunion [2, 6, 10].

Nowadays nonsurgical treatment is mainly reserved for non-displaced fractures and very fragile patients with ongoing medical issues which pose a high surgical risk. Other possible indications of conservative management would be patients with high-degree cognitive impairment or low-demand or nonfunctional upper extremities [2, 4, 12].

Recently, Atiken et al. reported on short- and medium-term functional outcomes in 40 elderly low-demand patients with distal humerus fractures treated conservatively ("bag of bones" strategy). Surviving patients (n = 20) had a mean Oxford elbow score of 30 points (7–48), and 95% of them reported a functional range of elbow flexion. The authors conclude that conservative management in a low-demand patient only gives a modest functional result but avoids the substantial surgical risks associated with primary ORIF or total elbow arthroplasty (TEA) [13].

Desloges et al. reviewed 32 low-demand, medically unwell, elderly patients with distal humerus fractures treated nonoperatively. Sixty-eight percent of patients reported good to excellent subjective outcomes, and the fracture union rate was 81% at a mean follow-up of 12 months. They conclude that satisfactory outcomes can be achieved after nonoperative management of distal humerus fractures in selected patients [14].

Nonoperative treatment often consists of a variable period of full-arm cast immobilization (usually 3 to 6 weeks) with the elbow in 60°–90° of flexion followed by early gentle motion [2].

9.5.2 Surgical Management

In active, fit for surgery, adult patients with reconstructible fracture patterns, open reduction and internal fixation are the gold standard of treatment [1, 2, 4, 6, 8, 10, 12, 15]. The main goal is to achieve an anatomic reduction of the articular surface, a correct alignment, and metaphyseal compression in order to secure a stable fixation which allows for early motion [1, 12].

As mentioned earlier, controversy still remains regarding surgical approaches, implants, fixation method, and handling of ulnar nerve [8].

9.5.3 Surgical Approaches

Several surgical approaches have been described with differences in terms of exposure and soft tissue aggression [6]. Different variants of a posterior approach are used, existing limited comparative data. Olecranon osteotomy is reported to offer the best articular exposure, but, even when performed, up to 40% of distal humerus articular surface cannot be visualized [16]. Wilkinson et al. demonstrated an exposed articular surface of 35% for the triceps splitting approach, for the triceps reflecting approach of 46% and for the olecranon osteotomy of 57% [6].

The olecranon and triceps act as obstacles to the visualization of the articular surface, so posterior approaches can be classified in two main groups: the ones that preserve the extensor mechanism and mobilize it and the ones that disrupt it [2].

9.5.3.1 Universal Posterior Incision

A posterior midline incision is made in a straight way or curved fashion around the olecranon according to the surgeon's preference. The mean length of the incision is usually 4–8 cm distal and at least 10 cm proximal to the tip of the olecranon. Special attention is paid to any skin injuries present (e.g., open fractures or previous scars) that can be incorporated into the incision [2, 12, 17]. Full-thickness fasciocutaneous flaps are developed medially and laterally to prevent skin necrosis and seroma formation. It is strongly recommended to identify the ulnar nerve along the medial border of the triceps, dissecting and elevating the fascia of the triceps for better visualization. For further mobilization of the nerve, it can be freed from proximal to distal, releasing the arcade of Struthers proximally (between 2.5 and 7 cm from the medial epicondyle) and the cubital tunnel retinaculum distally, trying to preserve the motor branches to the flexor carpi ulnaris and flexor digitorum profundus muscles [8, 17, 18]. The management of the released nerve will be discussed later.

The radial nerve needs to be dissected only when the approach is extended further proximally in order to apply longer plates (fractures with diaphyseal extension). In those cases, the posterior antebrachial cutaneous branch of the radial nerve, which is often located distal and laterally, should be identified [2, 17].

9.5.3.2 Bilaterotricipital Approach (Alonso-Llames)

Dissection is carried along the medial and lateral borders of the triceps which are elevated off the posterior periosteum of the humerus and the medial and lateral intermuscular septa. Medial and lateral windows are created, allowing the surgeon to work through either side of the muscle mass, achieving excellent visualization of the entire posterior humerus [8, 17].

This is a less aggressive approach in which the extensor mechanism is not disrupted, so there is no need to protect it postoperatively. The surgical time is shortened as well, thereby decreasing the risk of perioperative complications, and it allows for a more extensile exposure through the Kocher interval and/or an olecranon osteotomy if needed [17].

The bilaterotricipital approach is useful for supracondylar and transcondylar fractures and as well for AO C1 and C2 intra-articular fractures; for more complex and multifragmentary articular fractures, the distal exposure is limited, and this approach would be insufficient [4, 8].

9.5.3.3 Triceps-Reflecting Approach (Bryan-Morrey)

This approach was described by Bryan and Morrey in 1982 [19]. The extensor mechanism is reflected from medial to lateral in continuity with the forearm fascia, olecranon and ulnar periosteum [8]. The ulnar collateral ligament can be released as well to gain further exposure, but it must then be reattached [17]. After fracture fixation, the triceps tendon is repaired by reattaching it to the olecranon with nonabsorbable sutures through bone tunnels [8, 20].

This surgical approach has been extensively used for elbow arthroplasty. Iselin et al. conducted a retrospective study which included 31 patients with distal humerus fractures treated with this approach and concluded that it is a valuable choice for ORIF in distal intra-articular humerus fractures since it preserves the normal joint anatomy of the olecranon, and the clinical outcomes were excellent, without any objective or subjective functional impairment related to the surgical approach [20].

9.5.3.4 Triceps-Reflecting Anconeus Pedicle Flap (TRAP)

This approach described by O'Driscoll in 2000 is a combination of modified Kocher and Bryan-Morrey approaches in which the triceps and anconeus muscles are elevated off the posterior humerus and olecranon [8, 21]; the anconeus is completely dissected from its insertion onto the proximal ulna.

Similar to Bryan-Morrey approach, it avoids the complications associated with olecranon osteotomy. Conversely, it requires familiarity with the anatomy, and the distal exposure is limited compared to the one obtained with olecranon osteotomy [21].

Traditionally, these triceps-elevating exposures have been related to weakness of extension or triceps' rupture by some authors. However, Ozer et al. have reported no significant impairment of elbow function in 11 patients with AO type C fractures treated with a TRAP approach. Azboy et al. reviewed 40 patients with distal humerus intra-articular fractures treated with a TRAP approach as well and concluded that it is a successful approach that reduces reoperations and complications rates, with no triceps' rupture observed and only one patient with poor strength after the procedure [22].

9.5.3.5 Triceps-Splitting Approach (Campbell Approach)

The triceps' muscle mass and tendon are incised on its midline dividing the triceps in two halves which are dissected to either side. The incision carries down distally to the olecranon, leaving the anconeus laterally and the flexor carpi ulnaris medially. The radial nerve needs to be protected during proximal exposure [8, 17].

This approach can result in triceps weakness as a result of muscle and intramuscular nerve branches injury and requires a thoughtful closure of the triceps [6, 8]. Besides, it hinders the positioning of lateral plates because the lateral half of the triceps can get in the way when it comes to drilling and screw insertion [17]. It can be performed for supracondylar and transcondylar fractures, but it does not provide an adequate exposure of the distal articular surface [2].

9.5.3.6 Olecranon Osteotomy

This surgical approach offers the best articular surface visualization as mentioned before so it is widely used for intra-articular fractures of the distal humerus [2, 6, 8, 17], being especially useful in complex intra-articular fractures with severe comminution (AO type C3). Once the "bare area" of the proximal ulna is identified, approximately 3 cm distal from the tip of the olecranon, a Chevron osteotomy is performed, initially with an oscillating saw, finishing with an osteotome [6, 8, 9, 17]. This type of osteotomy is preferred by many authors, rather than a transverse one, because of its intrinsic stability. The proximal olecranon is mobilized along with the tricipital tendon proximally, and, if needed, the exposure may be extended with a bilaterotricipital approach [17]. After the procedure, the ulna is reduced and fixed with either a lag screw, an intramedullary nail, a plate, or tension band wires, depending on the surgeon's preference [8, 17]. According to Meldrum et al., fixation with a single screw is the technique that had the least complications in their review of different types of fixation for olecranon osteotomies [12, 23].

Disadvantages of this procedure are the risk of the nonunion at the site of the osteotomy (0–9%), further need for surgery to remove symptomatic hardware (6–30%), not easy conversion to TEA, and potential risk of intra-articular adhesions [2, 21]. Furthermore, if an olecranon osteotomy is not performed, the surgeon can use the olecranon, coronoid and radial head as a three-dimensional template upon which the articular bony fragments of the distal humerus can be reassembled until final fixation is achieved.

9.5.4 Implants

The main goal when treating distal humerus fractures in adults is to achieve an anatomic reconstruction of the articular surface with a rigid and stable internal fixation allowing early motion exercises, bone consolidation, and prevention of future osteoarthritis [2, 5, 8, 9]. There is unanimity in the literature on how a double plate construct is superior over single plating or screw fixation when fixing intra-articular distal humerus fractures involving both columns [24]. Many biomechanical and clinical studies highlight the advantages of double plating over other fixation methods [25–27]. Although there is general agreement on rigid fixation with dual plates as the gold-standard treatment when fixing bicolumnar distal humerus fractures, the most adequate plating configuration remains controversial [2, 6, 8, 10]. The debate mostly revolves around whether the plates should be applied in a parallel fashion or orthogonal to each other [8]. In the orthogonal configuration, the two plates are applied at 90 degrees, with a medial plate on the medial column and a posterior plate on the lateral column. The parallel configuration uses a medial plate on the medial column combined with a lateral plate on the lateral column [10].

Several biomechanical studies comparing the two configurations have proven that parallel plating provides more stability than perpendicular plating [6, 9, 10]. Stoffel et al. compared the biomechanical stability of perpendicular and parallel locking plating systems for the internal fixation of 24 simulated AO Type C2 distal humerus fractures in cadaveric osteoporotic bone. They concluded that the parallel locking system showed improved stability in axial compression as well as in external rotation although both locking plate systems would allow early mobilization of the elbow [28]. Arnander et al. conducted another biomechanical study and concluded that a parallel plate configuration is significantly stronger and stiffer than a perpendicular plate configuration when subjected to sagittal bending forces [29]. Zalavras et al. compared parallel to orthogonal constructs in an intra-articular distal humerus fracture model and reported that parallel plate constructs had significantly higher stiffness than orthogonal ones during cyclic varus loading without any screw loosening compared to screw loosening in all posterior plates of orthogonal constructs. Parallel constructs had as well significantly higher ultimate load in axial/sagittal loading to failure [10, 30]. However, recent clinical studies that have compared orthogonal to parallel plating found no difference between the constructs regarding functional outcome or complication rate [6].

Shin et al. compared perpendicular to parallel plate fixation in a prospective randomized comparative study of 35 patients and found no significant differences in clinical outcomes or range of motion between treatment groups (Level II evidence) [2, 31]. Lee et al. compared orthogonal versus parallel plating in a prospective randomized trial of 67 patients (Level II evidence). They found no differences between the two groups with regard to clinical outcomes, operating time, time to union, or complication rates at a minimum follow-up time of 2 years [2, 32].

Having no differences in clinical outcomes or complication rate, it is important to apply the plates according to the fracture pattern because, if properly applied, both parallel and orthogonal positioning can provide adequate stability. Plates should be placed in the most biomechanically adequate placement in relation to the fracture lines rather than in positions predetermined by the plate itself [33]. Parallel plating could be preferred for the fixation of fractures in the most distal end of the humerus, favored by the opportunity for additional distal screw fixation; meanwhile perpendicular plating is preferred in cases of coronal shear fractures, where anterior to posterior fixation gaining additional stability in the coronal plane is desirable [5, 8, 9].

The cornerstone to achieve stable fixation is an adequate reduction of the fracture. Without successful reconstruction of the triangular anatomy of the distal humerus and the olecranon fossa-tip relationship, solid anatomical fixation cannot be achieved [8, 33].

Different types of plates have been used for fixation of distal humerus fractures: limited contact dynamic compression plate (LC-DCP), 3.5 mm reconstruction plates, and anatomically precontoured plates. All have been proven successful to provide rigid fixation. Only one-third tubular plates are considered too weak to ensure adequate bone fixation and are no longer recommended for fixation of distal humerus fractures [8, 9, 33, 34]. Regarding the use of locking plates versus traditional compression plates, biomechanical studies have found that the use of locking screws is only superior when poor bone quality is present [35]. Otherwise, it has been shown no significant difference between both options with regard to clinical outcome, rate of nonunion, infection, and reoperation [36].

9.5.5 Fixation Methods

Once the fracture has been exposed, debris and hematoma clots are removed. We should be sure to preserve and to pay attention to the orientation of free small bony fragments which may be present and can be useful to reassemble the articular surface.

9.5.5.1 Reduction and Temporary Fixation

A traditional approach includes reducing first the articular fragments to each other with the help of reduction forceps, manipulation, and small-diameter Kirschner wires (0.035–0.045 inches) that can be used for provisional fixation. The surgeon must foresee that these K wires won't interfere with the placement of definitive fixation plates later on. Articular fragments may be held together as well with interfragmentary lag screws, threaded K wires, or resorbable pegs, always allowing future screw insertion and plate positioning [1, 33]. Alternatively, if one column presents a relatively simple fracture pattern, the surgeon may choose to reduce and fix it first (converting an AO type C fracture into a type B fracture), reducing afterwards the articular segment to this column [1, 8]. In case of significant cartilage loss at the joint level, special care must be taken at restoring the adequate width of distal humerus, avoiding compression at this location since it would lead to articular incongruence [33].

Once the articular surface has been rebuilt, it has to be reduced and fix to the humerus shaft at the metaphyseal level using provisional 0.065 K wires. As mentioned before, limited contact dynamic compression plate (LC-DCP), 3.5 mm reconstruction plates, or anatomically precontoured plates can be used for definitive fixation after an optimal reduction is achieved. The plates are applied to both columns and should have different lengths in order to reduce the stress riser effect and risk of peri-implant fracture [6, 8, 9].

The literature supports that each plate should have at least three screws proximal to the metaphyseal fracture line. A biomechanical study published by Zarifian et al. reported that the optimal configuration should include four screws in the distal segments of both plates, three screws in the medial plate proximal segment, and five screws in the lateral plate proximal segment, so the construct resists all bending, axial, and torsional forces [37].

A plate applied directly over the lateral column should be precontoured at its distal end, so it matches the anatomical tilt of the capitellum; the medial column does not angle forward distally, but, in low fractures, the medial plate should wrap around the medial epicondyle to maximize screw insertion in the articular fragments [1, 33].

9.5.5.2 Definitive Fixation

Once the plates have been placed in the desired position, the articular segment must be firmly secured. O'Driscoll enunciated eight technical principles that should guide the fixation of distal humerus fractures [34]:

1. Every screw in the distal fragments should pass through a plate.
2. Engage a fragment on the opposite side that is also fixed to a plate.
3. As many screws as possible should be placed in the distal fragments.
4. Each screw should be as long as possible.
5. Each screw should engage as many articular fragments as possible.
6. The screws in the distal fragments should lock together by interdigitation, creating a fixed-angle structure.
7. Plates should be applied such that compression is achieved at the supracondylar level for both columns.
8. The plates must be strong enough and stiff enough to resist breaking or bending before union occurs at the supracondylar level.

Additional implants should be available if definitive fixation of small articular fragments is needed: mini-fragment plates, 2.7-mm reconstruction plates, headless compression screws, and bioabsorbable pins [9].

Next, proximal fixation and supracondylar compression should be achieved, aided by reduction clamps and the dynamic compression holes in the plates. If there is extensive metaphyseal comminution and significant bone loss, shortening of the humerus is tolerable up to 2–3 cm [2, 33]; in some cases, bone grafting and bridge plating may be necessary. Autologous bone from the iliac crest, demineralized bone matrix allograft, and structural cadaveric allograft are some of the options available.

Prior to closure, elbow range of motion and stability should be assessed, checking there is no bony or soft tissue impingement. Under fluoroscopic examination, adequate fracture reduction and plates and screws position should be verified, ensuring that no screws penetrate the joint [1, 9] (Figs. 9.1 and 9.2).

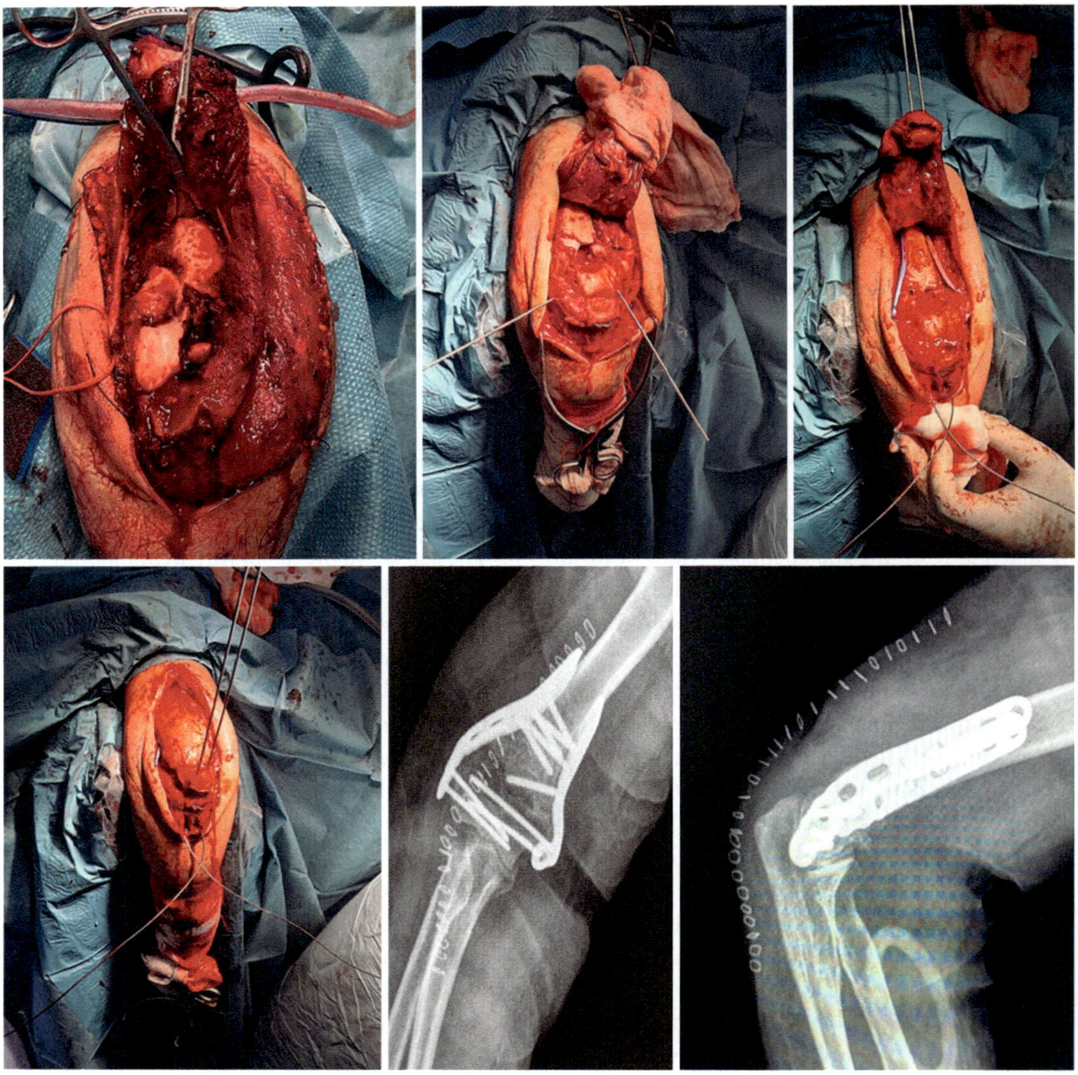

Fig. 9.1 Comminuted type C supracondylar fracture. From left to right, from up to down: Olecranon osteotomy provides extensile exposure to distal humerus, including part of the articular surface; provisional fixation with K-wires is helpful; fixation is best achieved by a combination of isolated lag screws and parallel anatomic precontoured 3.5 mm plates; olecranon osteotomy is closed with a cerclage; anteroposterior postoperative radiograph; lateral postoperative radiograph

9.5.6 Management of Ulnar Nerve

The operation protocol should clearly detail how the ulnar nerve was handled during surgery [1]. Although it is acknowledged that the ulnar nerve must be identified and protected during the procedure, controversy still remains regarding the best management of the nerve after the distal humerus fracture has been fixed. The options include returning the ulnar nerve to its initial location or to transpose it anteriorly [2, 6].

A 2018 meta-analysis by Shearin et al. included five retrospective studies, totaling 366 distal humerus fracture cases that underwent ORIF and either the ulnar nerve underwent in situ management or anterior transposition.

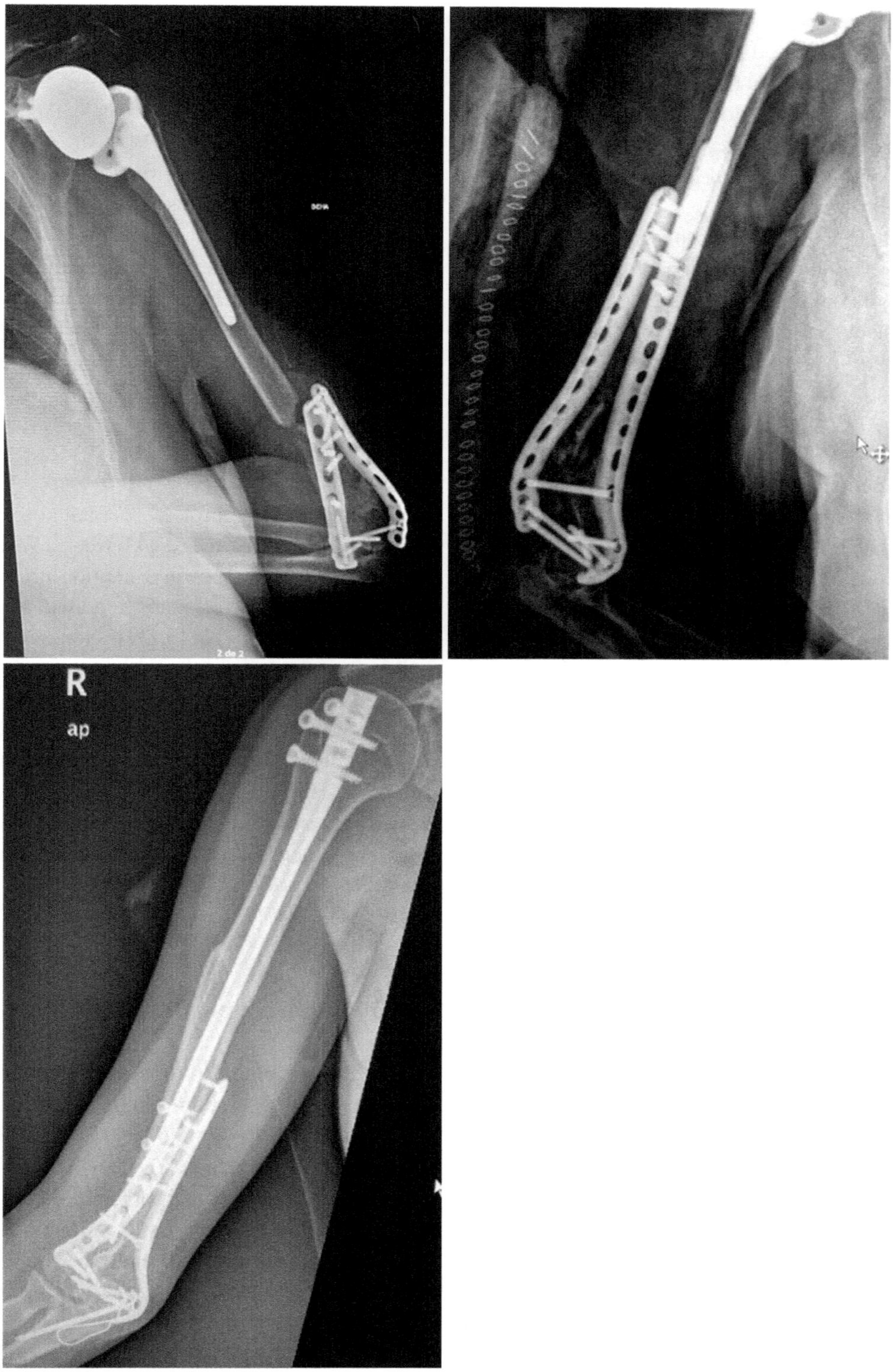

Fig. 9.2 In supracondylar fractures of the humerus, one plate should be larger than the other to avoid a stress riser point. It is especially important in case of previous implants such as shoulder prosthesis (top left), plates (top right), or nails (bottom left). Overlap in the proximal implant is also recommended to facilitate fracture consolidation

They observed that postoperative ulnar neuropathy was increased in patients who had transposition versus in situ management and concluded that transposition does not have a protective effect against the development of late ulnar neuropathy after distal humerus fracture repair surgery [38].

Either way, at the end of the procedure, ulnar nerve stability and relationship to the implants through complete elbow range of motion should be tested.

9.6 Postoperative Management

As mentioned before, early mobilization of the elbow after surgery is pursued in order to obtain the best outcomes [1, 2, 4–6, 9, 10, 14, 33, 39]; however, if the quality of the fixation is not optimal (i.e., due to fracture complexity or poor bone quality), it is advisable to immobilize and protect the elbow for 3–4 weeks to ensure the fracture consolidates in an adequate position. Although immobilization for more than 3 weeks has been associated with poorer outcomes, most patients will not develop significant stiffness, and if they do it is simpler to deal with stiffness rather than a loss of fixation [1, 9].

A posterior splint in neutral position can be applied for 24–48 h to protect the soft tissues; after it has been removed, active exercises of ipsilateral shoulder and wrist and active assisted exercises of the elbow are initiated. Light functional use of the extremity for daily live activities such as eating or personal hygiene is encouraged, not being allowed lifting weights over 1 kg. If an olecranon osteotomy has been performed, extension against gravity or resistance is banned for 6 weeks [33]. Exercises against resistance are initiated at approximately 6 weeks. Three months after surgery, full strengthening exercises are allowed, and, at 6 months postoperatively, patients can return to a preinjury activity level. Improvement can be achieved over the first year after surgery [1, 9, 12].

9.7 Complications of Surgical Management

9.7.1 Stiffness

Some degree of reduced elbow motion is often observed after ORIF in distal humerus fractures, particularly regarding extension. For some authors, this would be the most common complication. However, many studies in the literature report achieving a functional range of motion [2, 33].

9.7.2 Nonunion

Distal humerus fractures are estimated to attain union in an average time of 14.6 weeks. With current surgical techniques and fixation principles, exceptional union rates are reported, varying between 90% and 98% [9, 33]. Nonunion typically occurs in the metaphyseal region and, when present, in a 75% of the patients is thought to be caused by inadequate initial fracture fixation. Other factors that contribute to nonunion are infection, nutritional and smoking status, and underlying endocrine conditions [2, 6].

Management of nonunion includes contracture release, revision of the fixation, and bone grafting.

9.7.3 Heterotopic Ossification

The incidence of heterotopic ossification (HO) described in the literature is highly variable, with rates ranging from 0% to 50% according to different series [6, 9]. However, it is often not associated with functional problems. Some risk factors for heterotopic ossification have been described: head injury, multiples surgeries, delayed surgical treatment, bone grafting, high-energy injuries, or open fractures [2, 33].

Naut et al. reported a heterotopic ossification rate of 8.6% [40]. Recently, Foruria et al. reported in their retrospective study a symptomatic HO rate of 41%. HO was associated with significant loss of extension and overall decreased flexion–extension arc of less than 100° [41].

To date, there is no quality data regarding HO prophylaxis in the management of distal humerus fractures treated surgically. Radiation therapy and indomethacin treatment have been suggested. Shin et al. reported a 3% rate of symptomatic HO and a nonunion rate of 6% after radiation therapy and 2 weeks of indomethacin [31]. Similarly, Liu et al. reported a 3% rate of symptomatic HO as well and a nonunion rate of 3% after 6 weeks of celecoxib [42].

9.7.4 Ulnar Neuropathy

Ulnar neuritis can be present in up to 19% of patients. Management of this complication includes neurolysis or anterior transposition [2].

9.7.5 Other Complications [33]

- Fixation failure
- Hardware pain or prominence
- Superficial or deep infection
- Radial nerve palsy
- Malunion
- Posttraumatic osteoarthritis and avascular necrosis

9.8 Outcomes

Despite the controversies and complications previously discussed, when anatomic reduction of the articular surface, rigid bicolumnar internal fixation, and early motion are achieved, satisfactory outcomes can be expected [10]. Overall outcomes of ORIF in intra-articular fractures of distal humerus are satisfactory or better in 71–86% of patients. Overall arc of motion of approximately 100° can be expected, and patients should also expect approximately 75% return of strength in the distal humerus fractured arm versus their uninjured arm [33].

Doornberg et al. reported on 30 patients that were evaluated at an average of 19 years after open reduction and internal fixation of a fracture of the distal humerus, to assess the range of elbow motion and the functional outcome. The average final flexion arc was 106°, and the average pronation-supination arc was 165° [43]. The average American Shoulder and Elbow Surgeons (ASES) score was 96 points, with an average satisfaction score of 8.8 points on a 0 to 10-point visual analog scale. The authors concluded that the long-term results of open reduction and internal fixation of intra-articular fractures of the distal humerus are similar to those reported in the short term, suggesting that the results are durable.

9.9 Elbow Arthroplasty

Indications for prosthetic replacement after a distal humerus fracture include unreconstructible fractures, with high degree comminution and/or the presence of poor bone quality in low-demand elderly patients. Also, it can be beneficial in patients with preexisting inflammatory arthropathy. In this context, total elbow arthroplasty (TEA) is a recognized alternative treatment [2, 10, 12]. Contraindications include ipsilateral hand neurological impairment, noncompliant patient, acute open fracture, or active infection [12].

McKee et al. conducted a prospective randomized controlled trial to compare functional outcomes, complications, and reoperation rates in elderly patients with displaced intra-articular distal humeral fractures treated with open reduction and internal fixation or primary semiconstrained total elbow arthroplasty. Forty-two patients over 65 years were included and randomized. The Mayo Elbow Performance Score (MEPS) and Disabilities of the Arm, Shoulder, and Hand (DASH) score were determined at 6 weeks, 3 months, 6 months, 12 months, and 2 years. They reported that TEA resulted in more predictable and improved 2-year functional outcomes compared with ORIF and that TEA may result in decreased reoperation rates. The authors concluded that TEA is a preferred alternative over

ORIF in elderly patients with complex distal humeral fractures that are not amenable to achieve a stable fixation [44].

A systematic review and meta-analysis was performed by Githens et al. in order to compare outcomes and complication rates in elderly patients with intra-articular distal humerus fractures, being treated with either total elbow arthroplasty or open reduction and internal fixation with locking plates. They selected 27 studies including 563 patients with an average follow-up of 3.8 years. They concluded that TEA and ORIF for the treatment of geriatric distal humerus fractures provided similar functional outcome scores and range of motion, without significant complication rates [45].

Nonetheless, total elbow arthroplasty has its own limitations and complications. Patients should be warned about the postoperative restriction of lifting no more than 2–5 kg and no repetitive lifting more than 0.5–1 kg. Complications include prosthetic loosening, periprosthetic fracture, mechanical failure, and deep wound infection. Consequently, although TEA may provide similar outcomes when compared with ORIF in appropriately selected patients, it can cause terrible complications, and appropriate patients must be carefully selected [2, 4, 10].

9.10 Conclusions

Despite the controversies and complications previously discussed, when anatomic reduction of the articular surface, rigid bicolumnar internal fixation, and early motion are achieved, satisfactory outcomes can be expected. Overall outcomes of ORIF in intra-articular fractures of distal humerus are satisfactory or better in 71% to 86% of patients. Overall arc of motion of approximately 100° can be expected, and patients should also expect approximately 75% return of strength in the distal humerus fractured arm versus their uninjured arm.

Indications for prosthetic replacement after a distal humerus fracture include unreconstructible fractures, with high degree comminution and/or the presence of poor bone quality in low-demand elderly patients. Also, it can be beneficial in patients with preexisting inflammatory arthropathy. In this context, TEA is a recognized alternative treatment. Contraindications include ipsilateral hand neurological impairment, noncompliant patient, acute open fracture, or active infection.

TEA and ORIF, for the treatment of geriatric distal humerus fractures, provide similar functional outcome scores and range of motion, without significant complication rates. Nonetheless, total elbow arthroplasty has its own limitations and complications. Patients should be warned about the postoperative restriction of lifting no more than 2–5 kg and no repetitive lifting more than 0.5–1 kg. Complications include prosthetic loosening, periprosthetic fracture, mechanical failure, and deep wound infection. Consequently, although TEA may provide similar outcomes when compared with ORIF in appropriately selected patients, it can cause terrible complications, and appropriate patients must be carefully selected.

References

1. Buckley R, Moran CG, Appivatthakakul T. AO principles of fracture management. Thieme E-books; 2018. Print ISBN 9783132423091. Online ISBN 9783132423107. https://doi.org/10.1055/b-006-149767.
2. Lauder A, Richard MJ. Management of distal humerus fractures. Eur J Orthop Surg Traumatol. 2020;30:745–62.
3. Court-Brown CM, Caesar B. Epidemiology of adult fractures: a review. Injury. 2006;37:691–7.
4. Onizuka N, Switzer J, Myeroff C. Management of geriatric elbow injury. Orthop Clin North Am. 2021;52:381–401.
5. Amir S, Jannis S, Daniel R. Distal humerus fractures: a review of current therapy concepts. Curr Rev Musculoskelet Med. 2016;9:199–206.
6. Beazley JC, Baraza N, Jordan R, Modi CS. Distal humeral fractures—current concepts. Open Orthop J. 2017;11:1353–63.
7. Robinson CM, Hill RM, Jacobs N, Dall G, Court-Brown CM. Adult distal humeral metaphyseal fractures: epidemiology and results of treatment. J Orthop Trauma. 2003;17:38–47.
8. Lee H-J. Surgical treatment strategy for distal humerus intra-articular fractures. Clin Shoulder Elbow. 2019;22:113–7.

9. Pollock JW, Faber KJ, Athwal GS. Distal humerus fractures. Orthop Clin North Am. 2008;39: 187–200.
10. Zalavras CG, Papasoulis E. Intra-articular fractures of the distal humerus - a review of the current practice. Int Orthop. 2018;42:2653–62.
11. Nolan BM, Sweet SJ, Ferkel E, Udofia A-A, Itamura J. The role of computed tomography in evaluating intra-articular distal humerus fractures. Am J Orthop (Belle Mead). 2015;44:E326–30.
12. Morrey ME, Morrey BF, Sanchez-Sotelo J, Barlow JD, O'Driscoll S. A review of the surgical management of distal humerus fractures and nonunions: from fixation to arthroplasty. J Clin Orthop Trauma. 2021;20:101477.
13. Aitken SA, Jenkins PJ, Rymaszewski L. Revisiting the 'bag of bones': functional outcome after the conservative management of a fracture of the distal humerus. Bone Joint J. 2015;97-B:1132–8.
14. Desloges W, Faber KJ, King GJW, Athwal GS. Functional outcomes of distal humeral fractures managed nonoperatively in medically unwell and lower-demand elderly patients. J Shoulder Elb Surg. 2015;24:1187–96.
15. Al-Hamdani A, Rasmussen JV, Olsen BS. Good functional outcomes after open reduction and internal fixation for acute distal humeral fractures AO/OTA type 13 C2 and C3 in patients aged over 45 years. J Shoulder Elbow Surg. 2021:S1058-2746(21)00640-6. https://doi.org/10.1016/j.jse.2021.07.024. Online ahead of print.
16. Wilkinson JM, Stanley D. Posterior surgical approaches to the elbow: a comparative anatomic study. J Shoulder Elb Surg. 2001;10:380–2.
17. Antuña S, Barco R, editors. Essentials in elbow surgery: a comprehensive approach to common elbow disorders. London: Springer Verlag; 2014.
18. Caetano EB, Neto JJS, Vieira LA, Caetano MF. The arcade of Struthers: an anatomical study and clinical implications. Rev Bras Ortop. 2017;52:331–6.
19. Bryan RS, Morrey BF. Extensive posterior exposure of the elbow. A triceps-sparing approach. Clin Orthop Relat Res. 1982;166:188–92.
20. Iselin LD, Mett T, Babst R, Jakob M, Rikli D. The triceps reflecting approach (Bryan-Morrey) for distal humerus fracture osteosynthesis. BMC Musculoskelet Disord. 2014;15(1):406.
21. O'Driscoll SW. The triceps-reflecting anconeous pedicle (TRAP) approach for distal humeral fractures and nonunions. Orthop Clin North Am. 2000;31:91–101.
22. Azboy İ, Bulut M, Ancar C, Demirtaş A, Özkul E, Gem M, et al. The comparison of triceps-reflecting anconeus pedicle and olecranon osteotomy approaches in the treatment of intercondylar fractures of the humerus. Turkish J Trauma Emerg Surg. 2015;22:58–65.
23. Meldrum A, Kwong C, Archibold K, Cinats D, Schneider P. Olecranon osteotomy implant removal rates and associated complications. J Orthop Trauma. 2021;35:265–70.
24. Helfet DL, Hotchkiss RN. Internal fixation of the distal humerus: a biomechanical comparison of methods. J Orthop Trauma. 1990;4:260–4.
25. Jacobson S, Glisson R, Urbaniak J. Comparison of distal humerus fracture fixation: a biomechanical study. J South Orthop Assoc. 1997;6:241–9.
26. Scolaro JA, Hsu JE, Svach DJ, Mehta S. Plate selection for fixation of extra-articular distal humerus fractures: a biomechanical comparison of three different implants. Injury. 2014;45:2040–4.
27. Papaioannou N, Babis GC, Kalavritinos J, Pantazopoulos T. Operative treatment of type C intra-articular fractures of the distal humerus: the role of stability achieved at surgery on final outcome. Injury. 1995;26:169–73.
28. Stoffel K, Cunneen S, Morgan R, Nicholls R, Stachowiak G. Comparative stability of perpendicular versus parallel double-locking plating systems in osteoporotic comminuted distal humerus fractures. J Orthop Res. 2008;26:778–84.
29. Arnander MWT, Reeves A, MacLeod IAR, Pinto TM, Khaleel A. A biomechanical comparison of plate configuration in distal humerus fractures. J Orthop Trauma. 2008;22:332–6.
30. Zalavras CG, Vercillo MT, Jun B-J, Otarodifard K, Itamura JM, Lee TQ. Biomechanical evaluation of parallel versus orthogonal plate fixation of intra-articular distal humerus fractures. J Shoulder Elb Surg. 2011;20:12–20.
31. Shin S-J, Sohn H-S, Do N-H. A clinical comparison of two different double plating methods for intraarticular distal humerus fractures. J Shoulder Elb Surg. 2010;19:2–9.
32. Lee SK, Kim KJ, Park KH, Choy WS. A comparison between orthogonal and parallel plating methods for distal humerus fractures: a prospective randomized trial. Eur J Orthop Surg Traumatol. 2014;24:1123–31.
33. Miller AN, Beingessner DM. Intra-articular distal humerus fractures. Orthop Clin North Am. 2013;44:35–45.
34. O'Driscoll SW. Optimizing stability in distal humeral fracture fixation. J Shoulder Elbow Surg. 2005;14(1 Suppl S):186S–94S.
35. Hungerer S, Wipf F, von Oldenburg G, Augat P, Penzkofer R. Complex distal humerus fractures - comparison of polyaxial locking and nonlocking screw configurations—a preliminary biomechanical study. J Orthop Trauma. 2014;28:130–6.
36. Berkes M, Garrigues G, Solic J, Zeeland NV, Shourbaji N, Brouwer K, et al. Locking and non-locking constructs achieve similar radiographic and clinical outcomes for internal fixation of intra-articular distal humerus fractures. HSS J. 2011;7:244–50.
37. Zarifian A, Fough AA, Eygendaal D, Rivlin M, Shaegh SAM, Kachooei AR. Length of plates and number of screws for the fixation of distal humerus fractures: a finite element biomechanical study. J Hand Surg. 2021:S0363-5023(21)00438-X. https://doi.org/10.1016/j.jhsa.2021.07.010. Online ahead of print.

38. Shearin JW, Chapman TR, Miller A, Ilyas AM. Ulnar nerve management with distal humerus fracture fixation: a meta-analysis. Hand Clin. 2018;34:97–103.
39. Throckmorton TW, Zarkadas PC, Steinmann SP. Distal humerus fractures. Hand Clin. 2007;23:457–69.
40. Nauth A, McKee MD, Ristevski B, Hall J, Schemitsch EH. Distal humeral fractures in adults. J Bone Joint Surg. 2011;93:686–700.
41. Foruria AM, Lawrence TM, Augustin S, Morrey BF, Sanchez-Sotelo J. Heterotopic ossification after surgery for distal humeral fractures. Bone Joint J. 2014;96-B:1681–7.
42. Liu J, Ruan H, Wang J, Fan C, Zeng B. Double-column fixation for type C fractures of the distal humerus in the elderly. J Shoulder Elb Surg. 2009;18:646–51.
43. Doornberg JN, van Duijn PJ, Linzel D, Ring DC, Zurakowski D, Marti RK, et al. Surgical treatment of intra-articular fractures of the distal part of the humerus. J Bone Joint Surg. 2007;89:1524–32.
44. McKee MD, Veillette CJH, Hall JA, Schemitsch EH, Wild LM, McCormack R, et al. A multicenter, prospective, randomized, controlled trial of open reduction - internal fixation versus total elbow arthroplasty for displaced intra-articular distal humeral fractures in elderly patients. J Shoulder Elb Surg. 2009;18:3–12.
45. Githens M, Yao J, Sox AHS, Bishop J. Open reduction and internal fixation versus total elbow arthroplasty for the treatment of geriatric distal humerus fractures. J Orthop Trauma. 2014;28:481–8.

Controversies in the Management of Radial Head Fractures in Adults

10

Juan S. Ruiz-Pérez, Primitivo Gómez-Cardero, and E. Carlos Rodríguez-Merchán

10.1 Introduction

10.1.1 Epidemiology

Radial head fractures account for between 1.7 and 5.4% of all fractures and approximately one-third of bone injuries of the elbow. Classically, two clear peaks of incidence have been observed between the ages of 20 and 60 and a distribution by male-female gender of 1:2 to 1:1 [1]. However, more recent studies suggest an epidemiological distribution with slight differences. Kaas estimated an incidence of 2.8 cases per 100,000 inhabitants with a male-female ratio of 2: 3 and a different distribution in terms of age, with female cases being 10–15 years older (48–54 vs. 37–41 years) [2]. These data are corroborated by even more current references in a sample of more than 70,000 patients collected between the years 2007 and 2016 [3]. This last study shows an increase during that period of time in the number of surgical interventions in the management of these injuries, as well as the use of locking plate fixation of comminuted fractures and radial head arthroplasty (RHA); meanwhile radial head resections decrease.

J. S. Ruiz-Pérez · P. Gómez-Cardero
E. C. Rodríguez-Merchán (✉)
Department of Orthopaedic Surgery, "La Paz" University Hospital-IdiPaz, Madrid, Spain

10.1.2 Anatomy and Biomechanics

The proximal radius consists of the radial head and the neck, and there is a large variation in dimensions, angles, and curvatures. Radial head is not completely circular, nor does it have a uniform elliptical shape. It articulates with the capitellum and the peripheral rim contacts with the lesser sigmoid notch. Articular cartilage covers the concave surface of the radial head in an approximately 280° arc [4]. The term "safe zone" refers to the remaining 80° of the posterolateral margin for screw and plate fixation. Ries et al. states that this area can reach up to 133° expanding the horizon for the reconstruction of more complex fractures [5].

Radial head plays a fundamental role in stabilizing the elbow against valgus, axial, and posterolateral forces. The medial collateral ligament (MCL) resists valgus, and the lateral collateral ligament (LCL) does the same for varus and posterolateral instability [6]. Restoring the length of the radiocapitellar joint is essential to optimize load on the cartilage of the capitellum and to reconstruct both lateral and medial stability. This is a complex goal since the interobserver correlation of radiological studies is low even among experienced surgeons [7]. It may be helpful to aim for a height of the radial head corresponding to the proximal edge of the lesser sigmoid notch with the forearm in neutral rotation.

E. C. Rodríguez-Merchán, A. Moreno-Garcìa (eds.), *Controversies in Orthopedic Surgery of The Upper Limb*, https://doi.org/10.1007/978-3-031-04907-1_10

10.1.3 Classification

Currently, there is still controversy in the classification of radial head fractures. The most widely known is described by Mason [8]. Mason's original classification describes non-displaced fractures (type I), marginal fractures with displacement (≥2 mm) (type II), and comminuted fractures involving the entire radial head (type III). Morrey quantified the extent of articular fragment displacement (>2 mm) and fragment size (≥30% of the articular surface), and Johnston added a fourth type to the Mason classification when the radial head fracture is associated with the dislocation of the elbow [9, 10]. However, these modifications do not present great interobserver correlation. Hotchkiss [11] to better delimit the need for surgical treatment defined a *type 2* fracture as the one with a reconstructible radial head fracture presenting a blocked forearm rotation and a *type 3* fracture as a non-reconstructible radial head fracture.

Given the frequent presence of associated bone and ligament injuries, the Mayo Clinic [12] suggested another modification to the classic Mason classification based on clinical and intraoperative observations adding a suffix that shows the articular injury (c, coronoid; o, olecranon) and ligamentous injury (l, lateral collateral ligament; m, medial collateral ligament; d, distal radio-ulnar joint).

10.2 Diagnosis

10.2.1 Clinical Examination

The main injury mechanism of radial head fractures occurs as a consequence of indirect trauma in falls with the wrist in extension and pronation. This situation produces the contact of the radial head with the capitellum. In the initial inspection, we must evaluate the signs of any fracture such as inflammation, ecchymosis, and functional limitation. Palpation of the radial head, proximal ulna, distal humerus, medial collateral ligament (MCL), lateral collateral ligament (LCL), interosseous ligament, and distal radioulnar joint (DRUJ) should be performed. If the patient allows it, the stability of the elbow as well as flexion/extension and pronation/supination of the wrist must be assessed. Arthrocentesis of the elbow can be useful, in addition to confirming the diagnosis, for removal of the mechanical block when secondary to joint effusion. Finally, the neurovascular examination includes different structures such as the radial, ulnar, median, and posterior interosseous nerves.

10.2.2 Radiological Tests

Anteroposterior, lateral, and Greenspan (forearm in neutral position and the X-ray beam centered on the radiocapitellar joint) views should be obtained in the basic radiological study (Fig. 10.1).

When no fracture is seen on routine views, some physicians still rely on the fat pad sign, which, despite its high sensitivity for disease in the elbow joint, is not pathognomonic of a fracture due to its decreased specificity in relation to trauma (also seen in hemophilia and rheumatoid arthritis). The sitting axial mediolateral projection is well tolerated due to the arm's placement: elbow joint in an angle greater than 90°, which is more comfortable for patients with tender and swollen joints. This projection is performed with the forearm in supination. The imaging receptor is placed on the dorsal site of the forearm, whereas the central ray is directed at a 45° mediolateral angle over the middle of the elbow joint [13].

CT (computed tomography) scan may be utilized for characterization of the fracture pattern, in case of high suspicion of fracture not confirmed with the initial radiological study and for preoperative planning.

Magnetic resonance imaging (MRI) will rarely be requested, although it may be useful for confirming soft tissue injuries associated with radial head fractures, especially in the most complex cases of joint dislocation [14].

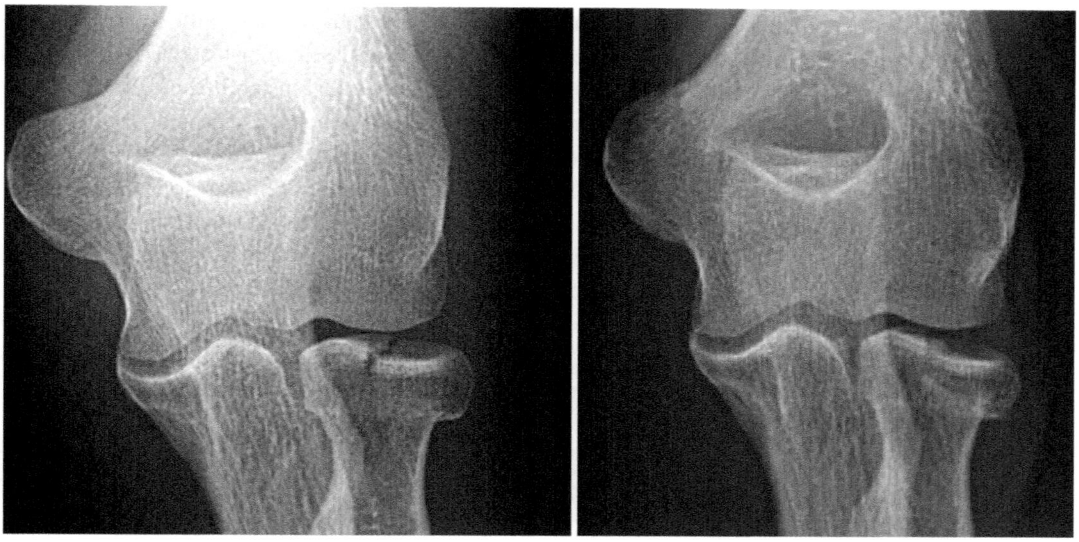

Fig. 10.1 A 22-year-old female patient with type I Mason fracture. Initial X-ray and 6 months after diagnosis. Excellent function without mobility restriction

Table 10.1 Main injuries associated with radial head fracture

Ligamentous injury	Lateral collateral ligament (LCL) 80%, medial collateral ligament (MCL), or both (MCL and LCL)
Essex-Lopresti injury	Interosseous membrane disruption and distal radioulnar joint (DRUJ)
Elbow fractures	Coronoid, olecranon, and capitellum
Elbow dislocation	"Terrible triad"(elbow dislocation, radial head fracture, coronoid fracture)
Carpal fractures (10%)	Hand and scaphoid fractures

10.2.3 Associated Injuries

In general, up to 35% of radial head fractures have associated injuries, depending on the intensity of the triggering trauma and ranging from 20% in undisplaced fractures to 80% in comminuted and displaced fractures [15]. Ring et al. [16] summarized the main injuries associated with radial head fractures in five groups (Table 10.1).

10.3 Management and Treatment

The definitive management of radial head fractures will depend on several factors. Displacement, comminution, stability, articular damage, and the existence of associated injuries in other locations (elbow, forearm, or wrist) will be taken into account. Classification of the type of fracture can be useful for treatment indication [17].

10.3.1 Nonsurgical Treatment

Conservative treatment consists of a short immobilization of 7–10 days with a sling or brachial splint limiting pronation/supination and flexion/extension followed by early mobilization. Patients are evaluated for clinical and radiological control at 2 weeks and to document if motion and pain is improving. By 6 weeks, the patient should have recovered full or nearly full elbow motion. If stiffness persists, a referral to the physiotherapists is indicated.

Nondisplaced or minimally displaced fractures (<2 mm), with minor articular involvement (<30%), without associated injuries or mobility blocks could be treated in this way. Herbertsson et al. [18] showed good or excellent results even in more complex cases. From our point of view, simple fractures with displacement between 2 and 5 mm may be treated nonsurgically or with internal fixation. Guzzini [19] reported 50/52 good or excellent results in his study in Mason type II fractures with a MEPS score of 94.5 (65–100) and DASH score of 12.4 (0–46). Controversy continues to exist regarding the management of this type of fracture, and there are no Level I/ II studies available to guide treatment in this uncommon scenario.

10.3.2 Surgical Treatment

Surgical treatment options include excision, internal fixation, and radial head arthroplasty. Goals of operative treatment include restoration of elbow stability and forearm rotation. The use of arthroscopy can be useful as an added value in cases where we decide to perform osteosynthesis. Figure 10.2 shows a good treatment algorithm for radial head fractures.

10.3.2.1 Surgical Approach and Arthroscopic Techniques

The preferred approaches for the vast majority of radial head fractures are those described by Kocher and Kaplan. In cases with greater comminution, a more posterior approach may be necessary.

Isolated fractures, especially those affecting the anterior half with intact collateral ligaments and without residual instability, can be treated by the Kaplan exposure performed between the extensor carpi radialis and the extensor digitorum muscle. The main risk of this approach is injury to the posterior interosseous nerve in the most distal area of the incision. It is advisable to perform the intervention with the forearm in pronation, and there is a "safe area" dissecting up to 29 mm from the radiocapitellar joint and up to 42 mm from the lateral epicondyle [20].

The Kocher approach exposes the joint in the interval between the anconeus and the extensor carpi ulnaris (ECU). It allows the reduction of fractures associated with instability, lesions of the LCL, and comminution. The radial nerve is protected by the muscular flap of the ECU; we can even perform the synthesis of coronoid fractures detaching the extensors from the humerus and elevating the anterior capsule [21].

In recent years, the use of arthroscopic techniques has gained popularity. Rolla et al. first described a standard approach for arthroscopic fixation of radial head fractures with cannulated screws in a case-series of six patients [22]. A study with a series of 20 patients with arthroscopically assisted radial head fractures revealed discrepancies in fracture classification regarding conventional imaging studies. Classification inconsistencies were found in 70% of the X-Ray cases and in 9% of the CT or MRI ones. Besides that, in 60% percent of the cases, arthroscopy revealed a larger number of loose bodies than described in CT/MRI, and osteochondral lesion of the capitellum was found in 80% of cases. It

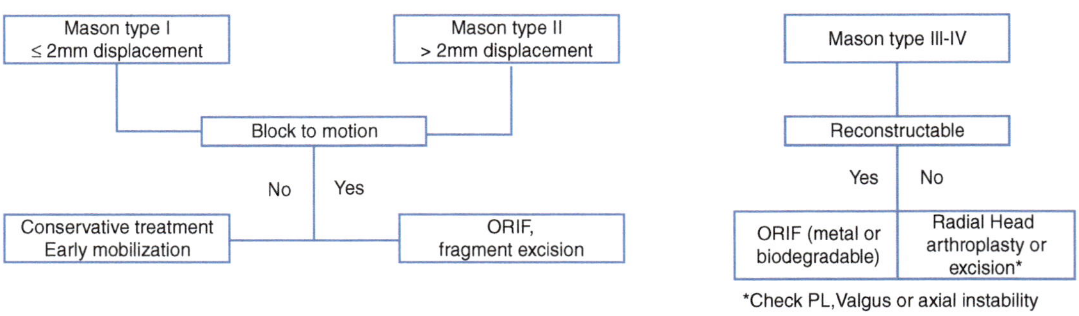

Fig. 10.2 Treatment algorithm for radial head fractures

can also be very useful in cases of LCL involvement and posterolateral rotational instability (PRLI). The authors conclude that arthroscopically assisted fracture reduction and internal fixation reduces invasiveness and reliably allows for excellent clinical outcomes [23]. New accessory portals have been described to facilitate reduction and screw placement in the radial head, and good reproducibility of Kirschner wire placement from distal AM and AL portals was observed among different surgeons [24].

10.3.2.2 Open Reduction and Internal Fixation (ORIF)

Mason type II fractures with>2 mm displacement and block to motion and Mason type III reconstructable fractures are the main indications for open reduction and osteosynthesis (Fig. 10.3).

From the current literature [12], clear indications for surgery are mechanical block after aspiration of the hematoma, two-part fractures with displacement >5 mm (head fragment) or >4 mm (neck), and fractures with comminution (>2 parts). The main objective is anatomical reconstruction and maintaining joint stability. In addition to the conventional radiological study, a CT scan may be useful in preoperative planning. At the time of surgery, examination of the lateral ulnar collateral ligament (LUCL), for injury and instability, is mandatory. The temporary use of Kirschner wires can be useful to promote reduction. As we said in the previous section, new arthroscopic techniques can provide information on the existence of associated injuries and assist in fracture reduction. Headless screws (1.5–2.4 mm) are typically used to fix head fragments with or without involvement of the radial neck. In fractures with extension toward the neck, low profile plates of 1.5 or 2.0 mm should be preferred for osteosynthesis. They must be positioned in the "safe zone" area described in the introduction as approximately 100° centered on the equator of the radial neck in neutral position. These plates may need to be removed in more than half of the cases once the fracture has healed according to Neumann et al. [25]. A recent study of 28 patients with Mason type II-III fractures shows excellent results in 85% of cases, returning to full activity after osteosynthesis. They indicate as good prognostic factors for open reduction and

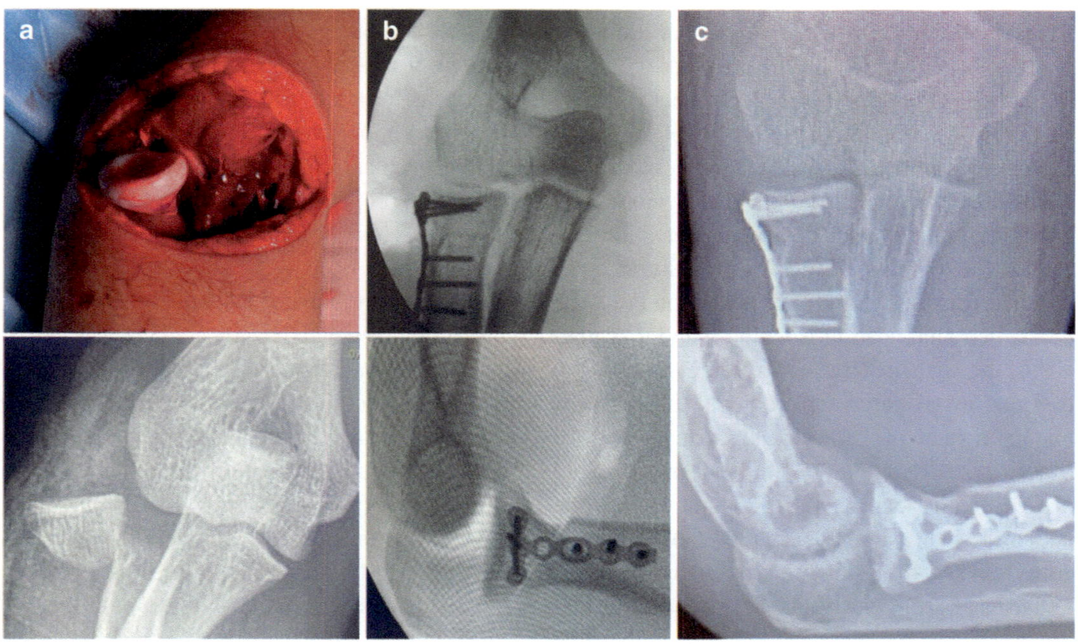

Fig. 10.3 (**a**) Traumatic open radial head fracture treated with open reduction and internal fixation (ORIF); (**b**) anteroposterior (AP) and lateral intraoperative fluoroscopic control; (**c**) AP and lateral radiographs at 6 months

synthesis cases in which the size of the fragment is large enough and there is little bone loss and metaphyseal resorption [26].

Cepni et al. [27] also advocate reconstructive treatment for Mason type II–III fractures whenever possible. In their recent study with 28 patients, they collected good results with a Mayo Elbow Performance score of 92 (range 60–100) and a disability of arm, shoulder, and hand (DASH) score of 15.5 (range 2.5–55.2). However, complications appear up to 25.9%, and 22.2% of the patients underwent a revision surgery. For comminuted fractures in which adequate reduction is difficult to obtain, the "on-table" reconstruction technique may be used. This technique consists in carrying out the reduction and osteosynthesis of the fracture with the main fragments on the surgical table to later proceed to anatomical reconstruction in the patient. Bosinger [28] used this technique in six patients for Mason type III and IV fractures with excellent clinical results, although one of the patients had symptoms of degenerative changes. Controversy regarding the advantage of surgical treatment of these fractures still exists. Hermena et al. [29] in a systematic review of the current literature comparing open reduction and osteosynthesis vs. radial head arthroplasty for Mason type III fractures conclude that radial head arthroplasty may be a better option when treating these complex fractures, but the current evidence is weak. Isolated fractures or that involving only part of the radial head should be treated with ORIF. Nevertheless, this option is prone to failure due to nonunion, loosening of the fixation device, restricted forearm rotation, and elbow stiffness, especially in comminuted fractures. Another valid option could be to fix the radial head in isolation without synthesizing the shaft in order to preserve vascularization and avoid hardware problems. In this way, nonunion rates of 70% have been registered for Mason type III fractures with a mean follow-up of 76 months (range, 12–152 months), but the patients remain asymptomatic [30]. Gokaraju et al. collected data from 46 patients comparing ORIF, radial head arthroplasty or excision with similar functional results, and range of motion in the three groups. The complication rate is around 39% in the group treated with osteosynthesis with indications for revision in his series including nonunion and prominent hardware causing impingement. Current designs including radial head specificity and low-profile implants with locking option may be helpful in reducing the risk of reoperations [31]. Perhaps the greatest controversy exists for type II Mason fractures. Lindenhovius classic study [32] included 16 patients with a 22-year follow-up and demonstrated no appreciable advantage over the long-term results of nonoperative treatment of Mason type II fractures. Along the same lines and for this specific type of fractures, a recent systematic review did not find statistically significant differences in favor of ORIF vs. nonsurgical treatment; however, in this second group the development of osteoarthritis in the radiocapitellar joint appears to be more likely [33]. In order to improve the results of surgical treatment, new implants are being developed, such as polylactide pins, proving the feasibility of ORIF of unsalvageable radial head fractures. Smaller diameter pins (1.5 mm) allow the fixation of each fragment from different directions handling in a simpler way than screws and plates. Tarallo et al. [34] demonstrated good clinical and functional results in their series of 82 patients treated with resorbable pins, although there was up to 8.5% redisplacement of the fracture fragments vs. 1.6% in the mini-screws group. Similarly, another retrospective study shows excellent results with this technique in a series of 17 patients for fractures considered unsalvageable [35]. Other more current alternatives carried out in biomechanical studies in cadavers find superior mechanical properties with the use of magnesium pins [36].

10.3.2.3 Excision of Radial Head

This technique would be indicated in cases of isolated and displaced and with great comminution radial head fractures. Given the frequent associated ligamentous injury with secondary instability, a thorough evaluation is required before selecting this option. It can be a valuable alternative in patients with low functional demand, intercurrent infection, or failure of previous reconstructions. The radius pull test described by Smith et al. [37] makes it possible to assess longitudinal instability by applying traction (shoulder at 90° abduction and internal rotation-90° elbow flexion and neutral rotation) or by using a bone reduction clamp. With the aid of the fluoroscope, radial migration greater than or equal to 3 mm of increase in ulnar variance is verified, confirming the lesion of the interosseous membrane. Antuña et al. reviewed a long-term (15 years) series of 26 patients younger than 40 years with excellent clinical and functional results in 24 of them, and none required a new reoperation [38]. A recent study with only 11 patients with Mason type III–IV fractures and a follow-up of 47.6 months shows good results (Mayo Elbow Performance score: 83.2 points) in 81% of the cases; however, seven patients had a valgus deformity, and two of 11 cases had elbow instability in valgus stress [39]. Another retrospective series comparing arthroplasty vs. radial head resection in cases of instability and dislocation shows similar results in both groups, although a greater number of reoperations (25%) were observed in the second group, mainly associated with heterotopic ossification as a secondary complication [40]. Mahzar et al. concluded that the results were similar between these last two alternatives, even for injuries as complex as the terrible triad, with no statistically significant differences in visual analogue scale (VAS) for pain, Mayo Elbow Performance score (MEPS), and disabilities of arm, shoulder, and hand (DASH) score [41]. Finally, a recent systematic review analyzing the three possible types of surgical intervention (osteosynthesis, excision, and radial head arthroplasty) suggests that prosthetic replacement constitutes the best treatment of choice for efficacy and safety, although resection behaves as a safest choice to minimize postoperative complications and enable patients to perform all daily life activities [42].

10.3.2.4 Radial Head Arthroplasty (RHA)

In cases of comminuted fractures, with a large number of fragments or complicated reconstruction and with poor bone quality, radial head arthroplasty may be the treatment of choice (Fig. 10.4).

The concomitant existence of posterolateral instability (external collateral ligament complex injury), valgus instability (MCL injury), or axial instability (interosseous membrane injury) should be taken into account. However, the therapeutic approach should be individualized focusing not only on the above aspects but also on other characteristics such as age, dominant hand, and baseline activity of the patient. One of the most critical aspects is determining the correct size and height of the implant. Overestimating or underestimating height can lead to loosening and

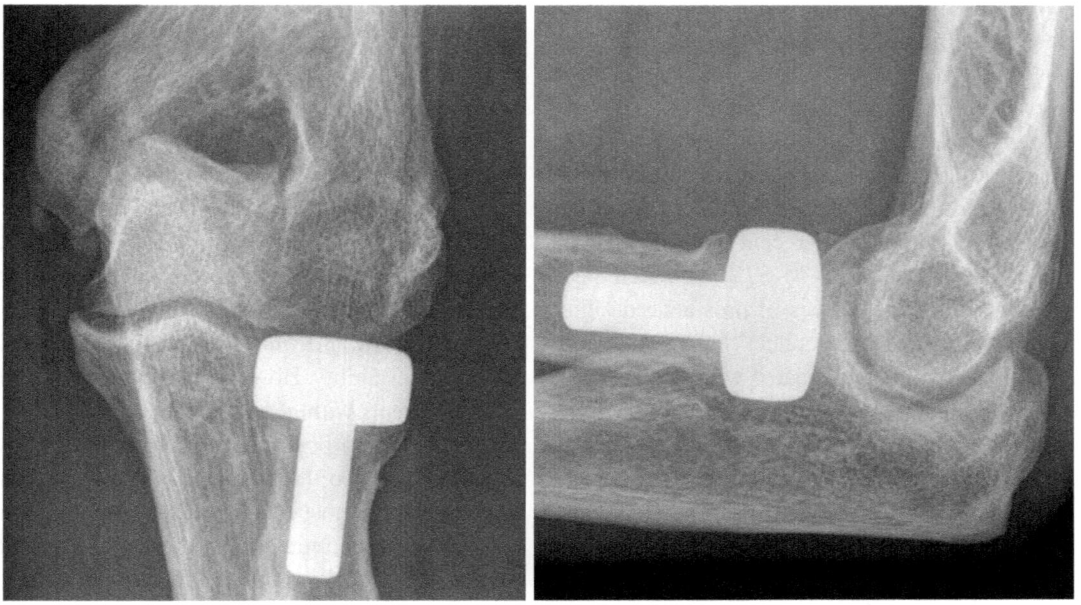

Fig. 10.4 X-ray control anteroposterior and lateral (EVOLVE prosthesis) at 12 years

early degenerative changes or instability, respectively. Morphologic parameters of the radiocapitellar joint (humeral condyle diameter, radial head diameter, and radial head height) measured with radiographic analysis could be useful to predict RHA size preoperatively [43]. The lesser sigmoid notch and the lateral coronoid edge [44] can be used as anatomical landmarks. The intraoperative radiographic study is very useful to avoid radial head overlengthening. Elbow and forearm motion and stability are tested using fluoroscopy after insertion of the trial implant. The medial ulnohumeral joint space should be parallel, and radiographic widening of this joint space is a sign of significant radial implant overlengthening, not the lateral ulnohumeral space widening since cartilage thickness is variable. Radial head overstuffing or overlengthening may produce pain and decreased range of motion making a second intervention necessary to remove the prosthesis. Maltracking may be due to an imperfect radial neck cut or a canal broached in a wrong direction.

Regarding the *type of implants*, we can differentiate unipolar (the most commonly used) or bipolar, anatomical or nonanatomical, and cemented stems, loose-stemmed, or press-fit ingrowth protheses. Despite the fact that anatomical implants reproduce biomechanical behavior in a similar way to the native radial head, they have not shown greater clinical relevance to date [45]. Bipolar prostheses are cemented into the radial neck and theoretically can provide improved congruency during elbow motion.

Loose stemmed implants have shown encouraging results in the reconstruction of complex radial head fractures [46]. An impeccable review by van Riet [47] includes recent studies with good or excellent results in 70–87% of radial head arthroplasties for all types of prosthetic designs. Laumonerie et al. [48] collect the experience of more than 146 patients treated with the EVOLVE Proline implant (modular, unipolar, loose-fitting radial head implant system), a mean follow-up of 4.8 years (range 1–14), concluding that outcomes are satisfactory, and associated complication rates are low (reoperation in 12 patients, with implant revision in 2 patients). A recent systematic review and meta-analysis for fixed-stem implants [49] shows that not all devices behave in the same way, with differences in revision rates, certain complications, and functional scores with worse outcomes in Essex-Lopresti or terrible triad injuries. This would imply an exquisite selection of the type of implant and individualization of each case. Other long-term studies conclude that press-fit radial head arthroplasty seems to become an alternative with satisfactory results in most patients with complex fractures despite finding an implant survival at 24 months of only 69.5% and a reoperation rate of 26.7% [50]. The greatest controversy continues to focus on Mason type III fractures. Chen et al. [4] showed better results for RHA (91%) compared to ORIF (65.2%) in their study with 45 patients and a follow-up of 2 years. With similar results, a systematic review [51] concluded that radial head replacement appeared to reach better outcomes in patients with Mason type III radial head fractures followed 5 years or less, finding a lower rate of complications (13.9%) in relation to osteosynthesis (58.2%). Following this line, another meta-analysis [52] indicated that RHA results in better function and reduced postoperative complications than ORIF-M (metal implants) and ORIF-B (biodegradable implants) over 2 years in the treatment of displaced radial head fractures. However, Kyriacou et al. [53] in a systematic review that includes 210 cases of “terrible triad” found no differences in results, risk of reoperation, and rate of complications between reconstruction and arthroplasty, suggesting that open reduction and internal fixation should be performed when a satisfactory reconstruction can be achieved as the longevity of RHA in young patients with terrible triad injury is currently questionable. Comparing radial head replacement versus excision in cases of previous instability, there are also studies that logically opted in favor of prosthetic reconstruction [54].

The main *complications* are stiffness, residual pain, and instability. However, it is quite common to find patients with neurological alterations secondary to the surgical intervention, an underestimated problem in the literature. The risk factors that have been most related to this complication are inappropriate retraction in the anterior aspect of the radial neck, a prolonged ischemia time, and concomitant coronoid, or olecranon fracture fixation [55].

Recent short- and medium-term studies such as that of Cho et al. [56] show good clinical results despite the appearance of radiological complications. Specifically, in their series of 24 patients with a mean follow-up of 58.9 months (range, 27–163 months), they found 16.7% heterotopic ossification, capital wear in 20.8%, and arthritic changes in 29.2% of the cases. For press-fit stems in the medium term, we can find up to 60–70% of proximal stress shielding regardless of the design, although no clinical correlation has been seen regarding stem loosening [57]. It is advisable to follow the patient with serial radiographs. A recent study including 24 patients operated on in the context of elbow fracture dislocation and a 10-year follow-up revealed the presence of osteolysis in all cases with moderate to high correlation to clinical outcomes, suggesting the need for close control of these cases [58] (Fig. 10.5).

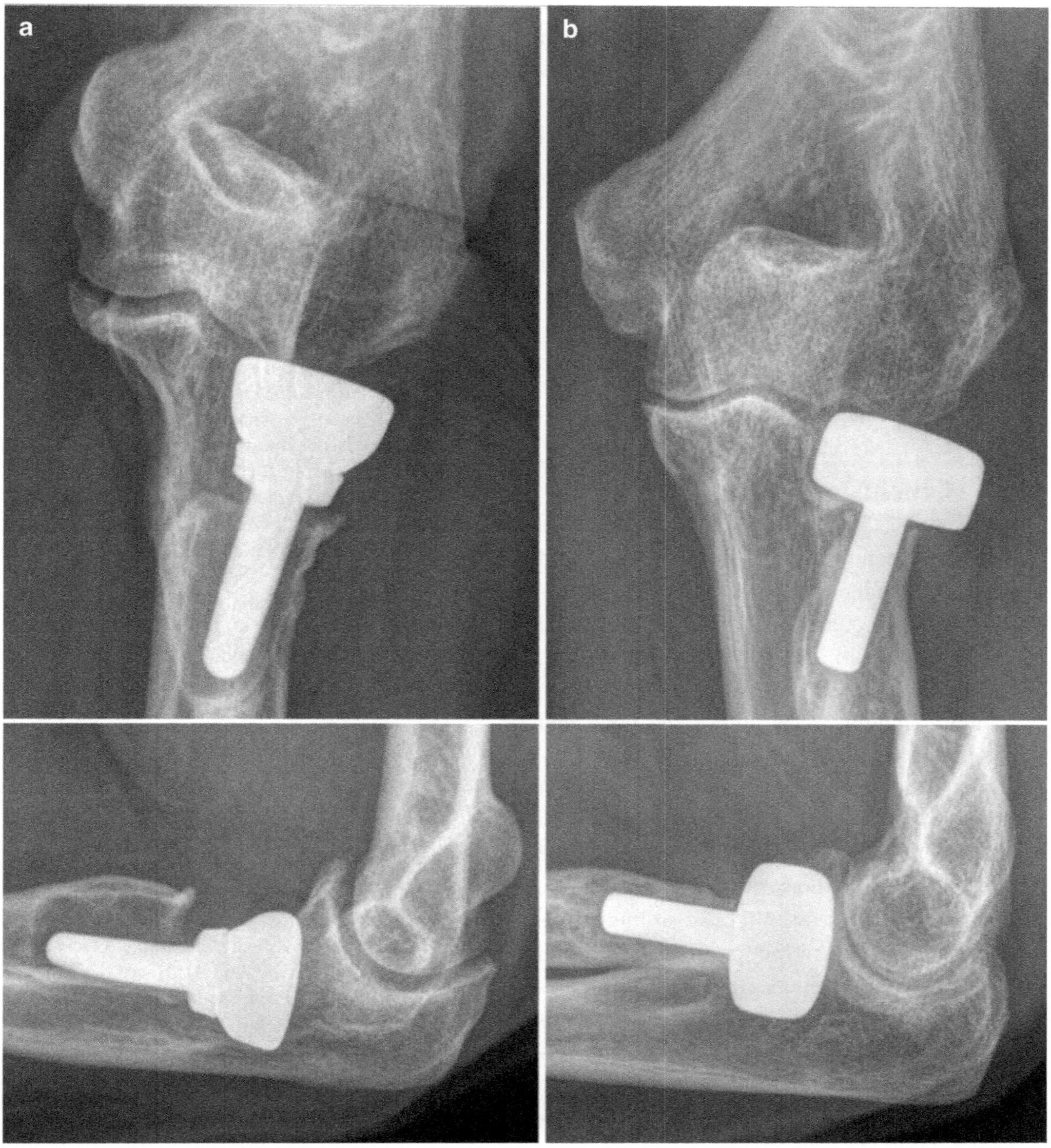

Fig. 10.5 (**a**) Radiographic control of the Acumed prosthesis at 13 years of follow-up (severe osteolysis in asymptomatic patient), (**b**) X-ray control of the EVOLVE prosthesis at 15 years of follow-up

Removal or revision of the implant would be indicated if the loosening becomes symptomatic with pain, instability, or striking radiological failure. The main causes of RHA revision were symptomatic loosening (30%), stiffness (20%), pain (17%), overstuffing (9%), dissociation of the prosthesis (5%), and symptomatic osteoarthritis (OA, 4%) [59]. Loss of range of motion both in flexion/extension and pronation/supination accompanied by pain should alert the surgeon. One of the factors that have been associated with a greater risk of failure and revision of the RHA is the delay of the initial surgical intervention. In one series, 55% of failed radial head implants were implanted more than 6 weeks after the initial injury [60]. Given that the number of radial head arthroplasties has increased in recent years, the percentage of complications associated with it is up to 23% [61]. It is therefore necessary to know the diagnosis and the possible causes of failure of RHA as well as the treatment alternatives. An excellent review raises an interesting algorithm with the existing technical solutions on this matter at the present time [62].

10.4 Conclusions

Radial head fractures account for up to one-third of elbow joint bone injuries. Mason's classification with the modifications of Hotchkiss and Morrey is still valid and is the most used today. Diagnosis through clinical examination and complementary imaging tests allows the bone and ligament structures involved to be identified. Following the criteria of displacement, joint block, possibility of reconstruction, and stability of the fracture, a treatment algorithm can be established. Within conservative management, early mobilization is essential. Regarding surgical treatment, the use of low-profile implants and the development of biodegradable alternatives can be useful for osteosynthesis. Arthroscopy is an additional and less invasive tool than traditional alternatives. Radial head excision should only be the technique of choice for non-reconstructable cases without associated instability, chronic infections, and patients with low functional demand. Radial head arthroplasty, through the wide range of solutions offered by the industry, has gained ground in recent years to support the management of the most complex cases, although a close monitoring of the possible medium and long-term complications and survival of the different implants is necessary.

References

1. Davidson PA, Moseley JB, Tullos HS. Radial head fracture. A potentially complex injury. Clin Orthop Rel Res. 1993;297:224–30.
2. Kaas L, van Riet RP, Vroemen JP, Eygendaal D. The epidemiology of radial head fractures. J Shoulder Elb Surg. 2010;19:520–3.
3. Klug A, Gramlich Y, Wincheringer D, Hoffmann R, Schmidt-Horlohé K. Epidemiology and treatment of radial head fractures: a database analysis of over 70,000 inpatient cases. J Hand Surg Am. 2021;46:27–35.
4. Chen X, Wang SC, Cao LH, Yang GQ, Li M, Su JC. Comparison between radial head replacement and open reduction and internal fixation in clinical treatment of unstable, multi-fragmented radial head fractures. Int Orthop. 2011;35:1071–6.
5. Ries C, Muller M, Wegmann K, Plau DB, Müller LP, Burkhart KJ. Is an extension of the safe zone possible without jeopardizing the proximal radioulnar joint when performing a radial head plate osteosynthesis? J Shoulder Elb Surg. 2015;24:1627–34.
6. Galik K, Baratz ME, Butler AL, Dougherty J, Cohen MS, Miller MC. The effect of the annular ligament on kinematics of the radial head. J Hand Surg Am. 2007;32:1218–24.
7. Bexkens R, Claessen F, Kodde IF, Oh LS, Eygendaal D, van dem Bekeron MPJ. Interobserver reliability of radiographic assessment after radial head arthroplasty. Shoulder Elbow. 2018;10:121–7.
8. Mason ML. Some observations on fractures of the head of the radius with a review of one hundred cases. Br J Surg. 1954;42:123–32.
9. Morrey BF. Functional evaluation of the elbow. In: Morrey BF, editor. The elbow and its disorders. Philadelphia: WB Saunders; 1985. p. 73–91.
10. Johnston GW. A follow-up of one hundred cases of fracture of the head of the radius with a review of the literature. Ulster Med J. 1962;31:51–6.
11. Hotchkiss RN. Displaced fractures of the radial head: internal fixation or excision? J Am Acad Orthop Surg. 1997;5:1–10.
12. van Riet RP, Morrey BF. Documentation of associated injuries occurring with radial head fracture. Clin Orthop Relat Res. 2008;466:130–4.
13. Vampertzis T, Barmpagianni C, Vavilis T, Nitis G, Fotiadis A, Papastergiou S. Traumatic elbow medio-

lateral investigatory screening: The value of the sitting axial mediolateral projection in the diagnosis of radial head fractures. J Clin Orthop Trauma. 2020 Feb;11(Suppl 1):S42–5.
14. Tarallo L, Merolla G, Porcellini G, Amorico MG, Micheloni G, Novi M, et al. Acute elbow dislocation: comparison between magnetic resonance imaging and intra-operative finding of ligament injury. Int Orthop. 2021;45:265–73.
15. Tejwani NC, Mehta H. Fractures of the radial head and neck: current concepts in management. J Am Acad Orthop Surg. 2007;15:380–38.
16. Ring D. Displaced, unstable fractures of the radial head: fixation vs. replacement—what is the evidence? Injury. 2008;39:1329–37.
17. Swensen SJ, Tyagi V, Uquillas C, Shakked RJ, Yoon RS, Liporace FA. Maximizing outcomes in the treatment of radial head fractures. J Orthop Traumatol. 2019;20(1):15.
18. Herbertsson P, Josefsson PO, Hasserius R, Karlsson C, Besjacov J, Karlsson M. Uncomplicated Mason type-II and III fractures of the radial head and neck in adults. A long-term follow-up study. J Bone Joint Surg Am. 2004;86:569–74.
19. Guzzini M, Vadal A, Agró A, Di Sanzo V, Pironi D, Redler A, et al. Nonsurgical treatment of Mason type II radial head fractures in athletes. A retrospective study. G Chir. 2017;37:200–5.
20. Schimizzi A, Maclennan A, Meier KM, et al. Defining a safe zone of dissection during the extensor digitorum communis splitting approach to the proximal radius and forearm: an anatomic study. J Hand Surg Am. 2009;34:1252–5.
21. Barco R, Antuña SA. Management of elbow trauma: anatomy and exposures. Hand Clin. 2015;31:509–19.
22. Rolla PR, Surace MF, Bini A, Pilato G. Arthroscopic treatment of fractures of the radial head. Arthroscopy. 2006;22(233):e231–6.
23. Haasters F, Helfen T, Böcker W, Mayr HO, Prall WC, Lenich A. The value of elbow arthroscopy in diagnosing and treatment of radial head fractures. BMC Musculoskelet Disord. 2019;20(1):343.
24. Cucchi D, Arrigoni P, Luceri F, Menon A, Guerra E, Müller LP, et al. ESSKA elbow and wrist committee 2016–2018. Modified anteromedial and anterolateral elbow arthroscopy portals show superiority to standard portals in guiding arthroscopic radial head screw fixation. Knee Surg Sports Traumatol Arthrosc. 2019;27:3276–83.
25. Neumann M, Nyffeler R, Beck M. Comminuted fractures of the radial head and neck: is fixation to the shaft necessary? J Bone Joint Surg Br. 2011;93:223–8.
26. Mangi IK, Abro AA, Memon MN, Siyal S, Khan N, Memon N, et al. Open reduction and internal fixation for radial head fractures: a prospective observational study. J Acute Dis. 2020;9:166–9.
27. Cepni S, Veizi E, Sahin A, AF, Kilicarslan K, Tahta M. Mason II–III radial head and neck fractures treated with locking plate fixation. Hand Microsurg. 2021;10:127–33.
28. Businger A, Ruedi TP, Sommer C. On-table reconstruction of comminuted fractures of the radial head. Injury. 2010;41:583–8.
29. Meacher H, Hermena S, Isaac S. Open reduction and internal fixation versus radial head arthroplasty for Mason III radial head fractures: appraising the current literature evidence. Cureus. 2020;12(4):e7501.
30. Gregori M, Zott S, Hajdu S, Braunsteiner T. Preserving the radial head in comminuted Mason type III fractures without fixation to the radial shaft: a mid-term clinical and radiographic follow-up study. J Shoulder Elb Surg. 2019;28:2215–24.
31. Gokaraju K, Domos P, Aweid O, Fisher R, White A, Van Rensburg L, Kang SN. Mid-term outcomes of surgical management of complex, isolated radial head fractures: a multicentre collaboration. Eur J Orthop Surg Traumatol. 2020;30:1369–76.
32. Lindenhovius AL, Felsch Q, Ring D, Kloen P. The long-term outcome of open reduction and internal fixation of stable displaced isolated partial articular fractures of the radial head. J Trauma. 2009;67:143–6.
33. Lanzerath F, Hackl M, Wegmann K, Müller LP, Leschinger T. The treatment of isolated Mason type II radial head fractures: a systematic review. J Shoulder Elb Surg. 2021;30:487–94.
34. Tarallo L, Mugnai R, Rocchi M, Capra F, Catani F. Comparison between absorbable pins and mini-screw fixations for the treatment of radial head fractures Mason type II-III. BMC Musculoskelet Disord. 2018;19(1):94.
35. Guo L, Li R, Yang X, Yu C, Gui F. Polylactide pins can effectively fix severely comminuted and unsalvageable radial head fracture: a retrospective study of 40 patients. Injury. 2020;51:2253–8.
36. Wagner FC, Polossek L, Yilmaz T, Jaeger M, Maier D, Feucht MJ, et al. Biodegradable magnesium vs. polylactide pins for radial head fracture stabilization: a biomechanical study. J Shoulder Elb Surg. 2021;30:365–72.
37. Smith AM, Urbanosky LR, Castle JA, Rushing JT, Ruch DS. Radius pull test: predictor of longitudinal forearm instability. J Bone Joint Surg Am. 2002;84-A:1970–6.
38. Antuña SA, Sánchez-Márquez JM, Barco R. Long-term results of radial head resection following isolated radial head fractures in patients younger than forty years old. J Bone Joint Surg Am. 2010;92:558–66.
39. Mebouinz FN, Kasse A, Habib SM. Results of radial head resection after Mason type 3 or 4 fracture of the elbow. Clin Shoulder Elbow. 2020;23:131–5.
40. Mikel AB, Javier AB, Fausto LM, Ángel PM, Irene LT, Carlos ÁG. A retrospective comparative cohort study of radial head arthroplasty versus resection in complex elbow dislocations. Injury. 2020;51(Suppl 1):89–93.
41. Mazhar FN, Ebrahimi H, Jafari D, Mirzaei A. Radial head resection versus prosthetic arthroplasty in terrible triad injury: a retrospective comparative cohort study: a retrospective comparative cohort study. Bone Joint J. 2018;100-B:1499–505.

42. Chaijenkij K, Arirachakaran A, Kongtharvonskul J. Clinical outcomes after internal fixation, arthroplasty and resection for treatment of comminuted radial head fractures: a systematic review and network meta-analysis. Musculoskelet Surg. 2021;105: 17–29.
43. Vaquero-Picado A, Núñez de Armas J, Antuña S, Barco R. Morphometry of the radiocapitellar joint: is humeral condyle diameter a reliable predictor of the size of the radial head prosthesis? J Shoulder Elb Surg. 2018;27:1092–6.
44. Doornberg JN, Linzel DS, Zurakowski D, Ring D. Reference points for radial head prosthesis size. J Hand Surg Am. 2006;31:53–7.
45. Bachman DR, Thaveepunsan S, Park S, Fitzsimmons JS, An KN, O'Driscoll SW. The effect of prosthetic radial head geometry on the distribution and magnitude of radiocapitellar joint contact pressures. J Hand Surg. 2015;40:281–8.
46. Dotzis A, Cochu G, Mabit C, Charissoux JL, Arnaud JP. Comminuted fractures of the radial head treated by the Judet floating radial head prosthesis. J Bone Joint Surg Br. 2006;88:760–4.
47. van Riet RP, van den Bekerom M, Van Tongel A, Spross C, Barco R, Watts AC. Radial head fractures. Shoulder Elbow. 2020;12:212–23.
48. Laumonerie P, Raad M, Tibbo ME, Kerezoudis P, Bonnevialle N, Mansat P. Midterm outcomes of 146 EVOLVE proline modular radial head prostheses: a systematic review. Shoulder Elbow. 2021;13:205–12.
49. Vannabouathong C, Venugopal N, Athwal GS, Moro J, Bhandari M. Radial head arthroplasty: fixed-stem implants are not all equal-a systematic review and meta-analysis. JSES Int. 2020;4:30–8.
50. Lobo-Escolar L, Abellán-Miralles C, Escolà-Benet A. Outcomes of press-fit radial head arthroplasty following complex radial head fractures. Orthop Traumatol Surg Res. 2021;107(2):102645.
51. Li N, Chen S. Open reduction and internal-fixation versus radial head replacement in treatment of Mason type III radial head fractures. Eur J Orthop Surg Traumatol. 2014;24:851–5.
52. Vannabouathong C, Akhter S, Athwal GS, Moro J, Bhandari M. Interventions for displaced radial head fractures: network meta-analysis of randomized trials. J Shoulder Elb Surg. 2019;28:578–86.
53. Kyriacou S, Gupta Y, Bains HK, Singh HP. Radial head replacement versus reconstruction for the treatment of the terrible triad injury of the elbow: a systematic review and meta-analysis. Arch Orthop Trauma Surg. 2019;139:507–17.
54. Kim BS, Cho CH. Radial head resection versus replacement for unreconstructable radial head fractures. Clin Shoulder Elb. 2020;23:117–8.
55. Carbonell-Escobar R, Vaquero-Picado A, Barco R, Antuña S. Neurologic complications after surgical management of complex elbow trauma requiring radial head replacement. J Shoulder Elb Surg. 2020;29:1282–8.
56. Baek CS, Kim BS, Kim DH, Cho CH. Short- to mid-term outcomes of radial head replacement for complex radial head fractures. Clin Shoulder Elbow. 2020;23:183–9.
57. Chanlalit C, Shukla DR, Fitzsimmons JS, An KN, O'Driscoll SW. Stress shielding around radial head prostheses. J Hand Surg. 2012;37:2118–25.
58. Chen AC, Cheng YH, Chiu CH, Cheng CY, Chan YS. Long-term outcomes of radial head arthroplasty in complex elbow fracture dislocation. J Clin Med. 2021;10(16):3488.
59. Heijink A, Kodde IF, Mulder PG, Veltman ES, Kaas L, van dem Bekeron MPJ, et al. Radial head arthroplasty: a systematic review. JBJS Rev. 2016;4(10):e3.
60. Laumonerie P, Reina N, Kerezoudis P, Declaux S, Tibbo ME, Bonnevialle N, et al. The mínimum follow-up required for radial head arthroplasty: a meta-analysis. Bone Joint J. 2017;99-B:1561–70.
61. Sershon RA, Luchetti TJ, Cohen MS, Wysocki RW. Radial head replacement with a bipolar system: an average 10-year follow-up. J Shoulder Elb Surg. 2018;27:e38–44.
62. Kodde IF, Viveen J, The B, van Riet RP, Eygendaal D. Management of the failed radial head arthroplasty. EFORT Open Rev. 2020;5:398–407.

Controversies in the Surgical Treatment of Distal Biceps Tendon Ruptures in Adults: To Fix or Not to Fix? Single Versus Double Incision?

11

Pablo Peñalver-Andrada, Jens Jared Cárdenas-Salas, and Julián Fernández-González

11.1 Introduction

The incidence of distal biceps tendon rupture is approximately 5.4 cases per 100,000 patients per year in adults [1]. Lately, the number of injuries and surgical procedures is increasing, probably related to a greater number of studies on the subject and the increased sporting activity [2]. We must take into account that, although most cases are seen in middle-aged active patients, ruptures in older patients are also increasing due to preexisting tendinopathy [3]. The main risk factors are weight lifting, contact sports, or the use of tobacco and anabolic steroids. According to several clinical studies, surgical treatment in young and active patients is appropriate. However, conservative treatment in certain cases is also correct [4]. In this chapter, we will discuss the surgical indications as well as the different techniques to perform it.

P. Peñalver-Andrada · J. J. Cárdenas-Salas
J. Fernández-González (✉)
Department of Orthopaedic Surgery, La Princesa University Hospital UAM, Madrid, Spain

11.2 Anatomy and Pathophysiology

Distal biceps tendon rupture usually occurs secondary to eccentric loading in extension associated with active flexion of the arm yielding to a load of 204 N [5].

The anatomical peculiarities of the muscle and the tendon with its insertion must be known in order to understand the causes of rupture and treatment.

The biceps is a two-headed muscle, behaving as functional unit but each head having a specific insertion zone. The long head inserts more proximally and the short head inserts more distally in the tuberosity and runs medially. The long head has more supinator function, and the short head is the flexor one. In up to 25% of patients, the tendon is bifurcated at its insertion [6, 7]. It is important to know the anatomy in order to perfectly recreate the insertion and recover the dual function. The medial part of the tendon must be reinserted in the distal part of the footprint. The *lacertus fibrosus* is a fascial reinforcement that connects the distal biceps tendon to the forearm flexor fascia. It prevents proximal migration, and it stabilizes primarily the short head. It is unclear whether it needs to be repaired in case of damage [8] and has also been used as graft in case of reconstruction [9].

E. C. Rodríguez-Merchán, A. Moreno-Garcìa (eds.), *Controversies in Orthopedic Surgery of The Upper Limb*, https://doi.org/10.1007/978-3-031-04907-1_11

11.3 Types of Injuries

An accurate diagnosis is important because there is a wide spectrum of distal biceps injuries. The most typical and easy to diagnose is the complete tendon rupture in a young patient. A second group would be the partial tendinous lesions, within which we would find isolated lesions of the short head of the muscle [10, 11], rare but with a specific diagnosis and treatment. The third group is degenerative lesions (bursitis/tendinosis). Complete or partial lesions can be divided according to the time of evolution into acute (less than 4 weeks) or chronic (more than 4 weeks).

11.4 Diagnosis

The diagnosis should be based mainly on clinical suspicion and physical examination, but complementary imaging tests are of great help for confirmation and in doubtful cases. Delayed diagnosis of these lesions is not uncommon.

11.4.1 Clinical Diagnosis

Patients usually feel a *"pop"* followed by pain and functional limitations. They usually present edema, hematoma, and greater deficit of supination than flexion [12]. In complete ruptures, the biceps usually loses its contour, increasing by more than 6 cm the distance between the muscle outline and the elbow crease (biceps crease interval) [13], and a positive Popeye the sailor sign.

Since its description in 2007, the Hook test [14] is the most used, with a very high sensitivity and specificity according to studies. However, its modification by placing the hand in resisted supination and elbow and shoulder at 90° helps to distinguish the biceps tendon and *brachialis* muscle.

Other tests used are the supination/pronation test in which the examiner observes the normal or pathological contour of the biceps when changing from supination to pronation [15] or the squeeze test which will not produce supination in case of rupture although it has limitations in cases of partial ruptures or pain [16].

To assess the integrity of the *lacertus fibrosus,* we use the biceps aponeurosis test [17] in which the patient must clench his/her fist, flex the wrist, and supinate the forearm with the elbow at 75° of flexion. The intact *lacertus fibrosus* should be palpated medially.

Partial lesions of the biceps tendon tend to have milder symptoms. They usually present with chronic pain from previous tendinopathy and without such an acute or painful event. Partial lesions of the short head of the biceps deserve a specific diagnosis because the hook test is usually negative, and, since it is so widespread used, it can be misdiagnosed. They present the characteristic symptoms of acute injuries with pain, edema, and hematoma, mild loss of flexion/supination, and asymmetry but a negative hook test. As the short head of biceps has more importance in flexion, it tears before the long head [18]. In fact, there are no isolated ruptures of the long head of biceps described in the literature.

11.4.2 Imaging Tests

If clinical tests show an obvious complete rupture, the need for an imaging test is arguable. However, they should be routinely performed when partial or chronic injury is suspected or when there is doubt in the diagnosis. Plain radiography provides little information unless there is a history of direct trauma or suspicion of associated fracture or in the rare cases of tendon insertion avulsion.

The gold standard is the magnetic resonance imaging (MRI) because it can detect tendinitis, complete and partial injuries, *lacertus fibrosus* lesions, and possible retraction in the event of partial ruptures [19]. According to Festa et al. [20], MRI has 100% specificity and up to 90% sensitivity to detect partial ruptures. Since the description of the optimal posture for performing MRI by Giuffre et al. [21], all MRI should be performed in FABS position (flexed, abducted, supinated) because it allows longitudinal assessment of the entire tendon in the same slice.

Ultrasound (US) is very useful if performed by an expert and to assess dynamic lesions. According to Lynch et al. [22], MRI is more accurate for detecting complete ruptures, while both MRI and US have the same accuracy for detecting partial midsubstance ruptures.

11.5 Treatment

We must differentiate the treatment depending on the type of rupture. It is important to discuss with the patient the pros and cons and surgical risks to make the decision, especially in borderline cases [23].

11.5.1 Partial Ruptures

The classical treatment of partial ruptures has been mainly conservative if they affect less than 50% of the thickness, with different protocols in terms of immobilization, rehabilitation, or corticosteroid injections. General treatment involves cold, rest, sling, and active mobilization according to pain tolerance, starting in supine position. In general, it has yielded good results as per the review by Bauer et al. [24]. According to this article, the failure rate of conservative treatment can be up to 56%, and therefore it could be advisable to consider surgical treatment in patients with a high functional demand. Another important issue is that changing from conservative to surgical treatment did not lead to worse results. There are few studies, except clinical cases, on the conservative treatment of partial ruptures with very good results. According to the article by Behun et al. [25], surgical treatment obtained 94% good results. If surgical treatment is decided, it will consist of completing the rupture and performing a complete reinsertion of the tendon as if it were a complete rupture.

In brief, the current recommendation is conservative management. Surgical management should be considered in patients with high functional demand and partial ruptures greater than 50% and in patients in whom symptoms persist despite nonsurgical treatment.

11.5.1.1 Partial Rupture of the Short Head of the Biceps

According to the review by Iqbal et al. [11], patients with isolated tears of the short head of the biceps do poorly when treated conservatively, but good outcomes with acute and delayed reconstruction have been reported. Partial reattachment of the short head or reattachment of the entire tendon after debridement has been described [26]. When treating these injuries, an anatomical reinsertion would be optimal; however, if the repair is performed by an isolated anterior approach, insertion must be lateralized without clinical repercussion [11].

11.5.2 Acute Complete Rupture

It is usually considered an acute tear up to 4 weeks. If the *lacertus fibrosus* remains intact, even up to 3 months, a primary repair could be achieved as it prevents tendon retraction.

Conservative treatment is recommended in elderly patients with low functional demand and in younger patients reluctant to surgical treatment or with contraindications for surgery. In general, it has good results [27], with loss of strength in supination of 40–50% but minimal in flexion no greater than 30% [28, 29]. It is important to explain to the patient the surgical risks and possible sequelae of conservative treatment in order to reach an informed decision.

Surgical treatment is reserved for young patients with medium to high functional demands. We will discuss the single and double approach, fixation methods, and anatomic vs. nonanatomic reinsertion.

The single approach can be considered a quicker technique in which the reinsertion achieved is not completely anatomical [30], being slightly more anterior to its actual footprint. It can be performed with direct transverse (Fig. 11.1), direct longitudinal, or extensile "lazy S" approach (Fig. 11.2).

In the double approach, the anterior window is performed to locate and prepare the stump and a posterolateral accessory approach for anatomical reinsertion (Fig. 11.3). Although from a

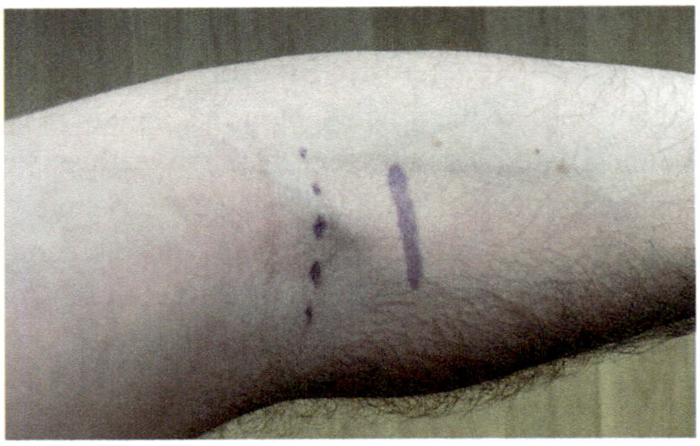

Fig. 11.1 Transverse incision (bicipital crease-dashed line)

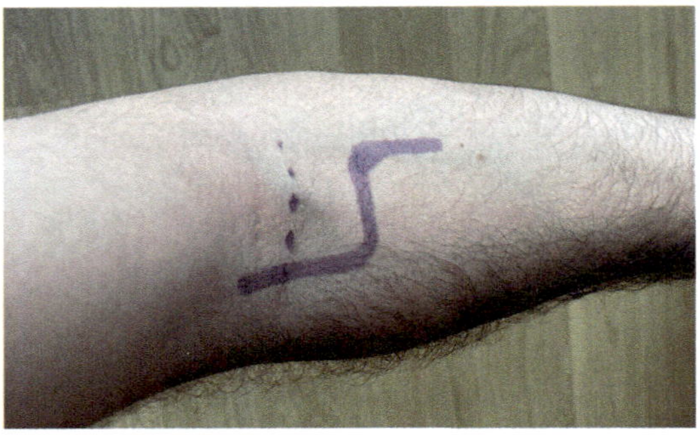

Fig. 11.2 Lazy S incision (bicipital crease-dashed line)

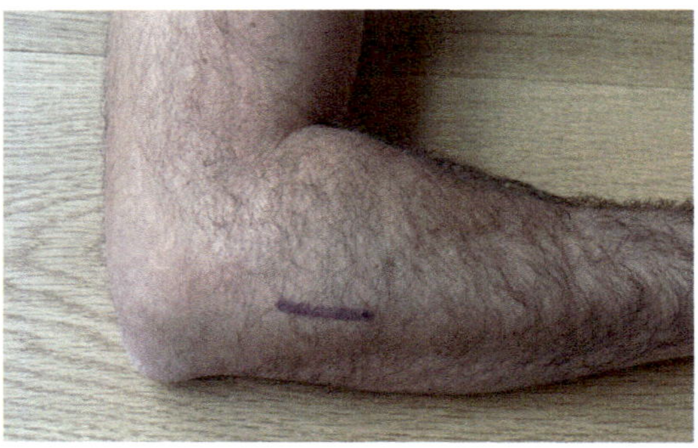

Fig. 11.3 Posterolateral incision (double approach)

biomechanical perspective the anatomical reinsertion improves supination strength [31], there are no clinical differences between single and double approach [32, 33], and regarding complications some authors have reported a higher degree of neurapraxia in the single approach group. Dunphy et al. found yet more complications in the double approach, especially in terms of heterotopic ossifications. There were no significant differences in rates of motor neurapraxia, infection, rerupture, and reoperation regarding surgeon's years of practice, fellowship training, or case volume [34].

When performing the double-incision technique, most authors use bone tunnels, but bone anchors or cortical buttons can also be used. These are commonly employed in the single-incision technique. Regarding the method of fixation, no differences have been found between any of them: bone tunnels, suture anchors, cortical buttons, or interference screws [35].

In short, and based on the available data, both techniques, single and double incision, provide successful outcomes. Therefore, the surgeon may choose depending on his/her experience, available material, and costs.

11.5.2.1 Surgical Technique

Anesthesia and Positioning

Patient in supine position with the arm in abduction and extended on a hand table, under regional anesthesia with axillary block.

Single-Incision Technique (Author's Preferred Method)

Approach

Transverse 2–3 cm incision at the level of the elbow crease or 1–2 cm (Fig. 11.4) distally at the level of the bicipital tuberosity. Secondary, dissec-

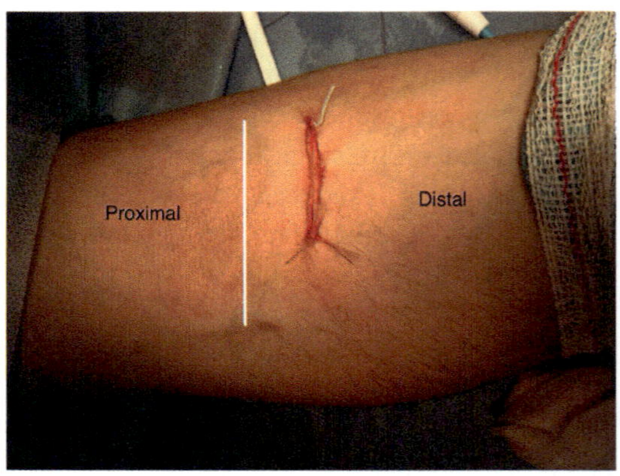

Fig. 11.4 Transverse anterior incision (white line bicipital crease)

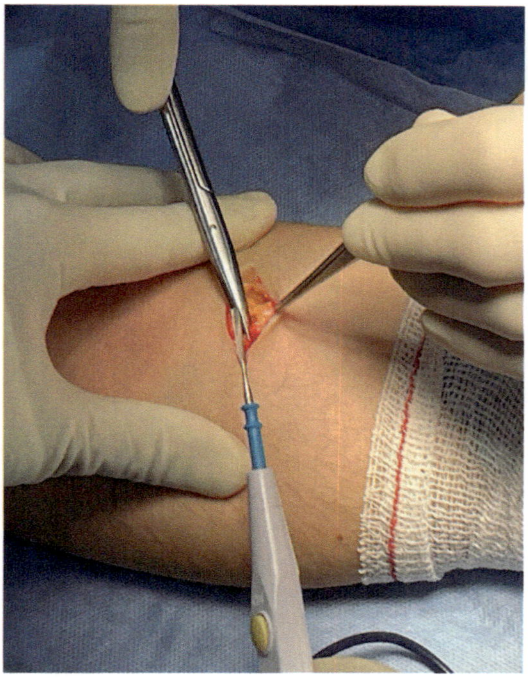

Fig. 11.5 Subcutaneous tissue

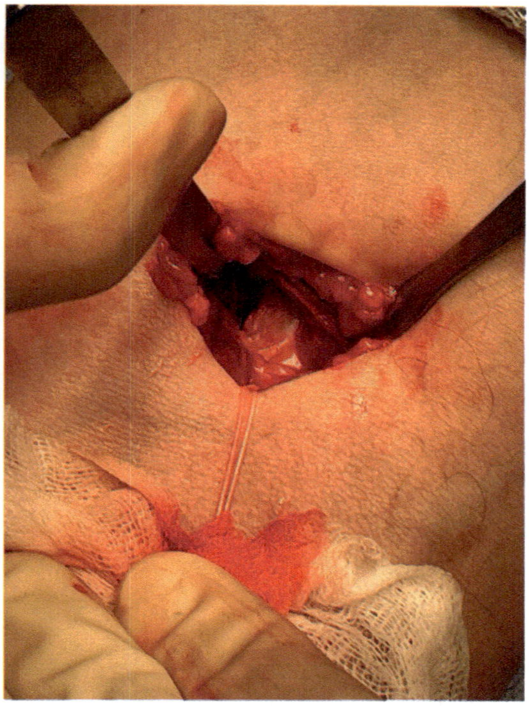

Fig. 11.6 Tendon footprint-bicipital tuberosity

tion of the subcutaneous tissue is done (Fig. 11.5) where the lateral antebrachial cutaneous nerve and the cephalic vein can sometimes be identified and must be preserved and protected in order to prevent paresthesia in the forearm [36]. Perform blunt dissection to the bicipital tuberosity. With the help of spreaders and the arm in maximum supination, the distal remnant of the tendon should be identified in the bicipital tuberosity [37] (Fig. 11.6). Do not apply too much tension with the spreaders to avoid injury to the posterior interosseous nerve (PIN). The PIN is located between 9 and 14 mm from the bicipital tuberosity [38, 39]; neuropraxia has been reported in up to 10% of patients [40].

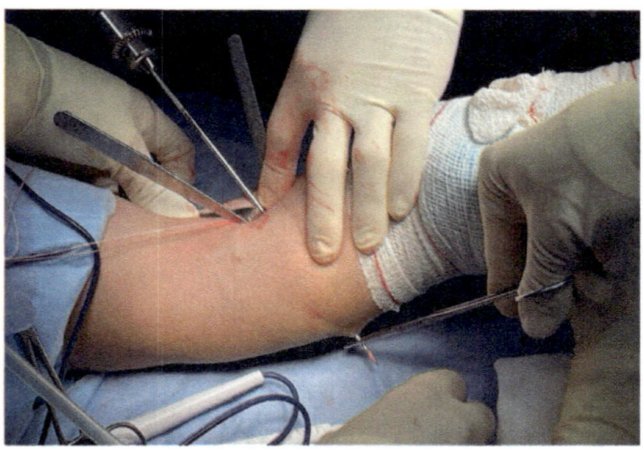

Fig. 11.7 Tunnel drilling over guide wire

Tuberosity Preparation

Once the bicipital tuberosity is exposed, all fibrotic debris should be removed. To perform the reinsertion technique with *endobutton*, a tunnel should be drilled at the level of the tuberosity (Fig. 11.7). The tunnel should be created in the most ulnar region of the tuberosity to recreate, as much as possible, its anatomical position [41, 42]. Place a guide wire in the central and ulnar region of the tuberosity (Fig. 11.8), and drill the anterior cortex with a drill bit of the same size as the biceps tendon (Fig. 11.9). The second cortex should be drilled with a thinner drill bit, only for the passage of the *endobutton*.

Tendon Preparation

Identify the tendon at the level of the arm through the transverse incision, applying traction release adhesions by blunt dissection at the level of the muscle belly. Resect the fibrotic and degenerate

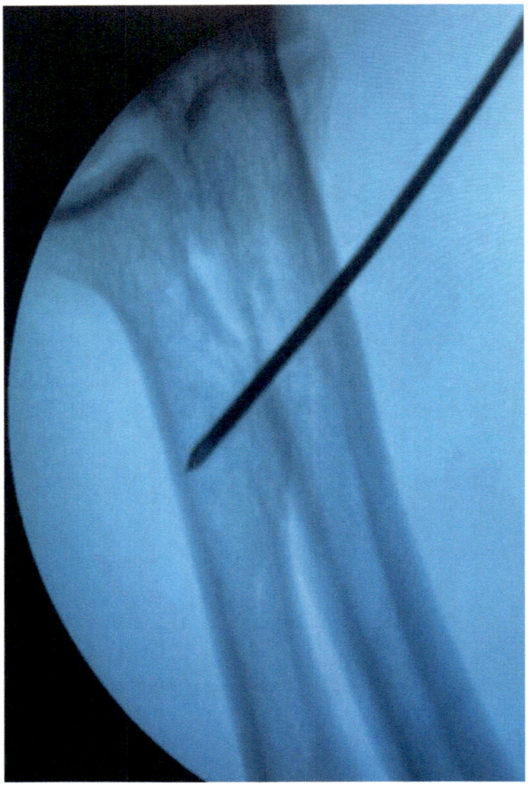

Fig. 11.8 Guide wire direction

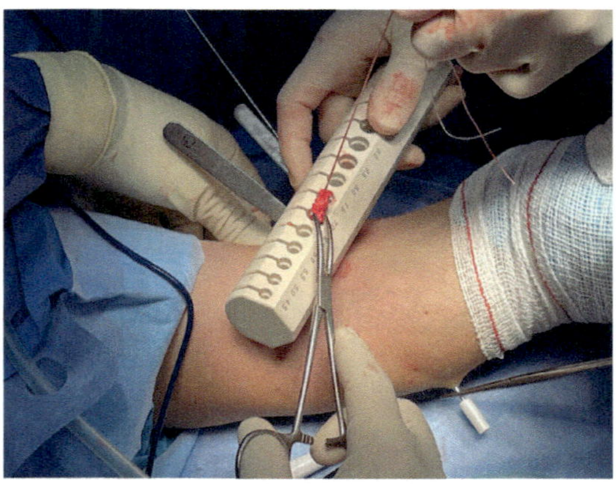

Fig. 11.9 Tendon measurement to choose drill size

tissue of the biceps stump (Fig. 11.10), perform a continuous type Krackow or Bunnell locking suture, or perform a combination of both [39, 40] (Fig. 11.11). The sutures must be knotted to the button with a small gap left between the tendon and the button to be able to turn the button for its

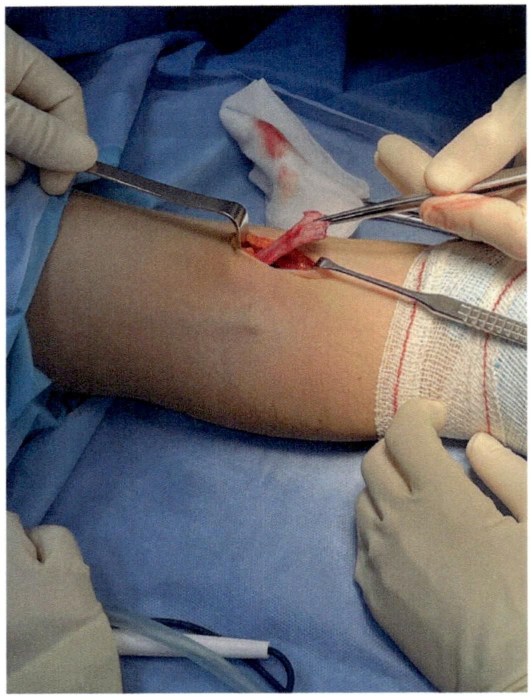

Fig. 11.10 Biceps tendon stump. Degenerated tissue

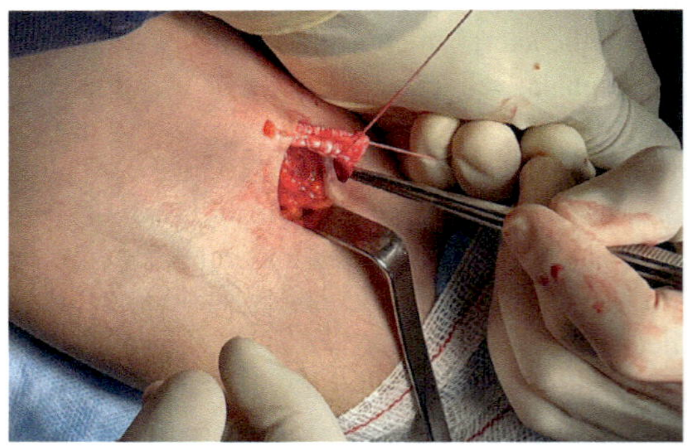

Fig. 11.11 Krakow suture technique

passage through the bony tunnel (Fig. 11.12). Some authors prefer not to leave any space between them even though it may be more difficult to perform the maneuver [36, 40, 43].

Fixation and Wound Closure

Place 2 threads of different colors on the ends of the button (Fig. 11.13), pass the 4 threads through the eyelet of the guide wire inserted in the tuberosity, and pull it to pass the 4 threads through the posterior cortex. With the arm in 90 degrees flex-

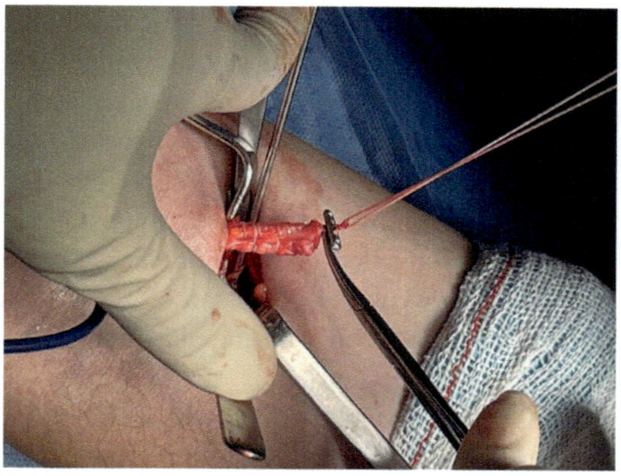

Fig. 11.12 Gap between tendon and endobutton

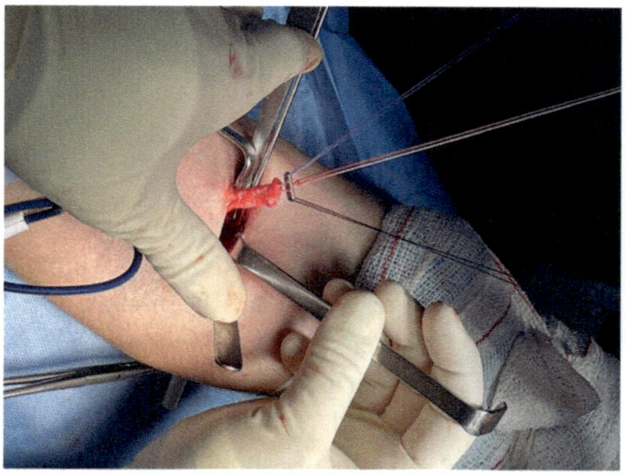

Fig. 11.13 Different color sutures to flip the endobutton

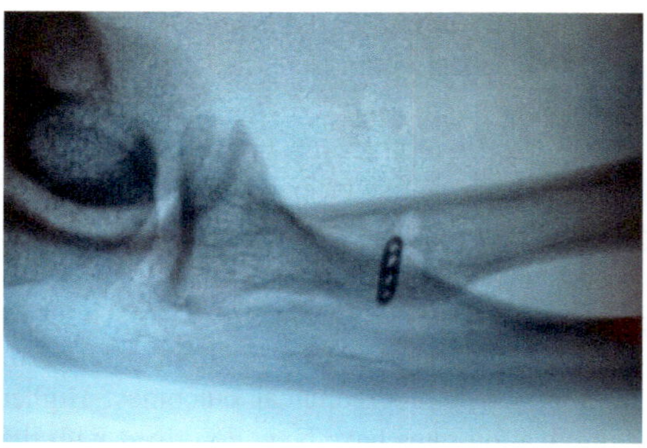

Fig. 11.14 Lateral x-ray to check correct position

ion, pull 2 threads of the same color to pass the button through the hole. Check for complete passage of the button with the aid of the scope (Figs. 11.14 and 11.15). Check mobility and tendon tension intraoperatively (Fig. 11.16). Perform wound closure in lawyers.

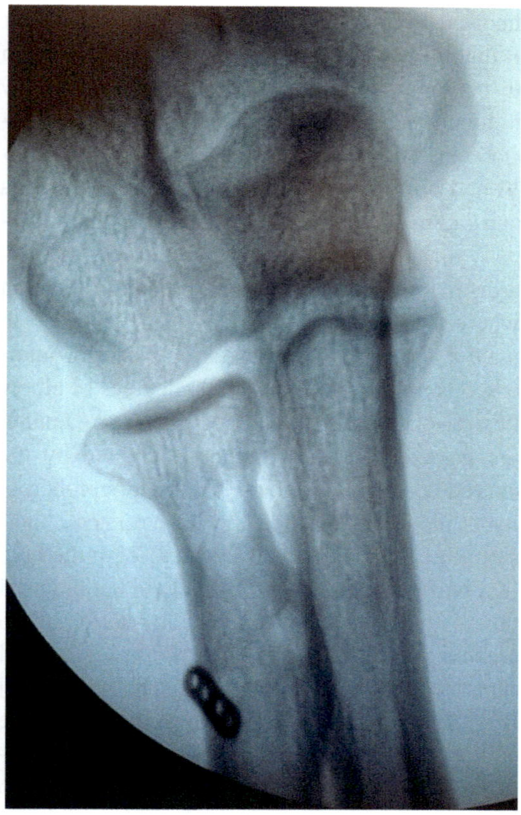

Fig. 11.15 Anteroposterior X-ray

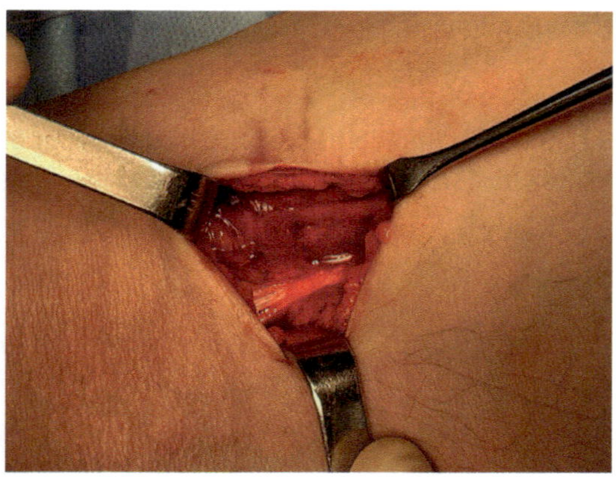

Fig. 11.16 Tendon reinserted. Tension checking

Double-Incision Technique

A 3–5 cm incision is made over the anterior elbow crease, the distal biceps tendon is identified, the fibrotic end is resected, and Krackow or Bunnell sutures are performed. With the forearm in maximum supination, the bicipital tuberosity is identified on the radius, and a curved hemostatic clamp is passed between the *brachioradialis* and *pronator teres* and then between the ulna and radius along the medial border of the tuberosity toward the posterolateral region of the forearm. A longitudinal incision is made in the skin where the clamp protrudes. With the forearm in maximal pronation to protect the posterior interosseous nerve [44] and with 90 degrees of elbow flexion, the suture threads of the biceps tendon are passed through the channel created by the curved hemostatic forceps. The bicipital tuberosity is identified through the posterolateral incision; the fibrotic debris is cleaned. With the help of a burr or a chisel, a pit is made in the bicipital tuberosity. Then, close to the lateral cortex of the created pit, 3 holes are made with 2 mm drill separated between them by 8 mm [28] (Fig. 11.17). Two threads are passed through the central hole and one on each side, the distal tendon of the biceps is approached and is fitted into the bicipital pit, and the central sutures are knotted with the lateral ones on the bony bridges left between the holes. Check mobility and tendon tension intraoperatively. Perform wound closure.

Postoperative Protocol

The elbow is immobilized with a plaster splint in 90° of flexion and in full supination. Depending on the patient's adherence to the postoperative indications, elbow mobilization can be started from the third postoperative day, allowing active extension, active pronation, and passive flexion and supination exercises, always with the use of a sling or removable splint during rest periods. The splint will be removed after the sixth postoperative week. If full extension was not reached intraoperatively, a weekly progression of 10 degrees of extension is started with the aid of an elbow brace until full extension is achieved. Muscle strengthening is started from week number 10, and unrestricted activities are allowed starting from the fourth to the sixth month [32, 40].

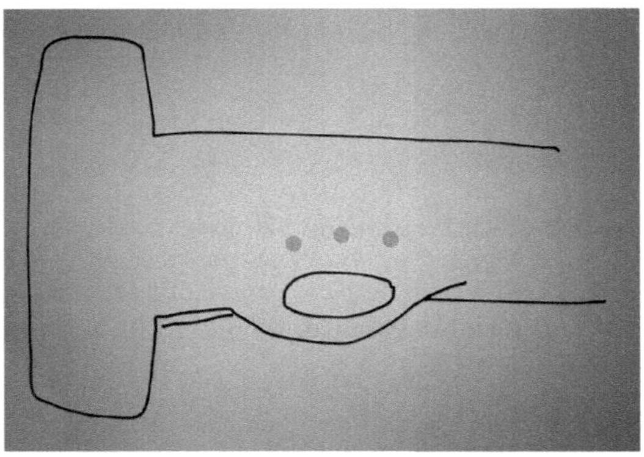

Fig. 11.17 Pit and drill holes over bicipital tuberosity in double-incision technique

Some authors recommend 25 mg of indomethacin orally three times a day for 3 weeks to prevent heterotopic ossifications [40].

11.5.3 Chronic Rupture

If surgical treatment is decided, primary repair should be attempted even if extension is limited at the end of surgery, as it has been shown that patients may recover nearly full extension postoperatively [45]. If it is not possible due to tendon retraction and poor tissue quality, reconstructive treatment should therefore be planned.

Tenodesis of the biceps to the *brachialis* can be performed to reduce pain but not to restore strength. Regarding grafts, many choices can be used for reconstruction such as *tibialis anterior, gracilis, semitendinosus, Achilles, lacertus fibrosus, or flexor carpi radialis*. For the attachment of the graft to the native biceps, several possibilities have been described as end-to-end, Pulvertaft weave and onlay technique.

There are no significant differences in graft type or fixation method in relation to range of motion, strength, or clinical outcomes. Higher complication rates have been described with the use of the autografts (34%), mainly related to the donor site, when compared to allografts (14%). For the fixation method, higher complications have been reported for the weave technique than for the onlay one [46].

The incidence of general complications according to the review of Amarasooriya et al.

[23] is 5% of major complications and 20% of minor complications. There are differences in terms of the approach used, but not according to the method of fixation. Major complications reported were 1.6% PIN lesions, 1.4% rerupture, 0.3% median nerve injury, and 0.1% synostosis. The most common minor complication was lateral cutaneous nerve injury 9.2%, more frequent in single incision than in extensile approach.

11.6 Conclusions

Distal biceps tendon rupture incidence is increasing in recent years. Clinical suspicion is paramount for the diagnosis, supported by clinical tests and imaging. A good knowledge of the anatomy and the surgical techniques available is essential to achieve successful results, although complications are not rare. Ruptures may be divided into acute and chronic. One should always try a direct repair, and, if not possible, different graft techniques are available. Acute partial ruptures normally receive conservative treatment except in high demand patients, greater than 50% rupture, or conservative treatment failure. Isolated short head partial tears should be treated surgically when diagnosed. Acute complete tears may be surgically treated except in elderly people. There is no difference between the two main techniques or fixation methods. Both single incision and double incision provide good results, as well as bone tunnels or button fixation. Regarding complications, neuropraxias are the commonest ones.

References

1. Kelly MP, Perkinson SG, Ablove RH, Tueting JL. Distal biceps tendon ruptures: an epidemiological analysis using a large population database. Am J Sports Med. 2015;43:2012–7.
2. Srinivasan RC, Pederson WC, Morrey BF. Distal biceps tendon repair and reconstruction. J Hand Surg Am. 2020;45:48–56.
3. Luokkala T, Sidharthan SK, Karjalainen TV, Paloneva J, Watts AC. Distal biceps tendon repairs and reconstructions-an analysis of demographics, prodromal symptoms and complications. Arch Orthop Trauma Surg. 2021; https://doi.org/10.1007/s00402-021-03750-1. Epub ahead of print.
4. Miyamoto RG, Elser F, Millett PJ. Distal biceps tendon injuries. J Bone Joint Surg Am. 2010;92:2128–38.
5. Idler CS, Montgomery WH 3rd, Lindsey DP, Badua PA, Wynne GF, Yerby SA. Distal biceps tendon repair: a biomechanical comparison of intact tendon and 2 repair techniques. Am J Sports Med. 2006;34:968–74.
6. Eames MH, Bain GI, Fogg QA, van Riet RP. Distal biceps tendon anatomy: a cadaveric study. J Bone Joint Surg Am. 2007;89:1044–9.
7. Athwal GS, Steinmann SP, Rispoli DM. The distal biceps tendon: footprint and relevant clinical anatomy. J Hand Surg Am. 2007;32:1225–9.
8. Landa J, Bhandari S, Strauss EJ, Walker PS, Meislin RJ. The effect of repair of the lacertus fibrosus on distal biceps tendon repairs: a biomechanical, functional, and anatomic study. Am J Sports Med. 2009;37:120–3.
9. Caputo AE, Cusano A, Stannard J, Hamer MJ. Distal biceps repair using the lacertus fibrosus as a local graft. J Shoulder Elb Surg. 2016;25:1189–94.
10. Voleti PB, Berkowitz JL, Konin GP, Cordasco FA. Rupture of the short head component of a bifurcated distal biceps tendon. J Shoulder Elb Surg. 2017;26:403–8.
11. Iqbal K, Leung B, Phadnis J. Distal biceps short head tears: repair, reconstruction, and systematic review. J Shoulder Elb Surg. 2020;29:2353–63.
12. Vishwanathan K, Soni K. Distal biceps rupture: evaluation and management. J Clin Orthop Trauma. 2021;19:132–8.
13. ElMaraghy A, Devereaux M, Tsoi K. The biceps crease interval for diagnosing complete distal biceps tendon ruptures. Clin Orthop Relat Res. 2008;466:2255–62.
14. O'Driscoll SW, Goncalves LB, Dietz P. The hook test for distal biceps tendon avulsion. Am J Sports Med. 2007;35:1865–9.
15. Metzman LS, Tivener KA. The supination-pronation test for distal biceps tendon rupture. Am J Orthop (Belle Mead NJ). 2015;44:E361–4.
16. Ruland RT, Dunbar RP, Bowen JD. The biceps squeeze test for diagnosis of distal biceps tendon ruptures. Clin Orthop Relat Res. 2005;437:128–31.
17. ElMaraghy A, Devereaux M. The "bicipital aponeurosis flex test": evaluating the integrity of the bicipital aponeurosis and its implications for treatment of distal biceps tendon ruptures. J Shoulder Elb Surg. 2013;22:908–14.
18. Bain GI, Johnson LJ, Turner PC. Treatment of partial distal biceps tendon tears. Sports Med Arthrosc Rev. 2008;16:154–61.
19. Nguyen ML, Rosenthal J, Karas S, Gottschalk M, Daly C, Wagner E, et al. A comprehensive review of the normal, abnormal, and post-operative MRI appearance of the distal biceps brachii. Skelet Radiol. 2020;49:1695–707.
20. Festa A, Mulieri PJ, Newman JS, Spitz DJ, Leslie BM. Effectiveness of magnetic resonance imaging

in detecting partial and complete distal biceps tendon rupture. J Hand Surg Am. 2010;35:77–83.
21. Giuffrè BM, Moss MJ. Optimal positioning for MRI of the distal biceps brachii tendon: flexed abducted supinated view. AJR Am J Roentgenol. 2004;182:944–6.
22. Lynch J, Yu CC, Chen C, Muh S. Magnetic resonance imaging versus ultrasound in diagnosis of distal biceps tendon avulsion. Orthop Traumatol Surg Res. 2019;105:861–6.
23. Amarasooriya M, Bain GI, Roper T, Bryant K, Iqbal K, Phadnis J. Complications after distal biceps tendon repair: a systematic review. Am J Sports Med. 2020;48:3103–11.
24. Bauer TM, Wong JC, Lazarus MD. Is nonoperative management of partial distal biceps tears really successful? J Shoulder Elb Surg. 2018;27:720–5.
25. Behun MA, Geeslin AG, O'Hagan EC, King JC. Partial tears of the distal biceps brachii tendon: a systematic review of surgical outcomes. J Hand Surg Am. 2016;41:e175–89.
26. Cho CH, Song KS, Lee SM. Isolated short head component rupture of a bifurcated distal biceps tendon mimicking as a complete rupture. J Hand Surg Eur. 2011;36:333–4.
27. Freeman CR, McCormick KR, Mahoney D, Baratz M, Lubahn JD. Nonoperative treatment of distal biceps tendon ruptures compared with a historical control group. J Bone Joint Surg Am. 2009;91:2329–34.
28. Morrey BF, Askew LJ, An KN, Dobyns JH. Rupture of the distal tendon of the biceps brachii. A biomechanical study. J Bone Joint Surg Am. 1985;67:418–21.
29. Nesterenko S, Domire ZJ, Morrey BF, Sanchez-Sotelo J. Elbow strength and endurance in patients with a ruptured distal biceps tendon. J Shoulder Elb Surg. 2010;19:184–9.
30. Hansen G, Smith A, Pollock JW, Werier J, Nairn R, Rakhra KS, Benoit D, Papp S. Anatomic repair of the distal biceps tendon cannot be consistently performed through a classic single-incision suture anchor technique. J Shoulder Elb Surg. 2014;23:1898–904.
31. Prud'homme-Foster M, Louati H, Pollock JW, Papp S. Proper placement of the distal biceps tendon during repair improves supination strength—a biomechanical analysis. J Shoulder Elb Surg. 2015;24:527–32.
32. Grewal R, Athwal GS, MacDermid JC, Faber KJ, Drosdowech DS, El-Hawary R, et al. Single versus double-incision technique for the repair of acute distal biceps tendon ruptures: a randomized clinical trial. J Bone Joint Surg Am. 2012;94:1166–74.
33. Shields E, Olsen JR, Williams RB, Rouse L, Maloney M, Voloshin I. Distal biceps brachii tendon repairs: a single-incision technique using a cortical button with interference screw versus a double-incision technique using suture fixation through bone tunnels. Am J Sports Med. 2015;43:1072–6.
34. Dunphy TR, Hudson J, Batech M, Acevedo DC, Mirzayan R. Surgical treatment of distal biceps tendon ruptures: an analysis of complications in 784 surgical repairs. Am J Sports Med. 2017;45:3020–9.
35. Kodde IF, Baerveldt RC, Mulder PG, Eygendaal D, van den Bekerom MP. Refixation techniques and approaches for distal biceps tendon ruptures: a systematic review of clinical studies. J Shoulder Elb Surg. 2016;25:e29–37.
36. Patterson RW, Sharma J, Lawton JN, Evans PJ. Distal biceps tendon reconstruction with tendoachilles allograft: a modification of the EndoButton technique utilizing an ACL reconstruction system. J Hand Surg. 2009;34:545–52.
37. Bain GI, Prem H, Heptinstall RJ, Verhellen R, Paix D. Repair of distal biceps tendon rupture: a new technique using the Endobutton. J Shoulder Elb Surg. 2000;9:120–6.
38. Greenberg JA, Fernandez JJ, Wang T, Turner C. EndoButton-assisted repair of distal biceps tendon ruptures. J Shoulder Elb Surg. 2003;12:484–90.
39. Greenberg JA. Endobutton repair of distal biceps tendon ruptures. J Hand Surg. 2009;34:1541–8.
40. Wysocki RW, Verma NN. Distal biceps repair. In: Cole B, Sekiya J, editors. Surgical techniques of the shoulder, elbow, and knee in sports medicine. 1st ed. Elsevier; 2008. Chapter 41. Hardcover ISBN: 9781416034476. eBook ISBN: 9781437721195.
41. Pereira DS, Kvitne RS, Liang M, Giacobetti FB, Ebramzadeh E. Surgical repair of distal biceps tendon ruptures: a biomechanical comparison of two techniques. Am J Sports Med. 2002;30:432–6.
42. Cerciello S, Visonà E, Corona K, Ribeiro Filho PR, Carbone S. The treatment of distal biceps ruptures: an overview. Joints. 2018 Dec;6:228–31.
43. Sethi P, Obopilwe E, Rincon L, Miller S, Mazzocca A. Biomechanical evaluation of distal bíceps reconstruction with cortical button and interference screw fixation. J Shoulder Elb Surg. 2010;19:53–7.
44. Drosdowech DS, King GJW, Faber KJ. Distal biceps tendon repair: one- and two incision techniques. Tech Shoulder Elbow Surg. 2002;3:90–5.
45. Alentorn-Geli E, Assenmacher AT, Sánchez-Sotelo J. Distal biceps tendon injuries: a clinically relevant current concepts review. EFORT Open Rev. 2017;1:316–24.
46. Litowski ML, Purnell J, Hildebrand KA, Bois AJ. Surgical outcomes and complications following distal biceps tendon reconstruction: a systematic review and meta-analysis. JSES Int. 2020;5:24–30.

12 Controversies in Tennis Elbow in Adults: Should We Ever Operate?

Carlos A. Encinas-Ullán, Primitivo Gómez-Cardero, and E. Carlos Rodríguez-Merchán

12.1 Introduction

Lateral epicondylitis (LE), or tennis elbow, is a challenging problem that can lead to significant disability and limitation not only in athletics but also in activities of daily living, affecting 1%–3% of the general population each year. LE can cause significant pain and functional impairment, and despite its relatively high prevalence, there remains a multitude of treatments due to the lack of a single gold standard solution. In the majority (80%–90%) of cases, it can be successfully treated nonsurgically. However, 4%–10% of patients will have persistent symptoms, often leading to surgical intervention that produces "good" or "excellent" results in 80%–90% of cases.

12.2 Epidemiology

LE most commonly affects adults in the fourth and fifth decade of life and is more common in the dominant arm, with no gender differences [1]. It is generally considered an overuse injury involving repeated extension of the wrist against resistance. Up to 50% of all tennis players develop symptoms due to various factors, including poor swing technique or the use of heavy rackets. It is also seen in workers who use heavy tools or perform repetitive gripping or lifting tasks.

12.3 Etiology and Pathogenesis

LE is mainly due to overloading by repetitive movements in wrist extension. In LE, the most frequently affected muscle is the extensor carpi radialis brevis (ECRB), at its origin (Fig. 12.1). The enthesis of the extensor digitorum communis (EDC), the extensor carpi radialis longus (ECRL), or extensor carpi ulnaris (ECU) may also be affected, but less frequently. Any activity that involves repeated activation of these muscles (screwing, typing, playing tennis, etc.) for long periods of time favors muscle overload and the appearance of tendinosis. Overuse, obesity, and smoking have been identified as risk/aggravating factors [2].

C. A. Encinas-Ullán · P. Gómez-Cardero ·
E. C. Rodríguez-Merchán (✉)
Department of Orthopedic Surgery, "La Paz" University Hospital-IdiPaz, Madrid, Spain

E. C. Rodríguez-Merchán, A. Moreno-Garcìa (eds.), *Controversies in Orthopedic Surgery of The Upper Limb*, https://doi.org/10.1007/978-3-031-04907-1_12

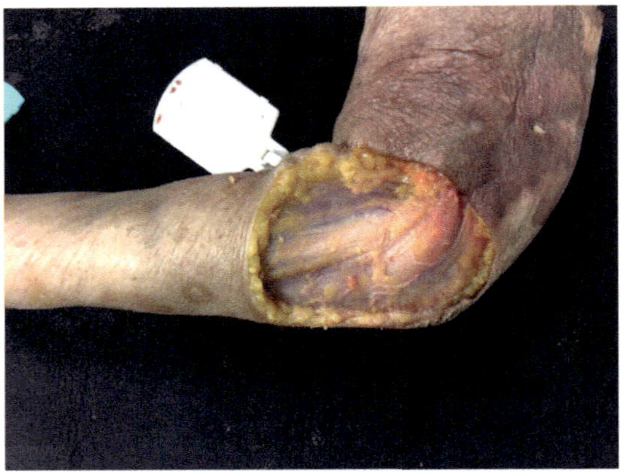

Fig. 12.1 Anatomical image of the epicondylar musculature

12.4 Clinical Symptoms

All patients with LE present with pain in the anterior and/or superior lateral epicondyle, radiating through the extensor musculature. The intensity of the pain can be highly variable: from pain only with certain gestures or activities to continuous disabling pain that is exacerbated at night. Typically, the pain is triggered when the patient is asked to perform wrist and finger extension against resistance. Generally, pain is less pronounced when wrist extension is performed with the elbow flexed and more when performed with the elbow extended. This is one of the most commonly used tests for the clinical diagnosis of LE.

Generally, joint balance is preserved in all patients. If this is not the case, the coexistence of added pathology should be considered [3]. The differential diagnosis should routinely rule out the following:

12.4.1 Posterolateral Instability

In all patients presenting with elbow pain, the joint should be checked for stability. A history of ulnar varus, previous surgery, or elbow dislocation should always be considered. Also, repeated corticosteroid injection may damage the lateral ligamentous complex and lead to elbow instability.

12.4.2 Posterolateral Plica

Its association with LE is very frequent. Usually, the pain is triggered by elbow extension while palpating the posterior part of the radiocapitellar joint.

12.4.3 Posterior Interosseous Nerve (PIN) Compression

Also known as radial tunnel syndrome, it produces pain of neuropathic characteristics in the lateral/posterior aspect of the forearm. Typically, the pain is not triggered by wrist extension, but it is triggered by wrist supination (due to compression of the supinator brevis over the PIN). A selective nerve block can be performed if there is any doubt about the diagnosis.

12.4.4 Other Pathologies

Other possibilities that should be considered in a patient with lateral elbow pain are cervical radiculopathies, overuse of the joint due to adjacent joint disease, low-grade infection, and capitellar osteochondritis.

12.5 Diagnosis

In most cases, LE can be diagnosed through anamnesis and physical examination.

However, it is not uncommon to perform complementary tests, aimed both at refining the diagnosis of tendinopathy and at ruling out the coexistence of other pathologies. In general, an anteroposterior and lateral X-ray should be requested in all patients. The presence of calcifications at the origin of the ECRB is suggestive of chronic evolution.

Ultrasonography has become an increasingly requested test that can demonstrate changes in the tendons (thickening, scarring, intrasubstance degeneration, microcalcifications, neovascularization) as well as facilitate the performance of infiltrations [4]. Magnetic resonance imaging (MRI) (Fig. 12.2) facilitates the observation of intrasubstance degenerative changes. However, the findings of the MRI do not always correlate with the severity of the clinical symptoms, and it is an expensive test, so its main indication is to rule out concomitant lesions [5]. Neurophysiological studies are indicated if there is a suspicion of a possible compression of the posterior interosseous nerve.

In general, the diagnosis of this tendinopathy relies on a good physical examination, with complementary tests being performed in case of doubt or to assess the presence of concomitant pathology.

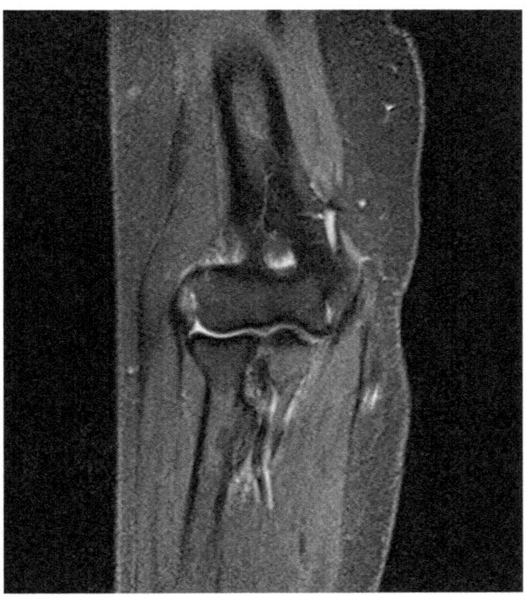

Fig. 12.2 MRI image showing signal changes of the lateral epicondyle, with thickening, irregularity, and slight edema of the extensor digitorum communis (EDC) and extensor carpi radialis brevis (ECRB) tendons

12.6 Conservative Treatment

As a rule, LE tends to self-resolve in the vast majority of patients and therefore nonsurgical treatments are recommended for the initial management of acute LE. Conservative treatment should be performed in all patients because of its low cost and high effectiveness (up to 90% of patients improve) [5]. Currently, there is no strong evidence for the efficacy of a single nonsurgical treatment option for LE. This may explain the numerous treatment options described in the scientific literature in the last decade.

12.6.1 Rest and Postural Reeducation

Rest improves symptoms in all patients. Postural reeducation is important especially in those cases due to overuse and is a fundamental part of treatment in work and sport-related cases. Reeducation should include the shoulder and periscapular musculature, both of which are important for proper elbow function. External supports that help relax the epicondylar musculature should also be included, such as wrist supports for computer keyboarding. Tennis players may benefit from additional sport-specific advice. Technique errors thought to predispose to LE etiology are (1) faulty backhand technique with the elbow forward, (2) excessive forearm pronation during an overhead forehand swing, and (3) excessive wrist flexion during a serve. Other potential risk factors include racquet type, grip size, string tension, court surface, and ball weight. These factors affect the biomechanical loading of the elbow during tennis.

12.6.2 Exercises

A 2015 systematic review included studies with low risk of bias. The conclusion was that home strengthening exercises are more effective than a wait-and-see policy. In addition, there is no difference in outcome after a specific type of exercise (stretching, concentric, or eccentric exercises). In addition, the supervised combined stretching and strengthening protocol is superior to a comparable at-home protocol [6].

12.6.3 Orthoses

The use of orthoses provides pain relief. They are based on decreasing the tension of the wrist extensors. No differences in results have been observed between the different types of orthoses [6]. The patient must be instructed in their proper use, since improper use can lead to compression of the posterior interosseous nerve.

12.6.4 Nonsteroidal Anti-Inflammatory Drugs (NSAIDs)

There has been no consensus on the superiority of oral versus topical NSAIDs in pain control, although oral NSAIDs may cause gastrointestinal adverse effects [7]. In a Cochrane review they found low-quality evidence showing that topical NSAIDs were more effective than placebo alone in the short term (up to 4 weeks) in reducing pain versus placebo, while the evidence on oral NSAIDs was conflicting. They concluded that there is limited data on the efficacy of topical or oral NSAIDs for LE treatment [8].

12.6.5 Shock Waves

It consists of the application of a sound wave of a specific frequency directly on the origin of the musculature, although the ultimate mechanism of action is unknown. They are a possible alternative to reduce pain and medical costs associated with more invasive therapy. A meta-analysis concludes that based on existing clinical evidence, extracorporeal shock wave therapy can effectively relieve pain and functional impairment (loss of grip strength) caused by LE, with greater overall safety than other methods, especially CS injections [9]. However, another meta-analysis suggests that shock wave therapy cannot significantly reduce pain compared with placebo or control group [10].

12.6.6 Injections

12.6.6.1 Corticosteroid (CS) Injections

Corticosteroid injections are one of the most frequently used treatments due to their low cost and ease of application, which is a concern given the evidence of low cost-effectiveness and potential long-term harm. They provide rapid and significant pain relief, but their long-term results are questioned in the literature [7]. Repeated CS injections can lead to iatrogenic tendon rupture and muscle atrophy. Therefore, clinicians should be wary of CS overuse in the treatment of LE because of poor long-term efficacy and potential adverse effects. Therefore, in principle, they would only be indicated in those patients who need rapid and intense short-term pain improvement (e.g., professional athletes). Therefore, while it appears that steroid injections are effective in relieving LE pain in the short term, there does not appear to be a lasting benefit.

12.6.6.2 Autologous Blood Injections

It has been shown that autologous blood injections could trigger an inflammatory reaction around the tendon to promote tissue healing with cellular and humoral mediators [11].

12.6.6.3 Platelet-Rich Plasma (PRP) Injections

PRP contains growth factors that could be beneficial for the healing of soft tissue injuries. However, available studies have reported conflicting results, making it difficult to draw clear conclusions. A systematic review stated that the PRP injection has no obvious effects on the treatment of chronic LE [12]. They provide better medium-term pain control than CS infiltrations [13]. They also appear to have lower complication rates than corticosteroids and autologous blood injection [14]. Among its major drawbacks is the diversity of commercial kits and protocols, which makes it difficult to know which is the best formulation to use [15]. PRP injection has been shown in some studies to be effective in the management of chronic LE in the medium and long term. In a successive systematic review and meta-analysis of randomized controlled trials to compare the effectiveness of three commonly used injections – CS, PRP, and autologous blood – in the treatment of LE, Houck et al. found that corticosteroid improves functional outcomes and pain relief in the short term, while autologous blood and PRP are the most effective treatments in the medium term [13].

Tang et al.'s study concluded that PRP was associated with greater improvement in long-term pain intensity and function than corticosteroids or autologous blood. However, in the short term, CS was associated with the greatest improvement [16]. Linnanmäki et al. designed a randomized, placebo-controlled trial comparing PRP, autologous blood, and saline injections in the treatment of LE. The authors concluded that PRP or autologous blood injections did not improve pain or function at 1-year follow-up compared to those who received a saline injection, so they do not recommend their use [17]. Simental-Mendía et al. reviewed the effects of platelet-rich plasma (PRP) injection versus placebo (saline injection) on pain and joint function in LE, in five randomized placebo-controlled trials with a total of 276 patients. PRP injection was not superior to placebo. However, patients reported improvement after both interventions in clinical parameters. Further randomized trials are needed to determine whether PRP injection is clinically more effective than placebo (saline injection) [18].

A current Cochrane review concludes that PRP or autologous blood injection therapies are likely to provide little or no clinically important benefit for pain or function (moderate evidence of certainty) and cause pain and carry a small risk of infection. Without evidence of benefit, the costs and risks are not justified [19]. In addition, much more research is needed to determine the optimal PRP formulation (e.g., high or low leukocyte concentration) that is effective in providing long-term pain relief in chronic LE.

12.6.6.4 Stem Cell Injections

They can be fat-derived, bone marrow-derived, or allogeneic. All the studies are of less than 20 patients and of short follow-up, so no clear conclusions can be drawn.

12.6.6.5 Botulinum Toxin A Injections

Botulinum toxin A injections act by decreasing muscle tension at the tendon origin, which promotes pain improvement. Randomized studies show conflicting evidence of pain reduction, and all studies show reduced grip strength for several weeks after injection. Many patients also experience transient weakness in finger extension. This therapy does not improve quality of life and is therefore less favorable. Overall, the current evidence on the use of botulinum toxin is insufficient and further studies on optimal dosing and administration are needed.

12.6.6.6 Prolotherapy

It consists of an injection composed of a hypertonic glucose solution that is believed to stimulate healing and strengthening of degenerative tendon tissue by inciting inflammation followed by collagen deposition and remodeling. Multiple randomized studies have been conducted with conflicting evidence on efficacy, pain scores, and grip strength.

12.6.6.7 Percutaneous Radiofrequency

Percutaneous radiofrequency consists of the introduction of a radiofrequency electrode, usually guided by ultrasound at the origin of the musculature. The thermal lesion produces a micro-rupture of the tendon with subsequent repair. It shows promising results, comparable to those of open surgery [20].

12.7 Surgical Treatment

In general, surgical treatment is reserved for patients who do not improve after the application of several conservative treatment modalities (lasting more than 6 months) and provided that other concomitant pathology is ruled out. As mentioned above, the vast majority of patients tend to improve; however, 4%–10% of recalcitrant LE patients who are not satisfied with nonsurgical modalities may require surgical intervention, with "good" or "excellent" results in 80%–90% of cases.

All surgical techniques are based on debridement and resection of the angiofibroblastic tissue with or without subsequent tendon repair. This debridement can be performed open, percutaneously, or arthroscopically. There is still controversy and little evidence as to which technique is superior. Three factors affect the choice of treatment: (1) the ability to visualize the elbow joint (to rule out other pathologies), (2) the complication rate, and (3) the duration of the surgical procedure. Some surgeons perform hybrid techniques associating surgical techniques with injections.

12.7.1 Open Techniques

These are the most commonly used and aim to debride the origin of the ECRB tendon through an incision over the lateral epicondyle. In the classic Nirschl technique [21], a controlled debriding of the ECRB is performed, the fibers are divided longitudinally, and the angiofibroblastic tissue is resected. Subsequently, the tendon can be repaired or lengthened, along with various gestures such as decortication or epicondyle perforation to promote blood supply and healing. The author reported a 97.7% improvement in a series of 88 elbows.

In 2008 Dunn et al., in a retrospective study, demonstrated sustained high rates of long-term satisfaction for 139 procedures using the Nirschl mini-open surgical technique, with a 97% improvement rate over an average of 12.6 years of follow-up after surgery [22].

Coleman et al. reported their 15 years of experience in the treatment of refractory LE. Among 158 consecutive patients treated with open surgery, 94.6% achieved good or excellent results with a mean follow-up of 9.8 years [23]. However, these results were not compared with the control group.

The open technique provides direct visualization of the lesion and provides excellent results, decreasing the surgical time and the cost of surgery when compared with other surgical techniques. On the other hand, it has been observed that it presents a slight increase in the infection rate. Also, excessive tissue resection can affect the lateral ligamentous complex, producing joint instability.

12.7.2 Percutaneous Release

This procedure involves the release of the extensor carpi radialis brevis using local anesthesia at the point of origin at the epicondyle. Mill's manipulation (full elbow extension with full forearm pronation and full wrist flexion) is then performed [24]. Nazar et al. reported good results with this technique despite being a relatively simple procedure. It is performed as an outpatient procedure and no complications have been reported, with complete pain relief in 87% off the cases. However, this procedure remains controversial [25].

In recent years, a novel technique called ultrasound-guided percutaneous tenotomy (UGPT) has been reported as a safe and effective procedure for the treatment of LE, with lasting improvements in terms of symptoms, function, and ultrasound imaging at 1-year follow-up. Seng et al. demonstrated in a series of 20 patients that this procedure provides sustained pain relief and functional improvement for recalcitrant cases at 3-year follow-up. They state that it is one of the few procedures that demonstrates positive sonographic evidence of tissue healing response [26]. Recently, Chalian et al. saw in 37 patients that UGPT significantly improves symptoms and function in patients with LE, also with long-term follow-up over 3 years. Post-procedure rehabilitation was associated with improved response to treatment and the authors suggest it should be considered after UGPT [27]. Ang et al. have shown that these UGPT results are maintained over the longer term, 90 months in 20 patients [28].

12.7.3 Arthroscopic Technique

In recent years, the arthroscopic technique has become increasingly popular. The patient is placed in lateral or supine decubitus and two portals are usually used. Both debridement and tendon repair can be performed arthroscopically. The main advantage, in addition to the lower aggressiveness, is that it allows assessment and treatment of concomitant intra-articular pathology, such as plicae or osteochondritis dissecans. However, arthroscopy has a high learning curve, prolongs surgical time, and is not exempt from producing iatrogenesis (e.g., injury to the lateral ulnar collateral ligament or the posterior interosseous nerve). Also, tissue resection may be incomplete. Jerosch et al. reported good results for this technique in Germany [29]. Baker described improvement in 26 of 30 (97%) patients in whom pathologic tissue is debrided by arthroscopy at a mean follow-up of 130 months, suggesting that the long-term benefits of arthroscopic release are sustained over time [30]. Behazin and Kachooei described, in a prospective study of 11 patients, the use of a no. 11 scalpel to cut the ECRB tendon perpendicular to its fibers at the level of the radiocapitellar joint, which requires a shorter operating time compared to tissue debridement [31].

In general, excellent results have been reported with the arthroscopic technique, similar in effectiveness to those of open techniques [32]. The vast majority of patients who undergo surgery present good clinical results. However, there are a number of cases with no improvement despite the surgical treatment. Among the causes of surgical failure are infection, technical errors (over- or under-resection/repair), the patient's occupational interests, or failure to diagnose concomitant pathology.

12.8 Results

12.8.1 Surgical Versus Nonsurgical

The main dispute about surgical interventions for LE concerns their effectiveness compared to wait-and-see, conservative, or less invasive procedures. A recent systematic review by Bateman et al. suggests that surgical interventions are no more effective than nonsurgical and sham interventions. Procedural modifications may improve the comparative effectiveness of surgical interventions. High-quality randomized controlled trials are lacking, and specifically none has compared surgery with a placebo intervention [33].

Merolla et al. performed a prospective study of 101 patients randomized to PRP injection or arthroscopic ECRB release and found that PRP patients experienced significant worsening of pain at 2 years, while arthroscopic release ensured better long-term outcomes in terms of pain relief and recovery of grip strength [34]. Watt et al. performed a prospective study randomizing LE patients to open surgical release (41 patients) or leukocyte-rich PRP injection (40 patients). Leukocyte-rich PRP and surgery produced an equivalent functional outcome, but surgery may result in lower pain scores at 12 months. Seventy percent of patients treated with platelet-rich plasma avoided surgery [35]. Boden et al. retrospectively compared the effects of PRP versus UGPT procedures in the treatment of medial and lateral epicondylitis. No statistically significant differences were found between the two treatment modalities. They concluded that PRP and UGPT procedures were effective regarding pain relief, improvement of function, and quality of life [36].

12.8.2 Open Versus Arthroscopic

Overall, a small number of comparative studies suggest that open and arthroscopic techniques are comparable and highly effective for the treatment of chronic LE. Moradi et al. in a systematic review of clinical outcomes of open versus arthroscopic surgery for LE suggested that, despite no superiority for either technique in terms of pain relief, subjective function, and better rehabilitation, postoperative complications were significantly higher in the open group compared to the arthroscopic procedure (57.3% vs. 33.4%; $p = 0.001$) [37].

Wang et al. performed a systematic review and meta-analysis of trials comparing arthroscopic versus open debridement. There was no significant difference between arthroscopic and open surgery with respect to failure rate, functional outcome score, and complication rate. The meta-analysis found that arthroscopic surgery had a longer operative time than open surgery for LE [38].

12.8.3 Open Versus Arthroscopic Versus Percutaneous

All three surgical techniques for the treatment of LE demonstrate excellent results. There is moderate evidence that there are no clinically significant differences between the three surgical techniques (open, arthroscopic, and percutaneous) in terms of functional outcome (Disabilities of the Arm, Shoulder, and Hand [DASH]), pain intensity (visual analog scale [VAS]), and patient satisfaction at 1-year follow-up [39]. In contrast, Pierce et al. found that open and arthroscopic approaches resulted in higher DASH scores than the percutaneous approach, with no difference in satisfaction or complication rates. Of note, the open approach was also associated with more postoperative pain and a slightly higher risk of infection [40].

Some of the limitations of these studies include a small population size and lack of randomization. Overall, the current evidence suggests that all three surgical approaches are highly effective in the treatment of LE, and larger randomized clinical trials are needed to delineate any clinically meaningful differences between the approaches.

12.9 Conclusions

Conservative treatment resolves 90% of cases of LE. Conservative treatments can reduce the need for surgical intervention in LE. This has important cost-saving implications, as the surgical cost for LE is estimated to be between $10,000 and $12,000 [41]. NSAIDs, rehab, orthoses, and shock waves are less effective for chronic cases. CS injection, which was initially considered the gold standard treatment, may be effective in the short term, but has reduced benefit in the long term, which may be related to structural weakening of the tendon and inhibition of tenocytes. There is controversy about its effect on tendonocyte structure and healing. PRP and autologous blood are more effective in the medium term than steroids for the treatment of LE and have minimal side effects.

Controversy still persists over the best surgical approach for the management of LE. Current evidence demonstrates that open, arthroscopic, and percutaneous surgical approaches are all very effective. Arthroscopic and percutaneous approaches may provide faster recovery and earlier return to work. Open surgery is the most effective in the long term, but is the most invasive and has the longest recovery.

References

1. Smidt N, van der Windt DAWM. Tennis elbow in primary care. BMJ. 2006;333:927–8.
2. Shiri R, Viikari-Juntura E, Varonen H, Heliövaara M. Prevalence and determinants of lateral and medial epicondylitis: a population study. Am J Epidemiol. 2006;164:1065–74.
3. Orchard J, Kountouris A. The management of tennis elbow. BMJ. 2011;342:d2687.
4. Shergill R, Choudur HN. Ultrasound-guided interventions in lateral epicondylitis. J Clin Rheumatol Pract Rep Rheum Musculoskelet Dis. 2019;25:e27–34.
5. Sasaki K, Tamakawa M, Onda K, Iba K, Sonoda T, Yamashita T, et al. The detection of the capsular tear at the undersurface of the extensor carpi radialis brevis tendon in chronic tennis elbow: the value of magnetic resonance imaging and computed tomography arthrography. J Shoulder Elb Surg. 2011;20:420–5.
6. Menta R, Randhawa K, Côté P, Wong JJ, Yu H, Sutton D, et al. The effectiveness of exercise for the management of musculoskeletal disorders and injuries of the elbow, forearm, wrist, and hand: a systematic review by the Ontario Protocol for Traffic Injury Management (OPTIMa) collaboration. J Manip Physiol Ther. 2015;38:507–20.
7. Ma KL, Wang HQ. Management of lateral epicondylitis: a narrative literature review. Pain Res Manag. 2020;2020:6965381.
8. Pattanittum P, Turner T, Green S, Buchbinder R. Non-steroidal anti-inflammatory drugs (NSAIDs) for treating lateral elbow pain in adults. Cochrane Database Syst Rev. 2013;5:CD003686.

9. Yao G, Chen J, Duan Y, Chen X. Efficacy of extracorporeal shock wave therapy for lateral epicondylitis: a systematic review and meta-analysis. Biomed Res Int. 2020;2020:2064781.
10. Zheng C, Zeng D, Chen J, Liu S, Li J, Ruan Z, et al. Effectiveness of extracorporeal shock wave therapy in patients with tennis elbow: a meta-analysis of randomized controlled trials. Medicine (Baltimore). 2020;99(30):e21189.
11. Calandruccio JH, Steiner MM. Autologous blood and platelet-rich plasma injections for treatment of lateral epicondylitis. Orthop Clin North Am. 2017;48:351–7.
12. de Vos RJ, Windt J, Weir A. Strong evidence against platelet-rich plasma injections for chronic lateral epicondylar tendinopathy: a systematic review. Br J Sports Med. 2014;48:952–6.
13. Houck DA, Kraeutler MJ, Thornton LB, McCarty EC, Bravman JT. Treatment of lateral epicondylitis with autologous blood, platelet-rich plasma, or corticosteroid injections: a systematic review of overlapping meta-analyses. Orthop J Sports Med. 2019;7:2325967119831052.
14. Arirachakaran A, Sukthuayat A, Sisayanarane T, Laoratanavoraphong S, Kanchanatawan W, Kongtharvonskul J. Platelet-rich plasma versus autologous blood versus steroid injection in lateral epicondylitis: systematic review and network meta-analysis. J Orthop Traumatol Off J Ital Soc Orthop Traumatol. 2016;17:101–12.
15. Vaquero-Picado A, Barco R, Antuña SA. Lateral epicondylitis of the elbow. EFORT Open Rev. 2016;1:391–7.
16. Tang S, Wang X, Wu P, Wu P, Yang J, Du Z, et al. Platelet-rich plasma vs autologous blood vs corticosteroid injections in the treatment of lateral epicondylitis: a systematic review, pairwise and network meta-analysis of randomized controlled trials. PM R. 2020;12:397–409.
17. Linnanmäki L, Kanto K, Karjalainen T, Leppänen OV, Lehtinen J. Platelet-rich plasma or autologous blood do not reduce pain or improve function in patients with lateral epicondylitis: a randomized controlled trial. Clin Orthop Relat Res. 2020;478:1892–900.
18. Simental-Mendía M, Vilchez-Cavazos F, Álvarez-Villalobos N, Blázquez-Saldaña J, Peña-Martínez V, Villarreal-Villarreal G, et al. Clinical efficacy of platelet-rich plasma in the treatment of lateral epicondylitis: a systematic review and meta-analysis of randomized placebo-controlled clinical trials. Clin Rheumatol. 2020;39:2255–65.
19. Karjalainen TV, Silagy M, O'Bryan E, Johnston RV, Cyril S, Buchbinder R. Autologous blood and platelet-rich plasma injection therapy for lateral elbow pain. Cochrane Database Syst Rev. 2021;9(9):CD010951.
20. Lee J-H, Park I, Hyun H-S, Shin S-J. A comparison of radiofrequency-based microtenotomy and arthroscopic release of the extensor carpi radialis brevis tendon in recalcitrant lateral epicondylitis: a prospective randomized controlled study. Arthroscopy. 2018;34:1439–46.
21. Nirschl RT. Lateral epicondylitis/tendinosis. In: Morrey B, Sanchez-Sotelo J, Morrey M, editors. Morrey's the elbow and its disorders. Elsevier; 2018. p. 574–81.
22. Dunn JH, Kim JJ, Davis L, Nirschl RP. Ten- to 14-year follow-up of the Nirschl surgical technique for lateral epicondylitis. Am J Sports Med. 2008;36:261–6.
23. Coleman B, Quinlan JF, Matheson JA. Surgical treatment for lateral epicondylitis: a long-term follow-up of results. J Shoulder Elb Surg. 2010;19:363–7.
24. Yigit Ş. Medium-term results after treatment of percutaneous tennis elbow release under local anaesthesia. Acta Biomed. 2020;91:305–39.
25. Nazar M, Lipscombe S, Morapudi S, Tuvo G, Kebrle R, Marlow W, et al. Percutaneous tennis elbow release under local anaesthesia. Open Orthop J. 2012;6:129–32.
26. Seng C, Mohan PC, Koh SBJ, Howe TS, Lim YG, Lee BP, et al. Ultrasonic percutaneous tenotomy for recalcitrant lateral elbow tendinopathy. Am J Sports Med. 2015;44:504–10.
27. Chalian M, Nacey NC, Rawat U, Knight J, Lancaster T, Deal DN, et al. Ultrasound-guided percutaneous needle tenotomy using Tenex system for refractory lateral epicondylitis; short and long-term effectiveness and contributing factors. Skelet Radiol. 2021;50:2049–57.
28. Ang BFH, Mohan PC, Png MA, Allen JC Jr, Howe TS, Koh JSB, et al. Ultrasonic percutaneous tenotomy for recalcitrant lateral elbow tendinopathy: clinical and sonographic results at 90 months. Am J Sports Med. 2021;49:1854–60.
29. Jerosch J, Schunck J. Arthroscopic treatment of lateral epicondylitis: indication, technique and early results. Knee Surg Sports Traumatol Arthrosc. 2006;14:379–82.
30. Baker CL Jr, Baker CL 3rd. Long-term follow-up of arthroscopic treatment of lateral epicondylitis. Am J Sports Med. 2008;36:254–60.
31. Behazin M, Kachooei AR. Arthroscopic recession technique in the surgery of tennis elbow by sharp cutting the extensor carpi radialis brevis (ECRB) tendon origin. Arch Bone Jt Surg. 2021;9:174–9.
32. Savoie FH, O'Brien MJ. Arthroscopic tennis elbow release. Instr Course Lect. 2015;64:225–30.
33. Bateman M, Littlewood C, Rawson B, Tambe AA. Surgery for tennis elbow: a systematic review. Shoulder Elbow. 2019;11:35–44.
34. Merolla G, Dellabiancia F, Ricci A, Mussoni MP, Nucci S, Zanoli G, et al. Arthroscopic debridement versus platelet-rich plasma injection: a prospective, randomized, comparative study of chronic lateral epicondylitis with a nearly 2-year follow-up. Arthroscopy. 2017;33:1320–9.
35. Watts AC, Morgan BW, Birch A, Nuttall D, Trail IA. Comparing leukocyte-rich platelet-rich plasma injection with surgical intervention for the management of refractory tennis elbow. A prospective randomised trial. Shoulder Elbow. 2020;12:46–53.

36. Boden AL, Scott MT, Dalwadi PP, Mautner K, Mason RA, Gottschalk MB. Platelet-rich plasma versus Tenex in the treatment of medial and lateral epicondylitis. J Shoulder Elb Surg. 2019;28:112–9.
37. Moradi A, Pasdar P, Mehrad-Majd H, Ebrahimzadeh MH. Clinical outcomes of open versus arthroscopic surgery for lateral epicondylitis: evidence from a systematic review. Arch Bone Jt Surg. 2019;7:91–104.
38. Wang W, Chen J, Lou J, Shentu G, Xu G. Comparison of arthroscopic debridement and open debridement in the management of lateral epicondylitis: a systematic review and meta-analysis. Medicine (Baltimore). 2019;98(44):e17668.
39. Burn MB, Mitchell RJ, Liberman SR, Lintner DM, Harris JD, McCulloch PC. Open, arthroscopic, and percutaneous surgical treatment of lateral epicondylitis: a systematic review. Hand (N Y). 2018;13:264–74.
40. Pierce TP, Issa K, Gilbert BT, Hanly B, Festa A, McInerney VK, et al. A systematic review of tennis elbow surgery: open versus arthroscopic versus percutaneous release of the common extensor origin. Arthroscopy. 2017;33:1260–8.
41. Lai WC, Erickson BJ, Mlynarek RA, Wang D. Chronic lateral epicondylitis: challenges and solutions. Open Access J Sports Med. 2018;9:243–51.

Total Elbow Arthroplasty

13

Raul Barco and E. Carlos Rodríguez-Merchán

13.1 Introduction

Total elbow arthroplasty (TEA) is a rare intervention. In 2016, the Dutch Arthroplasty Register included about 400 elbow arthroplasties compared with 28,000 hip arthroplasties and 27,000 knee arthroplasties overall. TEA is usually performed after other treatments aimed at relieving pain and improving joint function have been tried: either conservative treatment with physical medicine and rehabilitation and analgesics or surgical such as arthroscopic joint debridement. In patients with mild to moderate elbow osteoarthritis (OA) and in young patients, these therapeutic options are preferable, as they delay the need for TEA. For each patient, the most appropriate implant should be chosen on the basis of its stability and extensibility; that is, a decision should be made whether to use an unlinked implant, which has less intrinsic stability, or a linked implant, which has more intrinsic stability; it should also be decided whether or not the replacement of the ulnohumeral joint should be accompanied by a replacement of the radiocapitellar joint [1].

Total joint replacements for the treatment of elbow arthritis were developed in the late 1960s, at the same time as total joint replacements for the treatment of knee arthritis. Since then, the number of arthritis patients treated with total knee joint replacements has been steadily increasing, in contrast to TEA, which has been decreasing since its peak in the 1990s. The main reasons for this decline are the continuing controversy over implant design, the relatively high rates of complications associated with TEA, the difficulties often encountered in revision surgery, and recent changes in the population of patients treated with TEA [2].

As published in 2021 by Poff et al., TEA is an effective treatment for multiple elbow pathologies. However, those authors identified a marked decline in the use of TEA after 2011. The article by Poff et al. also showed that from 2002 to 2017, TEA was primarily performed on fracture-related elbow problems. However, inflammatory arthropathy-related TEA steadily decreased during that time period, although it was the second most frequent diagnosis. The aforementioned article also showed that during the period 2002–2017, TEA was most frequently used in women over 65 years of age with various comorbidities [3].

The Australian Orthopaedic Association National Joint Replacement Registry (AOANJRR) was analyzed in 2019 by Vivieen et al. to determine trends in primary TEA use, types of prostheses used, primary diagnoses, causes and types of revision, and whether primary diagnosis or prosthetic design influenced

R. Barco · E. C. Rodríguez-Merchán (✉)
Department of Orthopedic Surgery, La Paz University Hospital-IdiPaz, Madrid, Spain

E. C. Rodríguez-Merchán, A. Moreno-Garcìa (eds.), *Controversies in Orthopedic Surgery of The Upper Limb*, https://doi.org/10.1007/978-3-031-04907-1_13

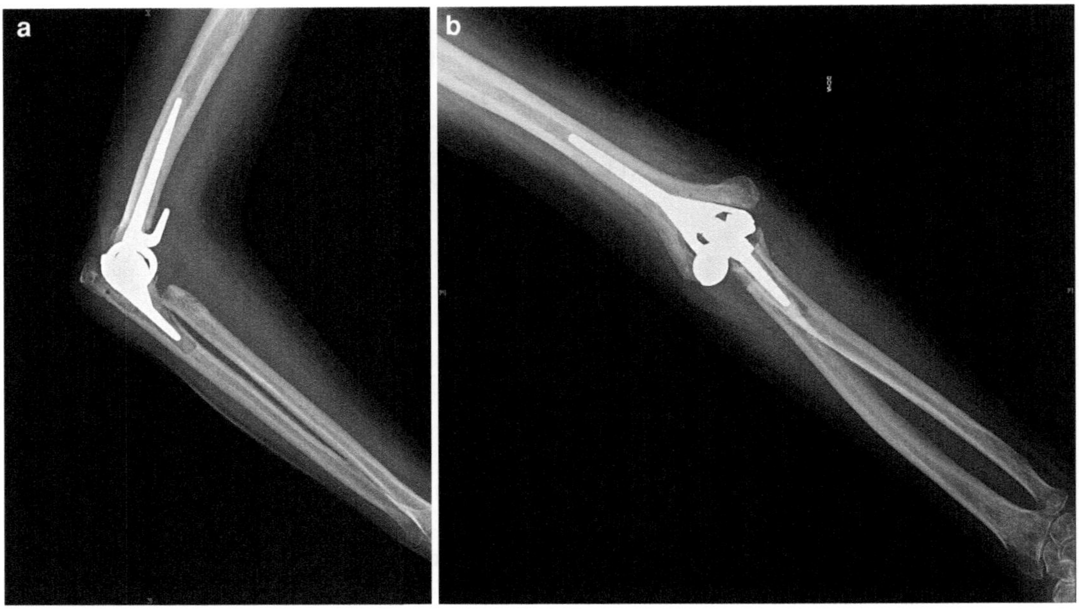

Fig. 13.1 (**a**, **b**) Loosening of both components. A major cause for loosening of both components is infection and should always be ruled out. When loosening affects only to one component, infection still remains the first cause to investigate but component loosening due to bushing wear or an incorrect cementing technique can be contributing factors. (**a**) Lateral view and (**b**) anteroposterior (AP) view

revision rate. During 2008–2018, 1220 primary TEAs were recorded, of which 140 were revised. Kaplan-Meier survival estimates were used to determine time to first revision and hazard ratios from Cox proportional hazard models, adjusted for age and sex, to compare revision rates. The annual number of TEAs performed was held constant. The three most frequent diagnoses for a primary TEA were fracture/dislocation (trauma) (36%), OA (34%), and rheumatoid arthritis (RA) (26%). The cumulative percentage of revision of all TEAs performed for any reason was 10%, 15%, and 19% at 3, 6, and 9 years, respectively. TEAs performed for OA had a higher revision rate than TEAs performed for trauma. The most commonly used prosthetic designs were Coonrad-Morrey (50%), Latitude (30%), Nexel (10%), and Discovery (9%). There was no difference in revision rates when comparing the four aforementioned designs. The most common causes of revision were infection (35%) and aseptic loosening (34%) (Fig. 13.1). Vivieen et al. also noted that the indications for primary and revision TEA in Australia were similar to those reported in other registries. However, revisions for trauma were lower than previously published in other registries [4].

In this chapter we will review the literature on primary and revision TEA in an attempt to clarify some of the current controversies surrounding these surgical interventions.

13.2 Primary TEA

13.2.1 Biomechanics

To optimize outcomes and minimize complications of a primary TEA, it is critical to understand its biomechanics. Nonconstrained TEA prostheses have little intrinsic stability and rely on soft tissue balance. The medial and lateral collateral ligaments are the main stabilizers of nonconstrained TEAs. The anterior capsule, posterior capsule, and surrounding muscles act as secondary stabilizers. There are implants not bound by a hinge mechanism that can be very constrained by virtue of their high degree of articular compliance. Semiconstrained TEAs use a hinge mechanism that allows small degrees of off-axis movement in order to reduce stress on the bone-cement interface of the components. During implantation, the components reproduce the alignment and rotation of the elbow axis. Malalignment of the components will increase the bending and torsional loading of the implant and may contribute to premature aseptic loosening and polyethylene wear. However, axis landmarks may not be present in some revision surgeries or fracture surgeries, which hinder proper implantation. Most current TEA systems employ Morrey's anterior flange design on the humeral implant, which reduces rotational stress at the bone-cement interface (as compared to a purely intramedullary humeral component) and counteracts extension forces at the elbow. If the flange does not have adequate contact with the anterior cortex, it should be augmented with a bone wedge. The anterior flange and the semi-constrained articulation are considered to be the main reasons why current designs outperform constrained hinged designs [5].

13.2.2 Patient Selection

Most of the existing TEA designs since the early 1970s have been successful in treating patients with severe degenerative changes secondary to RA, which was originally the main surgical indication. In the mid-1990s, the type of patients changed, as effective drugs against RA became available and, consequently, patients with RA became rare. The disease-modifying drugs have served to preserve normal bone architecture and, as a result, the elbows of RA patients increasingly resemble those of patients with OA. However, TEA has been less successful in treating patients with OA than in treating patients with RA. Consequently, since the mid-1990s, surgeons performing TEA have become increasingly aware that their results are less satisfactory than those they obtained in the past. Thus, despite further improvements in implant design, surgeons are increasingly reluctant to recommend TEA for the treatment of elbow arthritis. The use of TEA for fractures began in rheumatic patients with severe joint involvement who suffered a fracture of the columns. Good initial results facilitated its extension of use to patients without inflammatory disease [2, 6].

13.2.3 Preoperative Planning

The preoperative planning of a TEA is relatively handcrafted. There are several stem thicknesses, various stem lengths, and anterior lozenge (flange) lengths, providing hundreds of possible combinations. Component orientation is based on coarse bone references, although these are assumed to be predictable. The use of newer technologies for planning may help to improve component positioning and, perhaps, improve implant survival.

In 2018, Iwamoto et al. analyzed the role of computed tomography-based three-dimensional preoperative planning for unlinked TEA. In a basic science (computer modeling) study, they observed that 3-D surgical planning enabled accurate calculation of implant size and proper placement of implant components. They analyzed 28 patients operated on for TEA with an unlinked total elbow implant (unlinked-type K-NOW implant [Teijin-Nakashima Medical, Okayama, Japan]). With two-dimensional planning, humeral stem sizes were accurately estimated in 57% of patients and 68% of ulnar stems, compared with 86% for the humerus and 96% for the ulna with 3D planning. The mean differences between the prosthesis positions after surgery with respect to the planned positions were 0.8° of varus and 1.5° of flexion for the humeral component and 0.7° of varus and 2.9° of flexion for the ulnar component. Rotational position was not evaluated in this study. The method described by Iwamoto et al. could help reduce the complication rate of TEA and improve its long-term outcomes [7].

13.2.4 Surgical Approaches for TEA

Most elbow approaches use a posterior midline skin incision with full-thickness flaps and identify the ulnar nerve early. It is generally accepted that the nerve should be identified early and decompressed superficially and protected throughout the procedure. However, the nerve is at risk when manipulated, and whether or not to transpose it depends on the surgeon's preference. Transposition is recommended when there is a previous nerve deficit or when the prosthesis affects the usual nerve pathway. However, the risk of injuring the blood supply to the nerve has led some authors to advocate leaving it in its bed with its deep soft tissues, in order to reduce the risk of postoperative neuritis. Trans-olecranon osteotomy is rarely used due to the involvement of the ulna for insertion and fixation of the component. Approaches can be broadly classified into triceps-on and triceps-off. Triceps-on approaches maintain the triceps mechanism and its insertion into the ulna. Triceps-off approaches imply that part or all of the triceps is removed from its insertion into the ulna or that the triceps mechanism is cut at some point. Triceps-off approaches can be subdivided into triceps turndown, triceps elevating, or triceps splitting. A triceps turndown involves cutting the triceps tendon above the ulnar insertion. A triceps elevating approach elevates the triceps off the ulna subperiosteally. A triceps splitting approach splits the triceps tendon longitudinally along its length and across its insertion. The triceps-on approach has functional advantages over the other approaches, although it provides reduced exposure that may compromise the correct position of the implants [8].

Some patients with inflammatory disease may have a compromised triceps insertion and in these cases a triceps-on approach may be chosen, generally respecting the triceps tendon. The most commonly used are the Alonso-Llames bilaterotricipital approach and the lateral para-olecranial approach [9]. All of them affect in some way the comfort of implant placement, especially the ulnar component. Recently, Celli and Bonucci published their experience with the anconeus-triceps lateral flap approach for TEA in patients with RA. They suggested that the decision not to separate the medial insertion of the triceps influenced the risk of triceps insufficiency and allowed patients to begin an active, unrestricted rehabilitation program earlier. It also provided adequate surgical exposure of the olecranon articular surface, particularly in patients with severe elbow joint deformity. This type of approach allowed adequate alignment between the olecranon and the posterior surface of the ulna, without interfering with the entire triceps muscle tendon between the two planes. The relationship between the two aforementioned planes was an important landmark during the implantation of the ulnar component. Whichever triceps-on approach is used, two windows are used (one medial and one through the per se approach), and one must try to dislocate the elbow through the surgical window in the position where the ulnar nerve is protected and free of tension and the exposure is adequate to achieve the correct orientation of the implant [10].

In 2018, in a level IV therapeutic study (case series), Na et al. evaluated the clinical outcomes and extensor strengths of primary TEAs implanted with a modified triceps fascial tongue approach. They concluded that it was an easy and effective approach for primary TEA, which prevented triceps weakness after arthroplasty. Triceps strength was normal (Medical Research Council [MRC] grade V) in 10 elbows (48%) and good (MRC grade IV) in 11 (52%). Triceps strength after arthroplasty was significantly improved over preoperative strength. This approach is a modification of the classic Campbell approach. They share the advantage that suprafascial dissection is minimal compared to approaches in which the triceps is approached medially and laterally but carries the potential risk of fascial tongue necrosis [11].

According to a level IV therapeutic study reported by Cottias et al., the digastric olecranon osteotomy approach allowed excellent joint exposure and preserved the main vascular supply and continuity of the extensor apparatus. These authors evaluated the early clinical and radiological results after Coonrad-Morrey-type TEAs were implanted using the aforementioned approach. The mean age of the patients was 80 years (range: 50–96). The causes of the interventions were 20 fractures, 2 malunions, and 4 elbows with RA. The mean follow-up time was

30 months (range: 6–132). At the last evaluation, the mean flexion arc increased from 23° to 112°. The Mayo Elbow Performance Score (MEPS) was 92 points on average. Mean triceps strength in extension and flexion was 1.9 and 4.7 kg, respectively. All elbows were stable. There was a single wound infection in the immediate postoperative period, which did not require any surgical revision. Heterotopic ossifications were observed in one elbow. One patient suffered an elbow dislocation due to fracture of the axe's component. The clinical and radiological results encountered were considered promising and supported the use of the digastric olecranon osteotomy for the implantation of TEAs [12].

13.2.5 Outcomes of TEA

13.2.5.1 Thirty-Day Readmissions and Reoperations After TEA

Cutler et al. have published that the 30-day unplanned reoperation rate was 2.4%, and the unplanned readmission rate was 5.1%. A low BMI (body mass index) predicted readmission. Contaminated or dirty wounds were predictors of reoperation. Dependent functional status and contaminated wounds were predictors of local complications. The indication for TEA (fracture vs. OA vs. RA) was a risk factor for reoperation or readmission after TEA [13].

13.2.5.2 Long-Term Outcomes of TEA

Davey et al. published a systematic review of the literature (level IV evidence) in which they evaluated functional outcomes and dislocation and revision rates of TEA. The mean minimum follow-up was 10 years. They analyzed 23 publications that included 1429 elbows (60.4% linked TEA) that met the inclusion criteria. There were 1276 patients (79% female), with a mean age of 64.7 years (range: 19–93). The mean follow-up was 137.2 months (range: 120–216). At final evaluation, the mean MEPS, Oxford Elbow Score, and Quick DASH (Disabilities of the Arm, Shoulder and Hand) scores were 89.1, 64.4, and 39.2, respectively. Further, 63.3% of patients claimed to be pain-free. The rates of aseptic loosening, infection, implant dislocation, and nerve injury were 12.9%, 3.3%, 4.2%, and 2.1%, respectively. The overall complication and revision rates were 16.3% and 14.6%, respectively [14].

13.2.5.3 Risk Factors for Reoperation After TEA

A traumatic indication has a higher risk of reoperation than other indications according to several studies. The reason is unclear and may be related to a worse patient condition that may affect immune status, wound healing capacity, use of canes for ambulation, or increased frequency of falls.

In a level IV evidence therapeutic study (case series), primary TEAs performed in two hospitals were retrospectively reviewed. Perretta et al. identified 102 primary TEAs in 82 patients performed by nine surgeons. The mean age of the patients was 61 years. Women accounted for 81% of the TEAs performed. The mean follow-up was 6.1 years. The main diagnosis was inflammatory arthritis in 63 patients (62%), acute or posttraumatic trauma in 28 (27%) and primary OA in 9 (8.8%). The mean reoperation rate was 41%. The mean time to first reoperation was 1.8 years. The percentage of elbows in which one or both components were revised was 30%. The most frequent indication for reoperation was component loosening (Fig. 13.1). Six elbows were treated with resection arthroplasty, and in one elbow fusion was performed. The implant revision rate was 27% for inflammatory arthritis, 11% for OA, and 57% for trauma. Trauma-related TEA was more likely to require additional reoperation and implant revision [15].

13.2.5.4 Mid- to Long-Term Survivorship of Cemented Semiconstrained "Discovery" TEA

In 2021, Borton et al. presented a mid- to long-term survivorship study of the "Discovery" TEA, with a follow-up of 5–12 years. This implant contains a spherical bearing designed to minimize polyethylene wear. According to the Kaplan-Meier method, they demonstrated an implant survival of 76.8% at 119 months. Borton et al. analyzed 67 TEAs in 58 patients, with a mean follow-up since surgery of 98.5 months. Four cases (6%) were lost to follow-up. The implant was revised in 14 cases (20.9%). There was a significant difference in survival between dominant and nondominant elbows (Breslow test $p = 0.012$). Elbow dominance implied a 4.5-fold increased risk of revision [16].

13.2.6 Complications After TEA

13.2.6.1 Periprosthetic Infection: Resection Arthroplasty

Resection arthroplasty is sometimes the best or only effective alternative to treat some of the complications of failed implants. It is surprising how well some of these patients can function, in some cases with remarkable elbow stability and good hand grip strength.

In 2016, Rhee et al., in a level IV evidence therapeutic study (case series), published their results on the use of resection arthroplasty for the treatment of infections after TEA and the factors that influenced them. They stated that resection arthroplasty may be an acceptable salvage treatment for infections after TEA in low-demand patients. They published that to achieve a successful outcome, both columns of the distal humerus should be preserved at the time of implant removal. They analyzed 10 resection arthroplasties (nine patients) for infection after TEA. The mean follow-up was 52.4 months. According to the remnant distal humerus bone stock, the elbows were divided into three groups: lateral column, medial column, and both columns. The mean time to resolution of clinical infection symptoms and normalization of serologic markers after resection was 6.8 days and 68.5 days, respectively. The mean MEPS and DASH scores changed from 50 and 46.5 preoperatively to 73.5 and 53 at the end of follow-up ($p < 0.001$ and $p < 0.001$, respectively). Although not significant, the both-column group showed better functional outcomes (MEPS 80; DASH score 43.7) than either the lateral column (74, 54.6) or medial column (62.5, 63) groups. The mean satisfaction score at the end of follow-up was 70. Only one case required additional operations to treat recurrent infection. There were no refractory infections, no fractures, and no permanent nerve lesions. This work reflects the importance of the integrity of the columns in the stability of the ulnar remnant after resection. It is important to note that in distal fractures of both columns, many surgeons choose to resect the columns for the sake of quick and operative resolution. It is neither clear whether devoting surgical time to reconstructing the columns is an appropriate strategy, nor is it clear what the ideal method of achieving such fixation is [17].

13.2.6.2 Heterotopic Ossification Following TEA

In 2018, Robinson et al. analyzed the incidence of heterotopic ossification in 55 elective ($n = 29$) and traumatic ($n = 26$) TEAs (52 patients). Throughout follow-up 15 patients (17 TEAs) died of unrelated causes. There were 14 men and 38 women, with a mean age of 70 years. The mean clinical follow-up was 3.6 years and the mean radiological follow-up was 3.1 years. The overall incidence of heterotopic ossification was 84%. The overall incidence was higher in the trauma group (96%) than in the elective arthroplasty group (72%). In addition, patients in the trauma group had heterotopic ossification of higher Brooker class. The presence of heterotopic ossification did not significantly affect elbow range of motion (ROM) within the trauma or elective groups. These findings are not surprising and in general are not going to affect the evolution of the patients so it is not advisable to perform any associated medical (indomethacin) or physical (radiotherapy) treatment in the trauma group [18].

13.2.6.3 Component Fracture After TEA

Component fracture can be defined as a failure of the material to withstand cyclic loading (Fig. 13.2). This is more frequent in some designs with material changes, with wedges, notches, or different surface treatments on the same component. The presence of osteolysis in which the

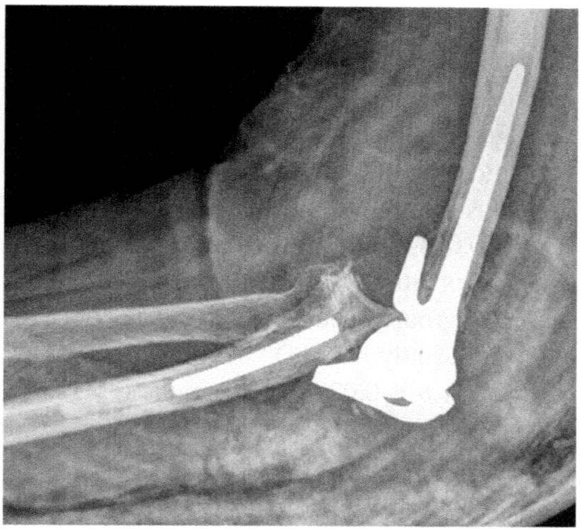

Fig. 13.2 Component fracture. The radiograph shows a broken ulnar component at the site of a notch of this particular ulnar component. The site of rupture occurs usually at the point where the ulnar component becomes unsupported from the ulna, typically at the olecranon in patients in which the ulnar component insertion was introduced slightly in flexion

implant is uncovered and has to bear the full mechanical load seems to favor this complication.

According to Lee et al., ulnar or humeral component stem fractures after TEA are serious complications. In a retrospective therapeutic level III evidence study, they reported that a component stem fracture after TEA appears to be caused by fatigue failure at or near the junction between an unsupported stem and well-fixed stem (Fig. 13.2). This area of unsupported stem occurs as a result of osteolysis caused by bushing wear. To avoid fracture of the components, bushing wear needs to be addressed. A total of 2637 primary and revision TEAs were analyzed. It was found that 47 operations (in 46 patients) were performed to treat component stem fractures. Bushing wear was graded according to percentage loss of polyethylene thickness and metal wear. In the 39 cases in which bushing wear could be quantified, it was severe in 34, moderate in 2, and mild in 3. All 47 cases showed evidence of periarticular osteolysis, which was found in zone 1 in 17 cases, in zones 1 and 2 in 29, and diffusely in 1 case. The mean length of the well-fixed stem, expressed as a percentage of the total length of the stem, was 63%. Stem fractures occurred most frequently (27 of 47 cases) at the junction between the well-fixed stem and unsupported stem. Some studies have associated bushing wear with the presence of osteolysis, but it is probably not the only cause. Measurement of polyethylene wear is sometimes complex because it is performed in static positions and may risk underdiagnosis. It is important to recognize that different designs have different degrees of freedom and it is necessary to be aware of these in order to correctly calculate polyethylene wear [19].

13.2.6.4 Humeral Amputation Following TEA

Claxton et al. analyzed the incidence and etiology of upper extremity amputations in patients who had previously undergone TEA implantation ($n = 1906$). Upper extremity amputation was performed in seven (0.36%) elbows (seven patients): five transhumeral amputations and two shoulder disarticulations. There were five women and two men, mean age 64 years. The TEAs had been implanted for RA ($n = 2$), for RA with acute fracture ($n = 2$), for radiation-associated nonunion ($n = 2$), and for metastatic cancer ($n = 1$). The mean follow-up after amputation was 3 years. The mean time between amputation and TEA was 5 years. Indications for amputation were uncontrolled deep infection in six (86%) elbows and tumor recurrence in one (14%) elbow. Only one (14%) elbow was fitted with a prosthesis. Six (86%) patients died after a mean of 3 years after amputation [20].

13.2.7 Inpatient Versus Outpatient TEA

There is a trend in the USA to transition arthroplasty procedures from inpatient to outpatient centers, generally in ambulatory surgical centers. The change is that the cost of the episode decreases dramatically and that there is a favorable alignment between the interests of providers and funders. Whether this benefit extends to patients is under study. In 2020, Furman et al. compared the outcomes and short-term complications of TEA in the inpatient and outpatient operative settings in a level III evidence-based retrospective therapeutic study using a large database. They analyzed 575 patients operated on for TEA (458 were inpatient procedures and 117 were outpatient procedures). Inpatient TEA had a higher rate of complications than outpatient TEA, including non-home discharge (14.9% vs. 7.5%, $p = 0.05$), unplanned hospital readmission (7.4% vs. 0.9%, $p = 0.01$), surgical complications (7.6% vs. 2.6%, $p = 0.04$), and medical complications (3.6% vs. 0%, $p = 0.04$). Obviously, the criteria to perform this procedure on an outpatient basis is stricter, so there is a bias in what type of patients go to the outpatient center, and generally patients with a higher risk of complications go to a center with hospital admission [21].

13.2.8 Elective TEA Versus TEA for Fracture in Elderly Patients

In 2009, McKee et al. published a prospective, randomized, controlled trial comparing functional outcomes, complications, and reoperation rates in elderly patients with displaced intra-articular fractures of the distal humerus treated with open reduction and internal fixation (ORIF) or primary semiconstrained TEA. Twenty-one patients were randomized to each treatment group. Inclusion criteria were age greater than 65 years; displaced, comminuted, intra-articular fractures of the distal humerus (Orthopaedic Trauma Association [OTA] type 13C) and closed or open Gustilo grade I fractures treated within 12 h of injury. Two patients died before follow-up and were excluded from the study. Five patients randomized to ORIF were intraoperatively converted to TEA because of extensive comminution and inability to achieve sufficiently stable fixation to allow early joint mobility. Finally, in the ORIF group, 15 patients (3 men and 12 women) with a mean age of 77 years were analyzed, while in the TEA group, 25 patients (2 men and 23 women) with a mean age of 78 years were analyzed. Baseline demographics regarding mechanism of injury, classification, comorbidities, fracture type, activity level, and ipsilateral injuries were similar in the two groups. The mean duration of surgery was 32 min shorter in the TEA group ($p = 0.001$). Patients who had a TEA implanted had significantly better MEPS at 3 months (83 vs. 65, $p = 0.01$), 6 months (86 vs. 68, $p = 0.003$), 12 months (88 vs. 72, $p = 0.007$), and 2 years (86 vs. 73, $p = 0.015$) than patients in the ORIF group. Patients operated on using TEA had significantly better DASH scores at 6 weeks (43 vs. 77, $p = 0.02$) and 6 months (31 vs. 50, $p = 0.01$), but not at 12 months (32 vs. 47, $p = 0.1$) or 2 years (34 vs. 38, $p = 0.6$). The mean flexion-extension arc was 107° (range, 42°–145°) in the TEA group and 95° (range, 30°–140°) in the ORIF group ($p = 0.19$). Reoperation rates for TEA (3/25 [12%]) and ORIF (4/15 [27%]) were not statistically different ($p = 0.2$). According to MEPS, TEA for the treatment of comminuted intra-articular distal humerus fractures provided better and more predictable functional outcomes than ORIF at 2-year follow-up. DASH scores were better in the TEA group in the short term, but were not statistically different at 2-year follow-up. Considering that 25% of fractures randomized to the ORIF group were not amenable to internal fixation, it appears that ORIF may cause the reoperation rate to decrease. Ultimately, McKee et al. concluded that in elderly patients with complex fractures of the distal humerus not amenable to stable fixation, implanting a TEA is preferable to performing an ORIF [22] (Fig. 13.3).

An additional question is what happens to these patients after some time. Given that ORIF complications are early and TEA complications occur throughout the history of the implant, with equal complications the only difference between the two indications would be the postoperative restrictions of TEA. In a long-term follow-up of 12.5 years in the surviving patients, the authors noted that there were 3/25 reoperations in the TEA group and 4/15 in the ORIF group. Only one patient with TEA required implant revision and 15 of the patients who died during follow-up did so with the implant in situ and functioning well [23].

It is important to appreciate that it is unclear what constitutes stable fixation in an osteoporotic patient. Additionally, the age range of the

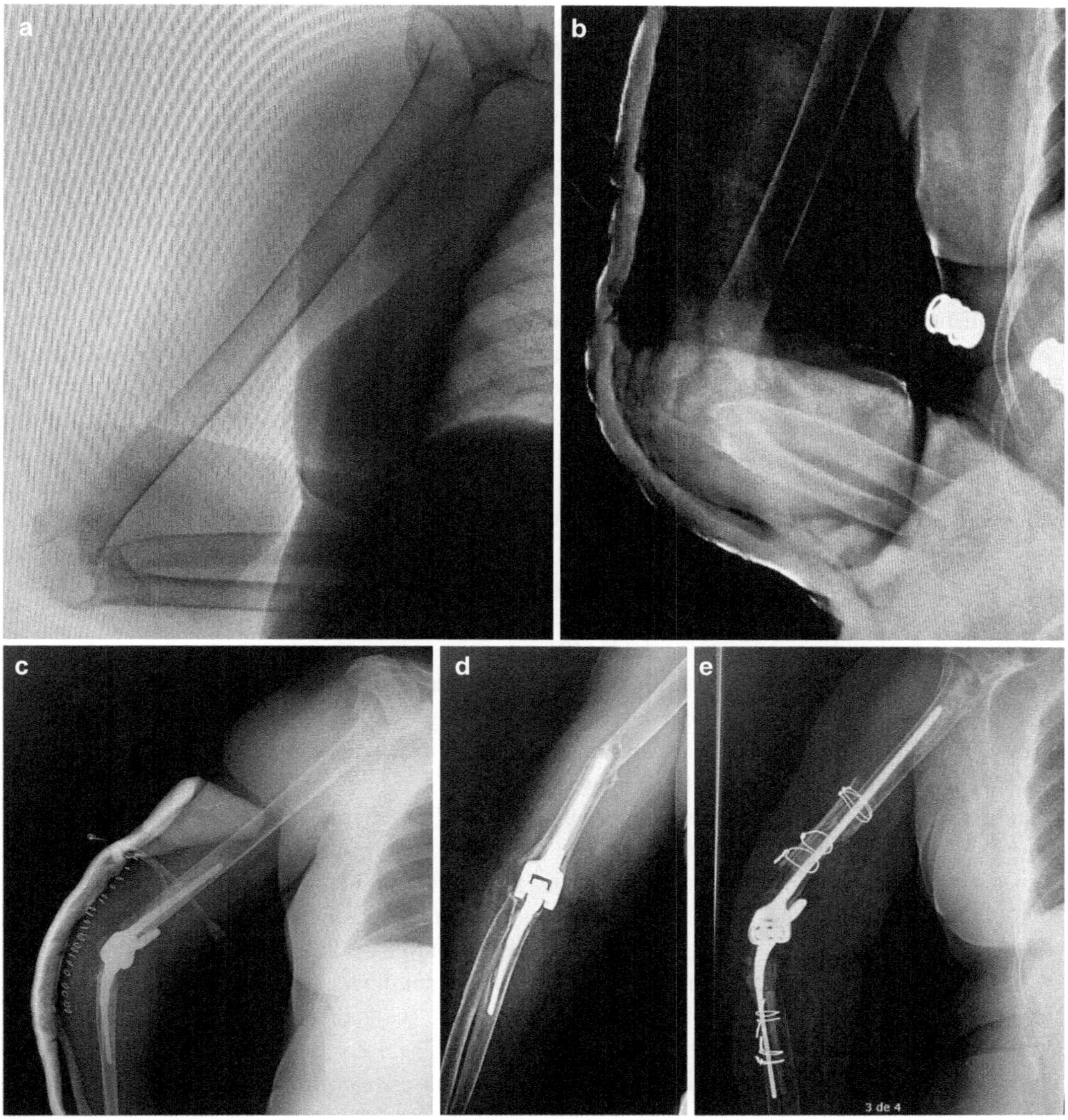

Fig. 13.3 (**a–e**) TEA for a distal humerus fracture is a good indication in cases where there is poor distal bone for fixation or extensive comminution and the patient is compliant with postoperative restrictions. However, TEA for fractures in elderly and weakened patients is subject to periprosthetic fractures which require complex revision surgery. (**a**, **b**) A patient with rheumatoid arthritis and elbow disease sustained a fall with a fracture of the proximal humerus and the distal humerus. (**c**) A linked TEA was implanted with a good outcome. (**d**) After 8 years the patient sustained a new fall with a humeral periprosthetic fracture at the tip of the humeral stem. (**e**) At revision the implant was found to be loose and a one-stage revision with longer implants and augmentation with strut allograft was performed with a good outcome

patients included is very wide and may not reflect well the different circumstances of an ORIF procedure in a 63-year-old patient versus an ORIF in an 82-year-old patient. It does seem clear that the best outcome is obtained from a single operation and that the outcome of a TEA after a failed ORIF is worse than that of a primary TEA [24].

In 2013, Mansat et al., in a case series (therapeutic study with level IV evidence), observed that reliable results can be obtained in patients with RA and in traumatic conditions and that the survival rate was similar or better than that published for unlinked implants. They analyzed 70 consecutive patients (78 elbows) who underwent implantation of a Coonrad-Morrey design TEA for inflammatory arthritis (45 elbows) or traumatic conditions (33 elbows: 18 acute distal humerus fractures, 10 nonunions, and 5 posttraumatic arthritis). Coonrad-Morrey-type TEA allowed treating a wide spectrum of indications with satisfactory results. Better results were obtained in patients with RA than in trauma patients. The complication rate was high, although the implant revision rate was low. However, with follow-up, there was an increased incidence of lucent lines around the ulnar component and bushing wear (which were of concern). After a mean follow-up of 5 years (range: 2–11 years), the mean MEPS for the RA group (89 points) was significantly higher than that of the trauma group (80 points). The QuickDASH score was not significantly different according to etiology. Radiolucencies were observed in 17 cases around the humeral component and in 14 cases around the ulnar component. Bushing wear was observed in 14 cases. There were 27 complications, 9 of which required revision surgery. Considering revision for aseptic loosening as an end point, the survival rate was 97.7% at 5 years and 91% at 10 years [25].

In 2016, Sánchez-Sotelo et al., in a therapeutic study with level IV evidence, published that elbow arthroplasty using a cemented linked semiconstrained design provided satisfactory clinical results in the treatment of RA, with a reasonable mechanical failure-free survival rate at 20 years. Although bushing wear was identified on radiographs in a quarter of the patients, revision for isolated bushing wear was infrequent. A total of 461 primary TEAs were performed with the Coonrad-Morrey prosthesis in 387 patients with RA. Fifty-five of the arthroplasties were performed to treat concurrent traumatic or posttraumatic conditions. A total of 305 women (365 elbows, 79%) and 82 men (96 elbows, 21%) underwent surgery. Ten patients (10 elbows) were lost to follow-up, 9 patients (10 elbows) died, and 6 patients (6 elbows) underwent revision surgery in the first 2 years. In the 435 elbows (362 patients, 94%) that had a minimum follow-up of 2 years, the median follow-up was 10 years (range: 2–30 years). At final evaluation, 49 (11%) of the elbows were found to have undergone surgical revision or component removal (10 elbows for deep infection, 39 elbows for mechanical failure). In another 8 elbows there was radiographic evidence of loosening. In the surviving implants, with a minimum follow-up of 2 years, the median MEPS was 90 points; in 71 (23%) of these implants bushing wear was identified radiographically; however, only 2% of the elbows had required surgical revision for isolated bushing wear. The rate of survivorship free of implant revision or removal for any reason was 92% at 10 years, 83% at 15 years, and 68% at 20 years. Survival at 20 years was 88% with revision for aseptic loosening as the end point and 89% with isolated bushing exchange as the end point. Risk factors for implant revision for any cause were male sex, history of concomitant traumatic pathology, and implantation of an ulnar component with polymethylmethacrylate surface finish [26].

In 2016, Prasad et al. published their experience with the Coonrad-Morrey TEA in distal humerus fractures in nonrheumatoid patients. The minimum follow-up was 10 years. Between 1996 and 2004 they performed TEAs through a triceps splitting approach in 37 nonrheumatoid patients with distal humerus fractures. One patient could not be located and 17 died before the tenth anniversary of surgery. Therefore, the study group consisted of 19 patients, with a minimum follow-up of 10 years. Of these, 13 patients were still alive at the time of the final assessment. The other 6 had died, but after at least 10 years of follow-up. The mean follow-up of the 19 patients was 156 months (range: 120–210). Two patients required revision surgery. Another patient underwent two-stage revision surgery for infection, but died before the 10-year follow-up. Six other patients showed signs of loosening or wear. Two were clinically symptomatic and were offered revision surgery. Male patients showed a higher incidence of loosening and wear. Survivorship, with revision and definite loosening as end points, was 89.5% at 10 years in patients with a minimum follow-up of 10 years and 86% in the entire group of 36 patients. Prasad et al. observed that only 53% of nonrheumatoid patients operated on for TEA for distal humerus fracture survived to the tenth anniversary of surgery. In those who survived, TEA provided acceptable results in terms of function and implant survival [27].

In 2017, in a level IV evidence study, Barco et al. evaluated the long-term outcomes of TEA after distal humerus fractures and compared elbows with or without inflammatory arthritis at the time of fracture. In surviving patients, they observed that the selective use of a TEA for the treatment of distal humerus fractures in elderly and less active patients and in patients with inflammatory arthritis had acceptable longevity, but with significant complications. Forty-four TEAs were performed on distal humerus fractures; minimum follow-up was 10 years. Pain, joint mobility, MEPS, complications, and reoperations were evaluated. Outcomes were compared between elbows with and without inflammatory arthritis and a Kaplan-Meier survivorship analysis was performed. TEA provided good pain relief and joint mobility. The mean visual analog scale for pain was 0.6. The mean joint flexion was 123° and the mean joint extension loss was 24°. The mean MEPS was 90.5 points, and three patients scored less than 75 points. Five elbows (11%) developed deep infection, which was treated surgically with component retention (three acute) or resection (two chronic). In eight elbows (18%) implant revision or resection was performed: three for infection (one reimplantation and two resections), three for ulnar loosening (associated with a periprosthetic fracture in one) and two for ulnar component fractures. Periprosthetic fractures occurred in five other elbows. Survival rates of TEAs in patients with RA were 85% at 5 years and 76% at 10 years. Survival rates for TEAs in patients without RA were 92% at both 5 years and 10 years. The most important risk factor for surgical revision was male sex. Since mechanical failure due to component fracture has been eliminated with the change in component design, the mechanical complications of the implant are small and most patients when they die during follow-up do so with the component "in place" [6].

In 2020, Strelzow et al., in a therapeutic study with level IV evidence, reviewed the results and complications of a cemented convertible TEA system in a linked configuration in patients with distal humerus fractures. Forty patients met the inclusion criteria (35 women, 5 men). The mean follow-up was 4 years (range: 2–13 years). The mean age of the patients at the time of surgery was 79 years. All implants were linked. Seven patients had heterotopic ossification. Lucent lines were observed mainly in the V-zone of the humeral implant. No lucent lines were observed around the ulnar component in any radiographic area. Complications occurred in nine patients (22%) and two surgical revisions were performed: one for infection and one for late periprosthetic fracture. Fracture TEA in elderly patients provided pain relief, functional range of motion, and good patient-reported outcome scores. No implant-related complications of this convertible implant system were encountered [28].

In 2021, Aziz et al. compared TEA in distal humerus fracture and arthritis cases. They analyzed in-hospital and postoperative complications 30 days after TEA implantation. A total of 646 TEAs were implanted, of which 149 (23.1%) were implanted in distal humerus fractures. Patients undergoing TEA for fracture had an overall complication rate of 13.42%, compared with a complication rate of 12.47% in patients undergoing elective primary TEA ($p = 0.76$). In univariate analysis, patients undergoing TEA for fracture were not significantly more likely to require reintervention within 30 days (1.34% vs. 4.63% for RA and 4.11% for OA, $p = 0.24$) or to require readmission within 30 days (5.37% vs. 4.63% for RA and 4.88% for OA, $p = 0.52$). Multivariable logistic analysis found that fracture TEA was not independently associated with readmission, reoperation, or major or minor complications. Increasing age was associated with an increased risk of minor complications. Female sex was associated with a lower risk of major complications, and higher ASA (American Society of Anesthesiology) classification was associated with higher odds of readmission. Ultimately, patients undergoing TEA surgery for distal humerus fracture did not have a higher risk of acute postoperative complications than patients undergoing elective primary TEA implantation [29].

13.2.9 TEA in Rheumatoid Arthritis Patients

The use of biologic medication has decreased the TEA implantation rate of these patients. At the same time, it has delayed their implantation and has decreased the severity of the lesions at the time of implantation. On the other hand, the increased activity that these patients engage in may not make valid the scientific papers describing the results of rheumatoid arthritis patients when such medication did not allow them to lead such an active lifestyle.

The fundamental controversy in patients with an inflammatory disease is which design to use. Although good results have been achieved with linked and unlinked systems, the pathogenesis of the disease would explain the failure of unlinked arthroplasties due to residual instability, making it a good option to opt for an unlinked but linkable implant (convertible system). The use of a linked, semiconstrained system has provided good results in the medium and long term and is the safest option with similar loosening figures to nonlinked implants. Obviously the decision depends on the degree and severity of joint and soft tissue involvement, assessed through the clinical and radiological examination. Implantation of a nonlinked implant requires accurate and balanced reconstruction of the collateral ligaments, which may be difficult to attain in practices with low annual case volume. The challenge in these patients depends on the degree of bone loss, the incidence of intraoperative fractures, the difficulty in component orientation due to lack of accurate bony landmarks, and the prevention of infection.

In 2005, Little et al. compared, in a level III evidence study, three TEA designs (Souter-Strathclyde, Kudo, Coonrad-Morrey) in patients with RA. The Souter is an unlinked implant with a highly congruous articulation with a metal distal humerus without an anterior flange and a polyethylene ulnar component. The Kudo is an unlinked elbow implant with less constraint than the Souter with a metallic unflanged humeral component and the option of a metallic or an all-poly ulnar component. The Coonrad-Morrey is a semiconstrained linked elbow arthroplasty through a loose hinge where there is a metal on polyethylene bearing. They found that all three implant types relieved pain. The sustained improvement in range of flexion was comparable among the three groups. No design drastically modified fixed flexion deformity and all three improved maximum flexion. Indications for revision surgery were infection, dislocation, and aseptic loosening. Survival of the Coonrad-Morrey implant was better than that of the other two implants. The 5-year survival rates, with revision and radiographic signs of loosening as end points, were 85% and 81% for the Souter-Strathclyde implant, 93% and 82% for the Kudo implant, and 90% and 86% for the Coonrad-Morrey implant. Although radiological signs of loosening of the Coonrad-Morrey implants were less frequent, adjacent focal osteolysis was observed in 16% of the ulnar components, and in fact, half of these cases progressed to clear loosening. All three implants were similar in terms of pain relief and elbow ROM. Little et al. considered that component linkage with the Coonrad-Morrey component prevented dislocation without increasing the risk of loosening [30].

In 2015, Mukka et al. investigated the outcomes and survival of the Discovery design of TEA in patients with RA. In a prospective cohort study, an elbow surgeon performed 31 TEAs in 25 consecutive patients. They had complete results in only 19 of the patients (25 elbows). The mean range of motion (ROM) improved in flexion/extension from 88° to 113° and in pronation/supination from 55° to 68° ($p < 0.05$). The mean QuickDASH score also improved from 66.5 to 40.2 ($p < 0.01$). The mean EQ-5D (EuroQol-5D) score improved from 0.68 to 0.75, but was not statistically significant ($p = 0.09$). Three patients were revised for loosening and two were reoperated. Thus, the Kaplan-Meier survival was 90%. The Discovery system showed satisfactory results in patients with RA, although the complication rate was relatively high [31].

In 2017, Kodama et al. evaluated the long-term results (more than 10 years of follow-up) of the Kudo type-5 elbow prosthesis in patients with RA. They analyzed 41 elbows (Larsen grade IV, $n = 21$; grade V, $n = 20$) in 31 patients with RA who had undergone such type of arthroplasty. In all patients the humeral component was cementless and the all-polyethylene ulnar component cemented. The clinical outcome was assessed using the MEPS. The revision rate was calculated and potential risk factors for revision were assessed. The mean follow-up was 141 months (range: 120–203). Aseptic loosening of the ulnar component occurred in 11 elbows. There was no radiolucency around any humeral component. There was one deep infection. The survival rate by Kaplan-Meier survival analysis was 87.8% at 5 years and 70.7% at 10 years. The mean extension/flexion amplitude was −38°/105° before surgery and −40°/132° at final evaluation. The mean MEPS was 43 before surgery and 80 at final assessment. Significant risk factors for revision or aseptic loosening were a duration of RA to TEA of less than 15 years and a preoperative ROM of >85°. The conclusion was that, although Kudo type-5 TEA provided satisfactory short-term results, aseptic loosening increased after 5 years. In most cases, elbow function was maintained in the long term, without implant loosening [32].

In 2019, Strelzow et al. compared in patients with RA the outcomes and complications of linked and unlinked TEA using a convertible system. They found that such type of TEA provided good patient-reported outcomes in the medium term. This study found no difference between linked and unlinked designs. Eighty-two patients with RA (27 with nonlinked TEA and 55 with linked TEA) were evaluated. The mean age at the time of surgery was 61 years. The mean follow-up was 6 years. Demographic characteristics were similar in the two groups, with the exception of longer follow-up in the unlinked group (8 years vs. 5 years, $p = 0.001$). No differences in ROM were observed. Elbow strength was similar except for pronation strength (74% in the unlinked group vs. 100% in the linked group, $p = 0.03$). The mean MEPS was 83; the Patient-Rated Elbow Evaluation score, 15; and the QuickDASH score, 34. There were no differences in reoperation (17% vs. 24%, $p = 0.4$), complication (32% vs. 31%, $p = 0.4$), or revision (13% vs. 17%, $p = 0.3$) rates between the unlinked and linked prostheses. Four patients presented instability, all of them with unlinked designs, and required revision to a linked design. Four patients, all with linked designs, required revision due to aseptic loosening of the smooth short-stem ulnar components [33].

In a systematic review (therapeutic study with level IV evidence) on TEA in patients with RA, Chou et al. found in general satisfactory results. However, TEA had a much higher implant failure and complication rates than hip and knee arthroplasties. Patient age and sex and whether a cemented fixation or an unlinked prosthesis was used influenced the results. Thirty-eight studies (2118 TEAs) were included in the study. The mean follow-up was 80.9 months. Implant failure and complication rates were 16.1% and 24.5%, respectively. Aseptic loosening was the most common cause of failure (9.5%). The mean post-operative ROM was flexion 131.5°, extension 29.3°, pronation 74°, and supination 72.5°; the mean postoperative MEPS was 89.3. Meta-regression analysis identified that younger patients and implants with unlinked design correlated with higher failure rates. In addition, younger patients had a higher complication rate, and female sex and unlinked prostheses were associated with aseptic loosening [34].

13.2.10 TEA in Juvenile Idiopathic Arthritis (Juvenile Rheumatoid Arthritis) Patients

Patients with juvenile idiopathic arthritis (JIA) have the problem of age of indication (under 16 years of age) and underlying deformity which poses a therapeutic challenge. Some of these patients may have systemic symptoms that require the use of interleukin inhibitors. Despite this, some of them develop severe elbow arthrosis. Technically, these patients are characterized by significant stiffness, even ankylosis, requiring shortening of the humerus, and narrow canals that can facilitate the creation of false pathways. Flexible drills are now recommended for endomedullary canal preparation and the tip of the stems may have to be shaped, cut, or bent to fit the canals and the preexisting deformity. Some of these patients postoperatively compromise their implants because of the need to use crutches or unloading systems to ambulate due to lower limb involvement.

In 2014, in a level IV therapeutic study (case series), Baghdadi et al. evaluated the clinical benefit and prosthetic longevity of primary semiconstrained linked TEA performed to treat patients with JIA. Between 1983 and 2005, 29 elbows were replaced in 24 patients (20 women and 4 men) because of JIA. Their mean age was 37 years. Because of the underlying deformity, the implant contour was modified in 9 elbows (31%) and a customized implant was inserted in 5 elbows (17%). The mean follow-up was 10.5 years. During the follow-up period, 8 elbows were reoperated, of which 6 (21%) underwent implant revision. At final evaluation, 22 elbows (76%) had subjectively satisfactory overall functional outcome. The mean MEPS was 78 points. In 18 elbows, the result was considered excellent or good. Compared with preoperative ROM, the mean extension-flexion arc improved from 65 to 89 ($p = 0.01$); mean flexion improved from 113 to 126 ($p = 0.02$); mean extension improved from 48 to 37 ($p = 0.08$). Using the Kaplan-Meier survivorship method, the rate of TEA survival from any revision was 96.4% and 79.9% at 5 and 10 years, respectively. In short, primary TEA in patients with JIA often required implant modification or the use of customized designs. In addition, these patients had high rates of complications and revisions. However, in the long term most of them benefited from the intervention [35].

13.2.11 TEA in Osteoarthritis Patients

Primary OA is a disease of functionally demanding adults (manual laborers or weightlifters) and is usually treated with debridement, osteophyte removal, and capsulectomy, which usually results in improvement. Some of these patients do not improve with this procedure and continue to manifest joint pain in addition to the typical terminal motion pain. If this occurs in patients who are not very active or older, TEA is a good option, but unfortunately few patients fit this profile, so it is a rare procedure in this indication.

Technically the most important characteristic of these patients is stiffness and the presence of osteophytes which can limit joint access. For this reason, the soft tissue dissection has to be extensive and it is generally recommended to perform a linked arthroplasty. If the soft tissues are in good condition and the patient has minimal deformity, the patient may be a candidate for an unlinked (linkable) arthroplasty. These patients may develop heterotopic ossification although it does not usually limit postoperative function.

In 2017, Schoch et al., in a therapeutic level IV evidence study (case series), stated that in patients with primary OA, TEA was a reliable surgical option to relieve joint pain. However, they did not always achieve extension recovery, which indicated that more aggressive soft tissue releases or even bony resection might be necessary. Twenty TEAs were performed. Two patients died before 2 years of follow-up. The mean age at the time of surgery was 68 years. The mean follow-up was 8.9 years. Three elbows suffered mechanical failure. Regarding complications, there was one intraoperative fracture, one wound irrigation and debridement, one bony ankylosis, one humeral loosening, one humeral component fracture, and one mechanical failure of radial head component. Fifteen elbows that had not suffered mechanical failure were analyzed. In them, pain improved from 3.6 to 1.5 ($p < 0.001$). ROM remained unchanged ($p > 0.05$), and preoperative flexion contractures did not improve. The mean MEPS of 13 elbows without mechanical failure was 81.5 points; in 5 elbows the results were considered excellent, in 2 good, and in 6 fair. All patients without mechanical failure were subjectively satisfied with the outcome [36].

13.2.12 TEA in Posttraumatic Arthritis

Posttraumatic OA is usually the result of persistent instability, joint incongruity maintained by malreduction of a fracture, or secondary to extensive chondral injury. Generally, patients have undergone an average of three operations before opting for a TEA so it is important to investigate and rule out infection, and it occasionally requires removal of the implants and sampling in a first operation and placement of the TEA implant in a second operation. Ulnar nerve involvement is common and usually needs to be identified, dissected, and transposed at surgery. Ideally in these patients with posttraumatic sequelae, a linked implant is used due to the frequent associated instability and bone loss or deformity. Bone loss, stiffness, and three-dimensional deformity necessitate extensive but selective soft tissue releases and the use of a linked implant is often advisable. It is important to make patients aware of the lifelong restrictions of having an elbow implant and patients must understand that longevity is linked to the use of their elbow.

In 2014, Barthel et al., in a retrospective level IV evidence study, stated that in posttraumatic conditions, semiconstrained TEAs provided ROM recovery and stable, pain-free elbows. However, age at the time of surgery was a risk factor for complications. Nineteen patients underwent a semiconstrained Coonrad-Morrey TEA, in 12 cases for posttraumatic elbow arthritis (group 1) and in seven cases for 7 distal humerus nonunions (group 2). The mean age at the time of surgery was 60 years (56 in group 1 and 67 in group 2). The mean delay between the initial trauma and arthroplasty was 16 years (group 1) and 22 months (group 2). In group 1, after a mean follow-up of 5.5 years, the QuickDASH score was 34 points, with results considered good to excellent in 75% of cases according to the MEPS. Radiographic progressive radiolucencies were identified in 33% of cases and moderate polyethylene insert wear in 17%. There were seven complications (58%) requiring revision in three cases (25%). In group 2, after a mean follow-up of 4.6 years, the QuickDASH score was 39 points, with good and excellent results in 86% according to the MEPS. Radiolucency was observed in 28% and moderate wear of the inserts in 14%. There were two complications (28%), one of which (14%) required surgical revision. The indication for TEA in patients younger than 60 years should be carefully considered in relation to other therapeutic options [37].

13.2.13 Outcomes Following TEA for Rheumatoid Arthritis Versus Posttraumatic Conditions

A systematic review and meta-analysis published in 2019 by Wang et al. compared the outcomes of TEA performed for RA with the outcomes of TEA performed in posttraumatic conditions. The parameters evaluated were implant failure, functional outcome, and perioperative complications. Of 679 TEAs, 482 operated for RA and 197 for posttraumatic conditions were analyzed. All TEAs were cemented with linked components. It was shown that the RA group had a higher risk of septic loosening after TEA. However, in the posttraumatic group there was a higher risk of bushing wear, axle failure, component disassembly, or component fracture. The MEPS was higher in the AR group. There were no significant differences in ROM, DASH questionnaire scores, and risk of aseptic loosening, deep infection, perioperative fracture, or ulnar neuropathy. After TEA, patients with RA had a better functional outcome [38].

13.2.14 Primary Versus Secondary TEA for Distal Humerus Fractures

In 2019, Ellwein et al., in a level III evidence study, analyzed 35 patients who had a semiconstrained, cemented total elbow prosthesis (Latitude, Tornier, Bloomington, IN, USA) implanted using a modified Campbell approach. It was observed that the primary TEA provided better functional results than the secondary TEA. Subjective assessment was better in the primary TEA group due to less pain than in the secondary TEA group. Despite the longer duration of surgery in secondary TEA, complication rates were comparable. Ellwein et al. stated that fracture reconstruction remains the treatment of choice due to the lifelong limitation of weight-bearing of up to 5 kg. Furthermore, revision options are limited and may result in complete loss of elbow function. When considering TEA, the 10- and 20-year survival rates are 81% and 61%, respectively, which are much lower than those of knee and hip arthroplasty. In view of the poor results after reconstruction, primary TEA should be recommended for elderly or selected patients, since primary TEA produces better functional results with less pain than secondary TEA. If complications develop after reconstruction, early revision to TEA should be recommended, as late conversion results in worse outcomes. Although secondary TEA requires removal of the implant in most cases, which implies a considerable prolongation of operative time, the rates of major complications were not significantly different [39].

13.3 Revision TEA

13.3.1 Outcomes After Revision TEA

In 2013, Plaschke et al. published the short- and midterm results of 20 Coonrad-Morrey revision TEAs. With a mean follow-up of 4.4 years, the results after revision TEA using the Coonrad-Morrey prosthesis were acceptable. The short- and midterm failure rate was low. Revision improved ROM and relieved pain. In one case there was a deep infection, which required further revision. In addition, two patients had ulnar nerve paresthesia postoperatively [40].

In 2016, De Vos et al. stated that revision surgery using the Latitude TEA improved elbow function, reduced joint pain, and provided greater elbow stability. Between 2006 and 2010, they used the Latitude TEA to revise 18 elbows (17 patients); their mean age was 53 years; 14 were women. Kudo TEAs were reviewed in 15 elbows and Souter-Strathclyde TEAs in three. Although the ulnar nerve was routinely identified during the operation, two patients (11.8%) had some sensory disturbance postoperatively. In one there was complete recovery 2 years postoperatively. In another patient there was a slight sensory loss of the radial nerve 2 months postoperatively, after removal of K-wires that had been used to fix a fracture of the medial epicondyle. Sensory loss was fully recovered at 6 months' follow-up. Intraoperative fracture occurred in seven patients (38%) [41].

In a systematic review (level of evidence IV) published in 2019, Geurts et al. stated that an improvement in functional outcomes is to be expected after revision TEA, but its complication rate remained high. Revision TEA should still be considered a salvage procedure of a failed TEA (Fig. 13.4). Linked designs of revision TEA give better results than unlinked designs in the medium term. Twenty-one articles with 532 cases were included in the study. The mean age at the time of review was 61 years. The mean interval between primary and revision arthroplasty was 77 months, and the mean follow-up period was 65 months. Different types of prostheses were included, with 69% of revision prostheses with linked designs and 31% with unlinked designs. The visual analog scale score, MEPS, Oxford Elbow Score, and ROM improved significantly after revision surgery. Complications occurred in 232 of 532 cases (44%), resulting in reoperations in 22%. After revision with linked prostheses, MEPS, flexion-extension, and pronation amplitude improved significantly more than with unlinked designs [42].

In 2020, DeBernardis et al. determined the impact that the cause of failure of a primary TEA could have on the failure rate of revision surgery (therapeutic level IV evidence study, case series). Forty-six patients were analyzed, whose mean age was 62.7 years. The minimum follow-up was 2 years. The causes of failure were infection (n = 20), aseptic loosening (n = 17), peripros-

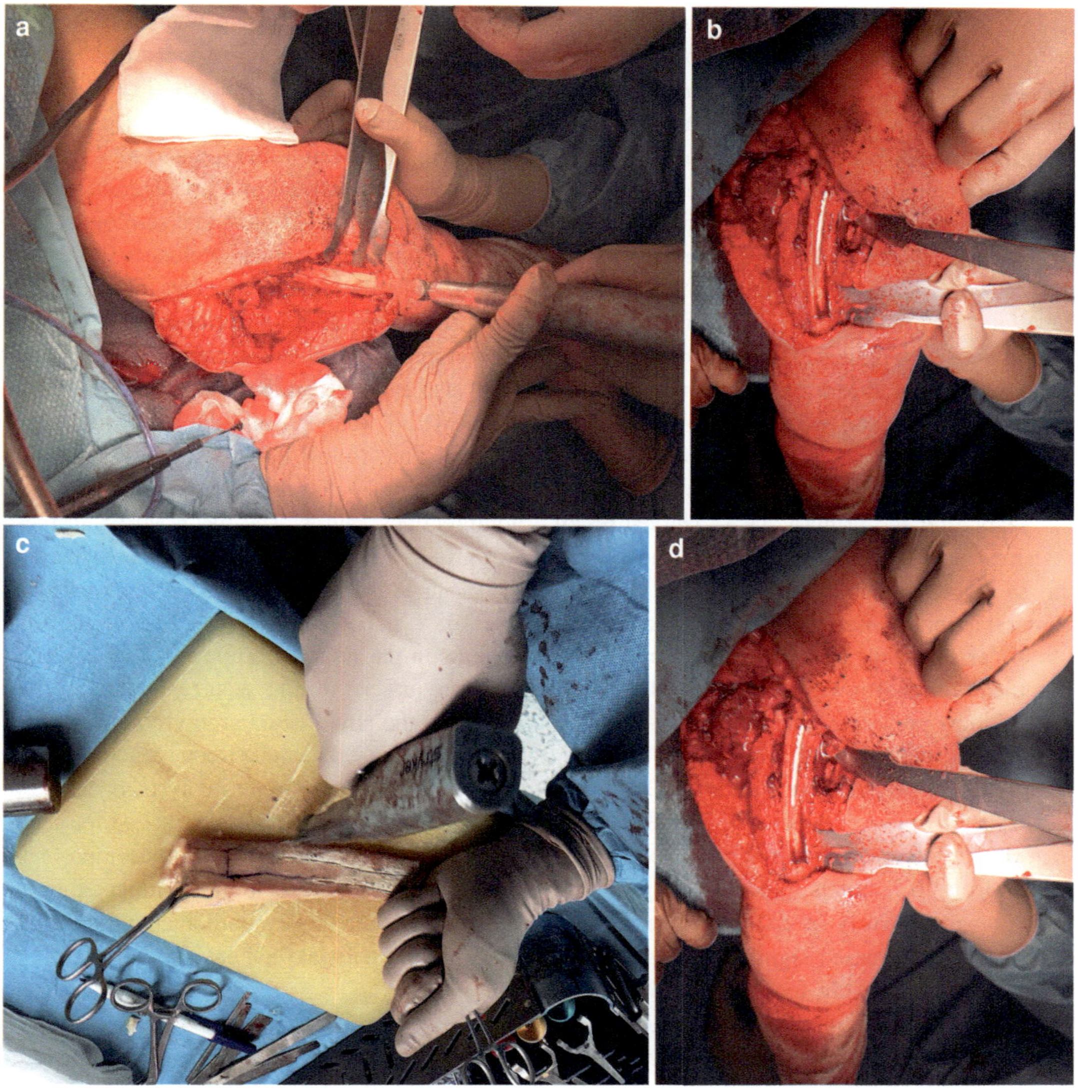

Fig. 13.4 (**a**–**d**) Revision total elbow arthroplasty surgery requires complex techniques including performing osteotomies for removal of the stem to decrease the risk of inadvertent fracture and allograft augmentation for appropriate reconstruction. (**a**) Longitudinal osteotomy with the aid of an oscillating saw and osteotomies is carried to the tip of the ulnar stem. (**b**) After opening the osteotomy, the stem is exposed, and after careful decortication, it can be easily extracted. (**c**) An allograft is prepared to obtain one or two struts. (**d**) After replacing the cortical window, strut allograft augmentation is performed with the use of wires, rather than cables

thetic fracture ($n = 6$), and bushing wear ($n = 3$). All noninfectious etiologies were grouped into an additional cohort. Patients who underwent revision for infection showed a significantly higher failure rate and number of new revisions per patient than those who underwent surgery for aseptic loosening, periprosthetic fracture, or noninfectious cause; they also showed a shorter time to failure than in the noninfectious group. Patients in whom primary TEA failed due to infection were more likely to have revision failure and required a greater number of subsequent operations than patients with other causes of primary TEA failure. This study questioned the efficacy of revision surgery in the treatment of infected TEA [43].

In 2021, in a level IV therapeutic study, Barret et al. evaluated the long-term outcomes of revision TEA using a single semiconstrained prosthesis design. They stated that revision TEA with this type of prosthesis could provide good clinical outcomes, which could be maintained during follow-up. However, the complication rate was high. They stated that proper evaluation of the risk-benefit ratio is essential for each revision TEA and the risk-benefit ratio should be discussed with each patient. Thirty-four revisions of TEA with Coonrad/Morrey prosthesis were performed in 32 patients; two patients were operated bilaterally. Their mean age was 61 years, and the revision TEA was performed at a mean time of 7.8 years after the primary TEA. The causes of revisions were humeral and ulnar aseptic loosening ($n = 14$), ulnar aseptic loosening ($n = 8$), humeral aseptic loosening ($n = 6$), septic arthritis ($n = 4$), and unstable unlinked prostheses ($n = 2$). The mean follow-up was 11.4 years. The MEPS at last follow-up was excellent in 6 cases, good in 18, fair in 8, and poor in 2, with a mean improvement between preoperative values of 42.4 points and postoperative values of 81.8 points ($p < 0.001$). Mean pain scores improved significantly from 6.7 points preoperatively to 1.4 points postoperatively ($p < 0.001$). The flexion-extension arc increased significantly ($p = 0.02$) from 74 preoperatively to 100 postoperatively. The total number of complications in 19 revision TEA was 29 (56%). Twenty of the 29 complications simply required management without surgical intervention. Six repeat surgical procedures were required and three implant revisions were performed (9%) [44].

13.3.2 Revision TEA: Comparison of Infected and Noninfected TEA

In 2019, Kwak et al. published the clinical and radiological results of revision TEA surgery according to the cause of failure (infection vs. noninfection). Those authors observed that revision TEA clinically improved elbow function and produced satisfactory results. Outcomes were worse in the infected group than in the noninfected group. Comorbidities and advanced age were risk factors for infected TEA. Twenty revision-operated patients were retrospectively evaluated. The mean follow-up was 52.7 months. Patients were classified into infected and noninfected based on radiological and serological evidence. Clinical outcomes included ROM and MEPS, and radiological outcomes included signs of loosening on anteroposterior and lateral plain radiographs at final assessment. Complications were also evaluated in both groups. Overall, the mean MEPS was 79.7 and the mean ROM was 97.9° at final follow-up. Nine patients required revision surgery due to infection, and 11 due to noninfectious causes. The mean MEPS in these two groups was 75.6 and 83.5, respectively, and the mean ROM for flexion-extension was 89.4° and 108°, respectively. Two (22%) of the nine patients in the infected group required a second revision surgery due to recurrent infection. No patient in the noninfected group required second revision surgery. The most frequent complication in the infected group was osteolysis, observed in five patients, four of them with symptomatic aseptic loosening and one with nonsymptomatic osteolysis. Two patients in the noninfected group showed a nonprogressive radiolucent line, which was asymptomatic at final evaluation [45].

13.3.3 Outcomes Following Revision of the Revision TEA

In 2020, Domos et al. published a level IV evidence-based therapeutic study (case series) in which they presented their results of the revision of revision TEA (RRTEA). Twenty-two patients operated on for RRTEA were identified. Of these, 14 were available for evaluation (2 died of unrelated causes, 2 could not be contacted, 2 declined to participate because of travel difficulties, and 2 had incomplete data). The mean age of the patients was 73 years. Follow-up since the last surgical procedure was 4.5 years. The mean number of previous revision arthroplasty procedures per patient was 3. The indications for RRTEA were aseptic loosening (60%), bushing wear (16%), fracture

(14%), and infection (10%). Of the patients, 30% required extra-long or custom-made implants and 50% required allograft augmentation. At final clinical evaluation, 56% of patients had triceps insufficiency, the mean flexion-extension arc was 90°, and the mean pronation-supination arc was 95°. Functional elbow scores revealed good results in most patients (mean visual analog scale score, 5; mean Oxford Elbow Score, 22; mean Mayo Elbow Performance Index score, 55; and mean QuickDASH score, 63). Eighty-one percent of patients were satisfied with their RRTEA. Encountered complications were infection in 2 patients (1 superficial and 1 deep), symptomatic aseptic loosening of the humeral component in 1, ulnar nerve sensory symptoms in 2, and radial nerve injury in 1. One patient required ulnar nerve release. Radiologic review revealed asymptomatic loosening in 1 patient (humeral component), and overall prosthesis alignment with cementation was adequate in 81%. Heterotopic ossification was present in 38% of cases. RRTEA was considered a satisfactory treatment option in these complex cases, with good short- and medium-term survival rates, but with a relatively high complication rate [46].

13.4 Conversion of a Surgical Elbow Arthrodesis to TEA

In 2015, Rog et al. published the first case in the English literature of conversion of a surgical elbow arthrodesis to a TEA. This was a 49-year-old man whose elbow had been surgically fused following trauma sustained 31 years earlier. However, the conversion of a surgically fused elbow had already been published in the German literature in 2013 by Burkhart et al. Rog et al. stated that in carefully selected patients who were dissatisfied with the functional limitations of elbow fusion, conversion of an elbow arthrodesis to a TEA was a feasible intervention. In addition, the duration of fusion and any anatomic alterations related to previous surgical interventions performed on the elbow had to be taken into account when performing preoperative planning [47, 48].

13.5 The Future for TEA

According to Pooley, TEA is now increasingly used to treat comminuted fractures of the distal humerus, especially in elderly patients. TEA has been shown to be superior to ORIF in such patients, which is why it is the most logical therapeutic choice, especially in type C distal humerus fractures of the OTA classification. However, complication rates associated with TEA remain much higher than those associated with replacement of other extremity joints (hip, knee). It seems logical to think that the improvements that are occurring in TEA design will reduce complication rates, especially implant wear and loosening [2].

TEA is a complex surgical technique, which when well indicated and in experienced hands can give excellent clinical results. The overall complication rate has decreased from 49% in 1993 to 25% in 2009. Some of the complications that occur may be facilitated by inadequate component orientation. Improved imaging and planning systems and possibly intraoperative navigation with or without virtual reality methods will improve proper component orientation. However, as with any arthroplasty surgery, soft tissue management is the key to achieving good functional outcomes. Lifestyle modifications after TEA are imperative to ensure optimal implant longevity. Patients should never lift 10 pounds or more and should not repeatedly lift weights of 2 pounds or more. To optimize the results of TEA, it is imperative to choose the right implant and patient type [49].

We know that patients do not remember postoperative restrictions after some time, which makes it extremely difficult for them to comply with them. Forty percent of patients perform high-demand activities, especially male patients and those who have undergone surgery for fracture or nonunion [50].

13.6 Conclusions

Currently, TEA is increasingly used for the treatment of traumatic elbow pathology (comminuted fractures of the distal humerus and posttraumatic OA), while the indication for inflammatory arthropathy has decreased due to the advance of medical treatments. TEA has proven to be a good option in elderly patients. It is therefore a logical therapeutic option, especially in type C distal humerus fractures of the OTA classification. The three most frequent indications for a primary TEA are fracture/dislocation (trauma) (36%), OA (34%), and RA (26%). The cumulative revision rate of all TEAs implanted for any reason is 10%, 15%, and 19% at 3, 6, and 9 years, respectively. TEAs performed for OA have a higher revision rate than TEAs performed for trauma, highlighting the importance of patient selection in achieving good results. The most commonly used prosthesis designs are linked (Coonrad-Morrey, Latitude) and linkable (Nexel and Discovery), with no differences between them in terms of revision rates. The most common causes of revision TEA are infection and aseptic loosening. A recent systematic review of the literature (level IV evidence) with a mean follow-up of at least 10 years showed that the rates of aseptic loosening, infection, implant dislocation, and nerve injury were 12.9%, 3.3%, 4.2%, and 2.1%, respectively. Moreover, the overall complication and revision rates were 16.3% and 14.6%, respectively. These figures are inferior to the ones reported with arthroplasties of other joints. We should reflect on the way forward in the evolution of these implants, including better patient selection, improvement of current designs, more refined preoperative planning, and more precise surgical technique with virtual, navigated, or robotic technical aids.

References

1. Prkic A, de Vos MJ, Wagener ML, The B, Eygendaal D. Total elbow arthroplasty: why and how. JBJS Essent Surg Tech. 2017;7(1–7):e5.
2. Pooley P. Total elbow replacement—patient selection and perspectives. Orthop Res Rev. 2019;11:23–40.
3. Poff CB, Kothandaraman V, Kunkle BF, Friedman RJ, Eichinger JK. Trends in total elbow arthroplasty utilization in the United States from 2002-2017. Semin Arthroplast. 2021; https://doi.org/10.1053/j.sart.2020.12.005.
4. Vivieen J, Van den Bejerom MPJ, Doornberg JN, Hatton A, Page R, Koenraadt KLM, et al. Use and outcome of 1,220 primary total elbow arthroplasties from the Australian Orthopaedic Association National Joint Arthroplasty Replacement Registry 2008–2018. Acta Orthop. 2019;90:511–6.
5. Zhang D, Chen N. Total elbow arthroplasty. J Hand Surg Am. 2019;44:487–95.
6. Barco R, Streubel PN, Morrey BF, Sanchez-Sotelo J. Total elbow arthroplasty for distal humeral fractures: a ten-year-minimum follow-up study. J Bone Joint Surg Am. 2017;99:1524–31.
7. Iwamoto T, Suzuki T, Oki S, Matsumura N, Nakamura M, Matsumoto M, et al. Computed tomography–based 3-dimensional preoperative planning for unlinked total elbow arthroplasty. J Shoulder Elb Surg. 2018;27:1792–9.
8. Booker SJ, Smith CD. Triceps on approach for total elbow arthroplasty: worth preserving? A review of approaches for total elbow arthroplasty. Shoulder Elbow. 2017;9:105–11.
9. Studer A, Athwal GS, MacDermid JC, Faber KJ, King GJ. The lateral para-olecranon approach for total elbow arthroplasty. J Hand Surg Am. 2013;38:2219–2226.e3.
10. Celli A, Bonucci P. The anconeus–triceps lateral flap approach for total elbow arthroplasty in rheumatoid arthritis. Musculoskelet Surg. 2016;100(Suppl 1):S73–83.
11. Na K-T, Song S-W, Lee Y-M, Choi J-H. Modified triceps fascial tongue approach for primary total elbow arthroplasty. J Shoulder Elb Surg. 2018;27:887–93.
12. Cottias P, Leclerc P, Zaoui A, Abouchaaya AM, Khallouk R, Anract P. Digastric olecranon osteotomy a new approach to the elbow: retrospective study of 24 Coonrad–Morrey total elbow arthroplasty at 30-month follow-up. Eur J Orthop Surg Traumatol. 2020;30:485–91.
13. Cutler HS, Collett G, Farahani F, Ahn J, Nakonezny P, Koehler D, et al. Thirty day readmissions and reoperations after total elbow arthroplasty: a national database study. J Shoulder Elb Surg. 2021;30:e41–9.
14. Davey MS, Hurley ET, Gaafar M, Molony D, Mullett H, Pauzenberger L. Long-term outcomes of total elbow arthroplasty: a systematic review of studies at 10-year follow-up. J Shoulder Elb Surg. 2021; https://doi.org/10.1016/j.jse.2020.11.014.
15. Perretta D, van Leeuwen WF, Dyer G, Ring D, Chen N. Risk factors for reoperation after total elbow arthroplasty. J Shoulder Elb Surg. 2017;26:824–9.
16. Borton ZK, Prasad G, Konstantopoulos G, Morgan ML, Cresswell T, Espag MP, et al. Mid-long term survivorship of the cemented, semi-constrained "discovery" total elbow arthroplasty. J Shoulder Elb Surg. 2021; https://doi.org/10.1016/j.jse.2020.12.007.
17. Rhee YG, Cho NS, Park JG, Song JH. Resection arthroplasty for periprosthetic infection after total elbow arthroplasty. J Shoulder Elb Surg. 2016;25:105–11.

18. Robinson PM, MacInnes SJ, Stanley D, Ali AA. Heterotopic ossification following total elbow arthroplasty: a comparison of the incidence following elective and trauma surgery. Bone Joint J. 2018;100-B:767–71.
19. Lee H, Vaichinger AM, O'Driscoll SW. Component fracture after total elbow arthroplasty. J Shoulder Elb Surg. 2019;28:1449–56.
20. Claxton MR, Shirley MB, Nauert RF, Morrey ME, Sanchez-Sotelo J, Houdek MT. Humeral amputation following total elbow arthroplasty. Int Orthop. 2021; https://doi.org/10.1007/s00264-020-04906-1.
21. Furman AA, Sherman AE, Plantz MP, Marra G, Saltzman MS. Differences in 30-day outcomes between inpatient and outpatient total elbow arthroplasty (TEA). J Shoulder Elb Surg. 2020;29:2640–5.
22. McKee MD, Veillette CJH, Hall JA, Schemitsch EH, Wild LM, McCormack R, et al. A multicenter, prospective, randomized, controlled trial of open reduction internal fixation versus total elbow arthroplasty for displaced intra-articular distal humeral fractures in elderly patients. J Shoulder Elb Surg 2009;18:3–12.
23. Dehghan N, Furey M, Schemitsch L, Ristevski B, Goetz T, Schemitsch EH, Canadian Orthopaedic Trauma Society (COTS), McKee M. Long-term outcomes of total elbow arthroplasty for distal humeral fracture: results from a prior randomized clinical trial. J Shoulder Elb Surg. 2019;28:2198–204.
24. Frankle M, Frankle MA, Herscovici D Jr, DiPasquale TG, Vasey MB, Sanders RW. A comparison of open reduction and internal fixation and primary total elbow arthroplasty in the treatment of intraarticular distal humerus fractures in women older than age 65. J Orthop Trauma. 2003;17:473–80.
25. Mansat P, Bonnevialle N, Rongieres M, Mansat M, Bonnevialle P. Experience with the Coonrad-Morrey total elbow arthroplasty: 78 consecutive total elbow arthroplasties reviewed with an average 5 years of follow-up. J Shoulder Elb Surg. 2013;22:1461–8.
26. Sanchez-Sotelo J, Baghdadi YMK, Morrey BF. Primary linked semiconstrained total elbow arthroplasty for rheumatoid arthritis: a single-institution experience with 461 elbows over three decades. J Bone Joint Surg Am. 2016;98:1741–8.
27. Prasad N, Ali A, Stanley D. Total elbow arthroplasty for non-rheumatoid patients with a fracture of the distal humerus: a minimum ten-year follow-up. Bone Joint J. 2016;98-B:381–6.
28. Strelzow JA, Frank T, Athwal GS, Faber KJ, King GJW. Results of linked convertible total elbow arthroplasty for the management of distal humeral fractures in the elderly. J Hand Surg Am. 2020; https://doi.org/10.1016/j.jhsa.2020.10.034.
29. Aziz KT, Kreulen RT, Best MJ, Nayar SK, Weiner S, Srikumaran U. Comparison of short-term outcomes in patients undergoing elective total elbow arthroplasty versus total elbow arthroplasty for fracture. Semin Arthroplast. 2021; https://doi.org/10.1053/j.sart.2020.12.006.
30. Little CP, Graham AJ, Karatzas G, Woods DA, Carr AJ. Outcomes of total elbow arthroplasty for rheumatoid arthritis: comparative study of three implants. J Bone Joint Surg. 2005;87-A:2439–48.
31. Mukka S, Berg G, Haj Hassany HR, Koye AK, Sjoden G, Sayed-Noor AS. Semiconstrained total elbow arthroplasty for rheumatoid arthritis patients: clinical and radiological results of 1–8 years follow-up. Arch Orthop Trauma Surg. 2015;135:595–600.
32. Kodama A, Mizuseki T, Adachi N. Kudo type-5 total elbow arthroplasty for patients with rheumatoid arthritis: a mínimum ten-year follow-up study. Bone Joint J. 2017;99-B:818–23.
33. Strelzow JA, Frank T, Chan K, Athwal GS, Faber KJ, King GJW. Management of rheumatoid arthritis of the elbow with a convertible total elbow arthroplasty. J Shoulder Elb Surg. 2019;28:2205–14.
34. Chou T-F A, Ma H-H, Wang J-H, Tsai S-W, Chen C-F, Wu P-K, et al. Total elbow arthroplasty in patients with rheumatoid arthritis: a systematic review and meta-analysis. Bone Joint J. 2020;102-B:967–80.
35. Baghdadi YMK, Jacobson JA, Duquin TR, Larson DR, Morrey BF, Sanchez-Sotelo J. The outcome of total elbow arthroplasty in juvenile idiopathic arthritis (juvenile rheumatoid arthritis) patients. J Shoulder Elb Surg. 2014;23:1374–80.
36. Schoch BS, Werthel J-D, Sánchez-Sotelo J, Morrey BF, Morrey M. Total elbow arthroplasty for primary osteoarthritis. J Shoulder Elb Surg. 2017;26:1355–9.
37. Barthel PY, Mansat P, Sirveaux F, Dap F, Molé D, Dautel G. Is total elbow arthroplasty indicated in the treatment of traumatic sequelae? 19 cases of Coonrad-Morrey reviewed at a mean follow-up of 5.2 years. Orthop Traumatol Surg Res. 2014;100:113–8.
38. Wang J-H, Ma H-H, Chou T-FA, Tsai S-W, Chen C-F, Wu P-K, et al. Outcomes following total elbow arthroplasty for rheumatoid arthritis versus post-traumatic conditions: a systematic review and meta-analysis. Bone Joint J. 2019;101-B:1489–97.
39. Ellwein A, Lill H, Smith T, Voigt C, Imrecke J, Katthagen JC. Primary vs. secondary total elbow arthroplasty for distal humerus fractures: clinical results of a retrospective case–control study. Obere Extremität. 2019;14:256–62.
40. Plaschke HC, Thillemann T, Belling-Sørensen AK, Olsen B. Revision total elbow arthroplasty with the linked Coonrad-Morrey total elbow arthroplasty: a retrospective study of twenty procedures. Int Orthop. 2013;37:853–8.
41. de Vos MJ, Wagener ML, Hannink G, van der Pluijm M, Verdonschot N, Eygendaal D. Short-term clinical results of revision elbow arthroplasty using the latitude total elbow arthroplasty. Bone Joint J. 2016;98-B:1086–92.
42. Geurts EJ, Viveen J, van Riet RP, Kodde IF, Eygendaal D. Outcomes after revision total elbow arthroplasty: a systematic review. J Shoulder Elb Surg. 2019;28:381–6.
43. DeBernardis DA, Horneff JG, Davis DE, Ramsey ML, Pontes MC, Austin LS. Revision total elbow arthro-

plasty failure rates: the impact of primary arthroplasty failure etiology on subsequent revisions. J Shoulder Elb Surg. 2020;29:321–8.
44. Barret H, Laumonerie P, Delclaux S, Arboucalot M, Bonnevialle N, Mansat P. Revision total elbow arthroplasty with the semiconstrained Coonrad/Morrey prosthesis: follow-up to 21 years. J Bone Joint Surg Am. 2021; https://doi.org/10.2106/JBJS.20.00889.
45. Kwak J-M, Kholinne E, Sun Y, Kim M-S, Koh K-H, In H-J. Clinical results of revision total elbow arthroplasty: comparison of infected and non-infected total elbow arthroplasty. Int Orthop. 2019;43:1421–7.
46. Domos P, Chelli M, Papanna MC, Gokaraju K, Stanley D, Ali AA. Outcomes following revision of the revision total elbow arthroplasty. J Shoulder Elb Surg. 2020; https://doi.org/10.1016/j.jse.2020.10.016.
47. Rog D, Zuckerman LM, Riedel B. Conversion of a surgical elbow arthrodesis to total elbow arthroplasty: case report. Case Reports Orthop. 2015:578189, 4 pages.
48. Burkhart KJ, Dargel J, Wegmann K, Müller LP. Conversion of elbow arthrodesis to total elbow arthroplasty. Unfallchirurg. 2013;116:371–5.
49. Shah PK. Patel CP, Total elbow arthroplasty. Evolution Biomech. 2021; https://doi.org/10.1016/j.jajs.2021.02.001.
50. Barlow JD, Morrey BF, O'Driscoll SW, Steinmann SP, Sanchez-Sotelo J. Activities after total elbow arthroplasty. J Shoulder Elb Surg. 2013;22:787–91.

Distal Radius Fractures in the Elderly: Current Controversies

14

E. Carlos Rodríguez-Merchán, Carlos A. Encinas-Ullán, and Primitivo Gómez-Cardero

14.1 Introduction

Distal radius fractures (DRFs) in the elderly population, above 65 years old, represent 18% of all fractures and are thereby the second most frequent fracture in the elderly [1]. These fractures are often the result of low-energy falls from a standing or seated position [2]. They are often comminuted and intra-articular fractures [3].

After hip fracture, DRF is the second most common fracture in the elderly. Peak incidence is in Caucasian women who are over 65 years of age. Osteoporosis is a common risk factor and occurs in 40% of postmenopausal women. Other significant risk factors for DRFs in patients older than 50 years include prior falls, prior fragility fractures, corticosteroid use, and advanced age. Dementia is also a risk factor in patients older than 75 years of age. In older patients, each additional risk factor conveys increased probability of suffering a DRF. DRFs extending into a joint space are twice as common in women with diabetes [4]. The incidence of DRFs is increasing as life expectancy grows, leading to a larger population of patients who are at risk for these injuries [3].

E. C. Rodríguez-Merchán (✉) · C. A. Encinas-Ullán
P. Gómez-Cardero
Department of Orthopaedic Surgery, "La Paz" University Hospital, Madrid, Spain

The purpose of this chapter is to revise the most important current controversies on DRFs in the elderly.

14.2 Conservative Treatment

14.2.1 Objective Outcome Measures Continue to Improve from 6 to 12 Months

In DRFs dislocation and comminution are often used to determine whether nonoperative or operative treatment is indicated. In a prospective case series of minimally displaced DRFs treated with closed reduction (CR) and cast immobilization, Thorninger et al. assessed the complication rate and patient-reported outcome measures. This study analyzed 50 conservatively treated DRF patients for 1 year [1]. Primary outcomes were complications and Quick Disability of Arm, Shoulder, and Hand (qDASH) score. Secondary outcomes were range of motion (ROM), grip strength and pain, and Patient-Rated Wrist/Hand Evaluation (PRWHE). Results showed only minor complications with a return to prior ROM, qDASH score, and pain after 12 months and amelioration in results after 6–12 months. Most DRF patients who were treated nonoperatively with CR and 5-week casting recovered fully after minimally displaced DRFs. Therefore, this approach was considered safe (Fig. 14.1) [1].

E. C. Rodríguez-Merchán, A. Moreno-Garcìa (eds.), *Controversies in Orthopedic Surgery of The Upper Limb*, https://doi.org/10.1007/978-3-031-04907-1_14

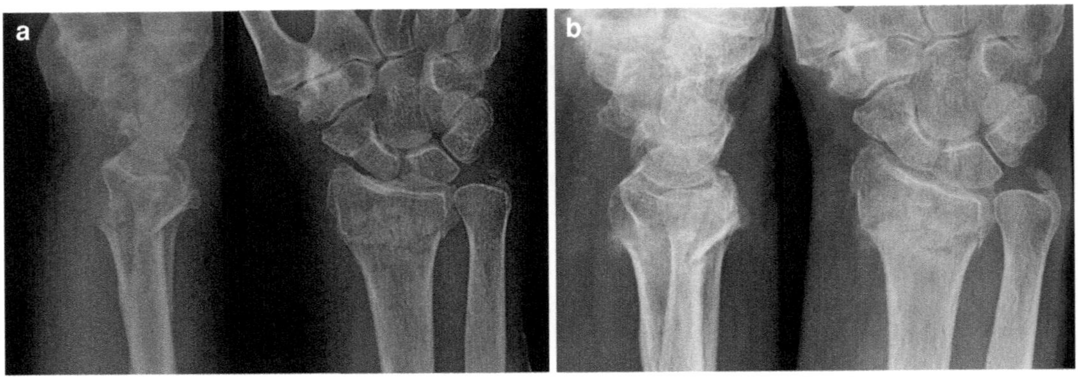

Fig. 14.1 (**a**, **b**) Distal radius fracture (**a**) treated conservatively with a cast for 6 weeks (**b**)

14.3 Surgical Treatment

14.3.1 Preoperative Planning

Yoshii et al. used a three-dimensional preoperative planning for the osteosynthesis of DRF (trial registration: registered as NCT02909647 at ClinicalTrials.gov). They evaluated the reproducibility of three-dimensional preoperative planning for the osteosynthesis of DRFs with three-dimensional reference points [5]. Sixty-three wrists of 63 DRF patients who experienced osteosynthesis with three-dimensional preoperative planning were assessed. After taking preoperative computed tomography (CT) scans of the injured wrists, 3D images of the distal radius were created. Fracture reduction, implant choices, and placement simulation were carried out based on the 3D images. One month after the surgery, postoperative CT images were taken. The reproducibility was assessed with preoperative plan and postoperative 3D images. The images were compared with the three-dimensional coordinates of the radial styloid process, volar and dorsal edges of the sigmoid notch, and the barycentric coordinates of the three reference points. The reproducibility of the preoperative plan was assessed by the distance of the coordinates between the plan and postoperative images for the reference points. The reproducibility of radial inclination and volar tilt on three-dimensional images were assessed by intraclass correlation coefficient (ICC). The distances between the preoperative plan and the postoperative reduction for each reference point were 2.1 mm, 1.9 mm, and 1.9 mm, respectively. The distance between the preoperative plan and postoperative reduction for the barycentric coordinate was 1.3 mm. ICCs were 0.54 and 0.54 for the volar tilt and radial inclination, respectively ($p < 0.01$). The conclusion of this study was that three-dimensional preoperative planning for the osteosynthesis of DRFs was reproducible, with an error of about 2 mm for each reference point and the correlations of reduction shapes were moderate. Therefore, the analysis method and reference points may be helpful to understand the accuracy of reductions for the three-dimensional preoperative planning in the osteosynthesis of DRFs [5].

14.3.2 Percutaneous Pinning Fixation

According to Zhao et al., percutaneous pinning (PP) fixation has been utilized for the treatment of DRFs for decades, especially in the elderly with fragile soft tissue. However, getting and maintaining a sound anatomic reduction prior to PP is difficult if we utilize the manipulative reduction method alone. In their study Zhao et al. utilized the Steinmann pin retractor for CR combined with PP [6]. Forty-nine patients were analyzed in this retrospective cohort study. Sixteen patients were treated with Steinmann pin retractor-assisted CR combined with PP (S-PP), 19 patients were treated with the manipulative reduction combined with PP (M-PP), and 14 patients were treated with the manipulative reduction combined with cast splint (M-C). All these patients received a positive postoperative radiological and clinical assessment. All the patients were followed up for a minimum of 2 years. The radiological parameters in each group improved significantly after surgery (post-treatment). In the S-PP group, the values of radial height (postoperative, 13.33 mm; first follow-up, 13.27 mm; last follow-up, 13.16 mm) and ulnar variance (postoperative, −0.10 mm; first follow-up, −0.05 mm; last follow-up, −0.12 mm) significantly improved as compared to the M-PP and M-C groups. While the patients in the M-C group experienced significant re-displacement at the first and last follow-ups, in the S-PP group the range of wrist motion including extension (89.94%), radial deviation (90.69%), and supination (90.25%), ulnar deviation (89.81%) and qDASH score (2.70), and grip strength (92.50%), pronation (90.50%), and Modified Mayo Wrist Score (MWS) (90.94, the excellent rate reached up to 75%) improved as compared to the M-PP group, M-C group, or both groups at the last follow-up. The conclusion was that S-PP improved fracture reduction and wrist function and can serve as an efficacious technique for A_2 (AO/OTA) and A_3 type of DRFs in the elderly with limited dorsal comminution, including intra-articular fractures with displacement less than 2 mm [6].

14.3.3 Dorsal Bridge Plate

In a systematic review (level IV of evidence) published in 2021, Fares et al. presented patient demographics, injury characteristics, results, and side events associated with dorsal bridge plating (DBP) in the treatment of DRFs [7]. Average age was 55 years, median follow-up was 24 months, and the most common indication was comminuted (92%), intra-articular (92%) DRF caused by fall (58%), or motor vehicle collision or motorcycle collision (27%). A minority of patients had open fractures (16%) and most of these were cases of polytrauma (65%). The median time from placement to DBP removal was 17 weeks (mean, 119 days). At the final follow-up, the mean wrist ROM was 45° flexion, 50° extension, 75° pronation, and 73° supination. The mean DASH score was 26.1, and the mean qDASH score was 19.8. The overall rate for any complication was 13%; the most common was hardware failure (3%) followed by symptomatic malunion or nonunion (3%) and persistent pain after hardware removal (2%). In this study, DBP was found to be utilized most commonly in intra-articular, comminuted DRF reporting overall functional wrist ROM, moderate patient-reported disability, and a 13% complication rate at follow-up [7].

14.3.4 IlluminOss System

Van Oijen et al. assessed the functional and clinical results after treatment of DRFs with the IlluminOss® System in adult patients. A retrospective case series was carried out in a single-level two-trauma center [8]. All consecutive adult patients with a DRF, treated with the IlluminOss® System between August 01, 2012, and August 15, 2015, were included in this study. Baseline patient characteristics and clinical data were retrospectively extracted from the medical records. Radial inclination, volar/dorsal tilt, ulnar variance, and radial length were measured on the latest available standard radiographs. Besides, patients were prospectively subjected to physical examination and were asked to complete the DASH, Patient-Rated Wrist Evaluation (PRWE), and Short Form-36 (SF-36) questionnaires. Twenty-six patients with 31 DRFs were included. The median age at the time of trauma was 77 years and 96% were females. Five patients developed a total of seven complications. Due to persisting pain, one reoperation was carried out, removing a small prominent part of the implant. Both patient-reported outcome scores and radiographic outcomes were good to excellent. It was stated that the IlluminOss® System appeared to be a feasible alternative to treat DRFs with seemingly good clinical and functional result. One out of seven complications required surgical intervention. These results justified more detailed prospective research [8].

14.3.5 Volar Locking Plate Preserving Pronator Quadratus Through the Minimally Invasive Approach

According to Fan et al., the VLP technique with an L-shaped incision of the pronator quadratus (PQ) muscle through the classic volar Henry approach is a popular technique for treating DRFs. Recently, they revised and improved this traditional technique by performing mini-invasive surgery [9]. They assessed the clinical effects after fixation of DRFs with VLPs while preserving the PQ through the minimally invasive approach. Fifty-eight patients (38 males and 21 females) with an age range of 22–72 years (mean age 44.6 years) and with DRFs underwent open reduction and internal fixation with VLPs. The patients were classified as 23A-2 through 23C-2 according to the AO/OTA fracture classification system. The group that received VLPs of distal radius performed with the traditional method through the Henry approach involved 33 patients (21 males and 12 females) and the group that received PQ through the minimally invasive approach group involved 25 patients (16 males and 9 females). Fan et al. compared the two groups for wrist pain, forearm ROM, grip strength, preoperative complications, and wrist functional recovery score. The minimum follow-up for the whole cohort was 1 year. The differences between the two groups were significant in terms of wrist pain, forearm ROM, grip strength, and wrist function at 1, 2, and 6 weeks postoperatively, but insignificant at 3 and 12 months postoperatively. In the minimally invasive group, a case of limited extension of the forefinger 3 months postoperatively was encountered. No significant differences were found for preoperative complications and radiographs postoperatively. The conclusion was that fixation with VLPs through the minimally invasive approach was a satisfactory and optional technique in the treatment of DRFs. This method yielded better early wrist function, shortened rehabilitation time, and high psychological satisfaction [9].

14.3.6 Bridge Plating with Bone Graft Substitutes in Combination with Systemic Romosozumab Administration

Uemura et al. have published a case report of a distal radius nonunion in which they used romosozumab (a humanized, anti-sclerostin monoclonal antibody used to treat osteoporosis, which augments bone formation and decreases bone resorption). It enhances fracture healing and systemic romosozumab administration may have therapeutic potentials for accelerating bone healing of nonunions. A 61-year-old heavy smoker male with distal radius nonunion who achieved successful bone union by combination therapy of romosozumab and spanning distraction plate fixation with bone graft substitutes was presented [10]. Through the dorsal approach, atrophic comminuted nonunion of the distal radius was sufficiently debrided. Reduction of the distal radius was performed using indirect ligamentotaxis, and a 14-hole locking plate was fixed from the third metacarpal to the radial shaft. A beta (β) tricalcium phosphate block was mainly packed into the substantial metaphyseal bone defect with additional bone graft from the resected ulnar head. Postoperatively, systemic administration of monthly romosozumab was continued for 6 months. Complete bone union was achieved 20 weeks postoperatively and the plate was, then, removed. During romosozumab treatment, bone formation marker levels increased rapidly and finally returned to baseline, and bone resorption marker levels remained low. In conclusion, the combination of systemic romosozumab administration and grafting β-tricalcium phosphate with bridge plating provided an efficacious treatment alternative for difficult cases of comminuted distal radius nonunion with risk factors such as smoking, diabetes, and fragility [10].

14.3.7 Combined Palmar and Dorsal Plating of Four-Part Distal Radius Fracture

In 2021, Kibar analyzed the radiological and clinical results of four-part intra-articular DRF treated with a volar anatomically locked plate and 2-mm low-profile plates using both the volar and dorsal approaches [11]. The retrospective study included 20 patients (8 males, 12 females; mean age 47; range, 25 to 67 years) who received open reduction and internal fixation with combined volar and dorsal plating to treat complex four-part DRFs (shaft, radial styloid area, dorsal medial facet, volar medial facet). According to the AO/OTA classification, all fractures were 2R3-C3. The mean follow-up time was 21 months. Union was achieved in all fractures. The mean tourniquet time was 103 min. The mean DASH questionnaire score was 10, and the mean Visual Analog Scale (VAS) score was 2.1. According to MWS, five patients had excellent, six had good, six had satisfactory, and three had poor outcomes. The mean grip strength was 25.2 (range, 15–40) kg and 78% of the opposite side. The mean wrist flexion was 48.7° (range, 30° to 80°), extension was 52.2° (range, 25° to 80°), the radioulnar deviation arc was 40.7° (range, 30° to 55°), and the mean forearm rotation arc was 152.3° (range, 130° to 170°). The conclusion was that this plating method with a dual approach may be an alternative for four-part intra-articular DRFs given its early mobility advantage and satisfactory functional and radiological outcomes [11].

14.3.8 Cobra Prosthesis in Complex Distal Radius Fractures

According to Benedikt et al., the Cobra prosthesis provides an alternative treatment option for complex fractures where conservative therapy seems not acceptable and osteosynthesis seems not possible [12]. In a retrospective follow-up study, they investigated the clinical and radiological midterm result of the Cobra implant in complex DRFs of elderly patients. Thirteen patients (mean age 73.5 years, range 65–87 years) were retrospectively assessed with at least a 1-year follow-up after surgery. Objective and subjective clinical parameters as well as the radiological results and side events were analyzed. The mean follow-up period was 31.2 months. Seven cases required a cemented prosthesis. The mean relative ROM compared to the healthy side was 72.3% and 51.8% for extension and flexion, respectively, and 87.9% and 85.7% for pronation and supination, respectively. The mean grip strength was 78.3% compared to the non-operated side. Eight patients were very satisfied, and five patients were partly satisfied with the outcome. The DASH, PRWE, Michigan Hand Outcome questionnaire (MHOQ), and Lyon Scores averaged 39.1, 36.2, 64.9, and 63.3 points, respectively. The mean VAS score for pain was 1.1 at rest and 3.2 during activities. Perioperative complications included one dissection of the extensor pollicis longus tendon, one heterotopic ossification, one radiocarpal dislocation, and two cases of an ulnar impaction syndrome due to implant subsidence. The conclusion was that the prosthetic treatment of complex DRFs in elderly patients with the Cobra implant led to clinically and radiologically satisfactory midterm outcomes. The Cobra prosthesis can be regarded as a feasible salvage option for complex DRFs when osteosyntheses may not be possible and nonoperative treatment will lead to further functional restrictions and wrist pain when performing activities of daily life in high functional demand patients [12].

14.4 Do We Need to Restore Anatomy to Have Satisfactory Clinical Result?

Marchewka et al. assessed the long-term results and complications associated with conservative and operative treatment of DRFs to determine if restoration of radiographic parameters influenced functional results [13]. They analyzed 207 patients with isolated DRFs (mean age 64 years, women 150 [72.5%], 101 treated operatively, 106 treated nonoperatively). There were no significant differences in sex, age, and AO/OTA-type fracture between study groups. After 3.9 years, clinical, functional, and radiological assessment was conducted using the DASH, PRWE, 9-Hole Peg Test (9-HPT), and grip and pinch strength tools. Marchewka et al. found higher rates of malunion in the nonoperative group ($p < 0.0001$) and worse radiologic parameters such as volar tilt ($p < 0.0001$) and teardrop angle ($p < 0.0001$) versus the operative cohort. Nevertheless, radiological parameters were not correlated with DASH and PRWE results. Moreover, patients aged 50 years and above treated operatively had similar functional outcomes (DASH, PRWE) to those treated nonoperatively. The conclusion was that restoration of anatomic and thus radiologic parameters of the radius may not be obligatory to get a satisfactory functional result in patients with DRF aged 50 years or above. The patient is the most important "factor" in determining the adequate and successful treatment technique for DRFs [13].

14.5 Treatment of Malunited Distal Radius Fracture

14.5.1 Corrective Osteotomy: 2D Imaging Techniques for Preoperative Alignment Planning Versus a Novel Patient-Specific Plate Which Features Navigation and Fixation of Bone Segments As Preoperatively Planned in 3D

According to Dobbe et al., corrective osteotomy of a malunited DRF conventionally relies on 2D imaging techniques for alignment planning and evaluation. However, this approach results in suboptimal bone repositioning, which is associated with poor patient outcomes. In a case series, Dobbe et al. assessed the utilization of novel patient-specific plates (PSPs), which feature navigation and fixation of bone segments as preoperatively planned in 3D (level of evidence IV) [14]. Ten participants with distal radius malunion underwent CT scans for preoperative alignment planning. Patient-specific guides and plates were designed, 3D-printed, and sterilized for utilization in corrective surgery of the distal radius. Pre- and postoperative outcomes were compared in regard to clinical, functional, and radiographic results. The application of a PSP was successful in seven of the ten cases. After treatment, the residual alignment error was diminished by approximately 50% compared with conventional treatment. The use of PSPs reduced pain significantly. Pre- and postoperative outcomes were pooled and showed significant correlations between pain and malpositioning; the range of pro- and supination motion, the MHOQ score, the EuroQol EQ-5D-5L questionnaire (EQ-5D-5L) score, and dorsovolar angulation; and MHOQ score and proximodistal translation. The conclusion was that the correlation between malalignment and MHOQ score, EQ-5D-5L score, pain, and ROM showed that alignment should be restored as well as possible. Compared to the conventional approach, which relies on 2D imaging techniques (Fig. 14.2), corrective osteotomy based on 3D preoperative planning and intraoperative fixation with a PSP has been shown to ameliorate bone alignment and diminish pain [14].

14.5.2 Corrective Osteotomy Through Planning with Prototyping in 3D Printing

According to Belloti et al., about one-third of DRFs can result in malunion with restriction of movement and pain in the wrist; the treatment in these cases consists of corrective osteotomy of the deformity. Due to its 3D complexity, careful preoperative planning is a paramount step in correction. The prototyping from the 3D reconstruction of the CT scan of the affected wrist allows the real understanding of the deformity. Patients with malunion of the distal radius with indication for surgical treatment were included in the group of corrective osteotomies through planning with prototyping in 3D printing [15]. The postoperative

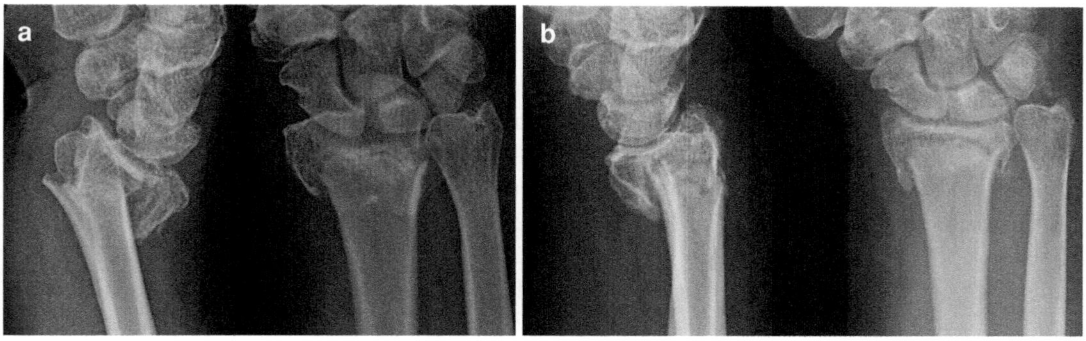

Fig. 14.2 (**a**, **b**) Conservatively treated wrist fracture (**a**) with malunion (**b**)

functional result was evaluated by the DASH and VAS. Radiographic data including radial inclination, volar tilt, and joint step were recorded from standard posteroanterior and lateral radiographic views. A total of nine patients were included. The mean age was 47 years. The average postoperative DASH value of the patients was 24.9 and VAS was 3.6. Radiographically, the palmar tilt had an average improvement of 25.22°, and the radial inclination had an average improvement of 2°. The conclusion was that corrective osteotomy through planning with prototyping in 3D printing was an efficacious technique of treating symptomatic distal radius malunions. The possibility of performing the osteotomy in a 3D model, simulating the surgery, makes the procedure more predictable [15].

14.6 Comparative Studies

14.6.1 Comparison of Surgical Effects Between Extension and Flexion Type of Distal Radius Fracture

Zhang et al. compared the therapeutic effects of internal fixation with VLP in treating extension and flexion type of DRF [16]. They analyzed 103 patients with DRF. According to the original fracture displacement direction, patients were divided into extension fracture (Colles) group and flexion fracture (Smith) group. In the Colles fracture group, there were 24 males and 44 females aged from 20 to 79 years old with an average of 59 years old; according to the AO/OTA classification, 9 patients were of type A2, 13 patients of type A3, 16 patients of type C1, 17 patients of type C2, and 13 patients of type C3; the time from injury to operation ranged from 2 to 9 days with an average of 3.9 days. In the Smith fracture group, there were 15 males and 20 females, aged from 27 to 87 years old with an average of 60.1 years old; according to the AO classification, 4 patients were of A2, 7 patients of A3, 14 patients of C1, 5 patients of C2, and 5 patients of C3; the time from injury to operation ranged from 2 to 6 days with an average of 4.1 days. Operation time, fracture healing time, and postoperative complications were recorded between the two groups. The DASH score at 6 and 8 weeks and 6 and 8 months were used to evaluate the functional recovery of the affected limbs during each follow-up. The volar tilt, radial inclination, and radius height were measured at 8 months after the operation. The Mayo score was measured at 8 months after the operation to assess the recovery of limb function. All patients were followed up for 8–30 months with an average of 14.8 months, and there was no difference in follow-up between the two groups ($p > 0.05$). There were no statistical differences in operation time, fracture healing time, and postoperative complications between groups ($p > 0.05$). The DASH scores at 6 and 12 weeks in the Colles fracture group were 37.24 and 19.68, while in the Smith fracture group were 39.05 and 23.44; the Colles fracture group results were better than that of the Smith fracture group ($p < 0.001$), while there were no differences in the DASH score at 6 and 8 months between the two groups ($p > 0.05$). The volar tilt of the Smith fracture group (11.1°) was better than that of the Colles fracture group (8.6°), and there were no significant differences in radial inclination and radius height between groups ($p > 0.05$). Moreover, there was no significant difference in the MWS ($p > 0.05$). The conclusion was that patients with Colles fracture and Smith fracture could receive good reduction and fixation through VLP. The radiographic parameters of both groups recovered satisfactorily after the operation. Recovery of the volar tilt of the Smith fracture group was better than that of the Colles fracture group, and early recovery function of the Colles fracture group was better than that of the Smith group, but there was no significant difference in long-term wrist joint function and incidence of postoperative complications between the two groups [16].

14.6.2 A Comparison of Six Outcome Measures Across the Recovery Period After Distal Radius Fixation: Which to Use and When?

According to Fang et al., many standardized outcome measures exist to measure recovery after surgical fixation of DRFs; however, choosing the optimal instrument is difficult. In a study with level II of evidence, Fang et al. assessed the responsiveness, ceiling/floor effects, and criterion validity over multiple time intervals across a 2-year follow-up period for six commonly utilized instruments [17]. A total of 259 patients who received open reduction and internal fixation for DRF between 2012 and 2015 were recruited. Patients were administered the PRWE, qDASH, Green and O'Brien score (Cooney modification) (CGNO), Gartland and Werley score (Sarmiento modification) (SGNW), flexion-extension arc (FEArc), and grip fraction test (GripFrac) at 1.5, 3, 6, 12, and 24 months postoperatively. Responsiveness was assessed by calculating the standardized response means (SRM) and Cohen's *d* effect sizes (ES) and by correlating each instrument's change scores against those of qDASH and PRWE, which were also utilized as external comparators to evaluate criterion validity. Ceiling/floor effects were calculated for all measures at each time point. The SRM (1.5–24 months) were 1.81, 1.77, 1.43, 1.16, 2.23, 2.45, and ES (1.5–24 months) were 1.81, 1.82, 1.95, 1.31, 1.99, and 2.90 for qDASH, PRWE, CGNO, SGNW, FEArc, and GripFrac, respectively. Spearman correlation coefficients against qDASH at 24 months were 0.809, 0.248, 0.563, 0.285, and 0.318 for PRWE, CGNO, SGNW, FEArc, and GripFrac, respectively. Significant (>15% of patients reaching maximum score) ceiling effects were observed before 6 months for PRWE and SGNW. This study supported the use of qDASH, PRWE, FEArc, and GripFrac up to 6 months postsurgery and qDASH and PRWE after 6 months [17].

14.6.3 Surgical Plating Versus Closed Reduction

In 2021, Lawson et al. evaluated whether current surgical treatment for displaced DRFs provided better patient-reported wrist pain and function than nonsurgical treatment in patients 60 years and older. In this multicenter randomized clinical trial and parallel observational study, 300 eligible patients were screened from 19 centers (trial registration, http://anzctr.org.au; identifier, ACTRN12616000969460) [18]. A total of 166 participants were randomized to surgical or nonsurgical treatment and followed up at 3 and 12 months by blinded assessors. Those 134 individuals who declined randomization were included in a parallel observational cohort with the same treatment options and follow-up. The primary analysis was intention to treat; sensitivity analyses included as-treated and per-protocol analyses. Surgical treatment was open reduction and internal fixation using a VLP. Nonsurgical treatment was CR and cast immobilization. The primary outcome was the PRWE score at 12 months. Secondary outcomes were the DASH questionnaire score, health-related quality of life, pain, major complications, patient-reported treatment success, bother with appearance, and therapy use. In the 300 study participants (mean age, 71.2 years; 269 [90%] female; 166 [81 VLP and 85 CR] in the randomized clinical trial sample and 134 [32 VLP and 102 CR] in the observational sample), no clinically important between-group difference in the 12-month PRWE scores (mean score of 19.8 for VLP and 21.5 for CR; mean difference, 1.7 points) was observed. No clinically important differences were found in the quality of life, wrist pain, or bother at 3 and 12 months. No significant difference was found in total complications between groups (12 of 84 [14%] for the CR group vs 6 of 80 [8%] for the VLP group; risk ratio [RR], 0.53; 95% CI, 0.21–1.33). Patient-reported treatment success favored the VLP group at 12 months (very successful or successful: 70 [89%] vs 57 [70%]; RR, 1.26; 95% CI, 1.07–1.48; p = 0.005). There was greater use of postoperative physical therapy in the VLP group (56 [72%] vs 44 [54%]; RR, 1.32; 95% CI, 1.04–1.69; p = 0.02). This randomized clinical trial found no between-group differences in improvement in wrist pain or function at 12 months from VLP fixation over CR for displaced DRFs in older people [18].

14.6.4 Plaster Immobilization Versus Anterior Plating for Dorsally Displaced Distal Radius Fractures

A prospective, multicentered, randomized trial analyzed results of 3- and 12-month follow-ups of 159 elderly patients aged more than 75 years with isolated DRF, treated by anterior locking plate or CR and cast immobilization (level III of evidence) [19]. The primary outcome was the PRWE score. The PRWE score at 12 months was not significantly different between the two groups; however, the radiological results and complications rates were worse in the CR group [19].

14.6.5 5 Cast Immobilization Versus Volar Locking Plate

Hasselund et al. compared operative and nonoperative treatment for displaced DRFs in patients aged over 65 years [20]. A total of 100 patients were randomized in this non-inferiority trial, comparing CR and cast immobilization with operation with a VLP. Patients with displaced AO/OTA A and C fractures were eligible if one of the following were found after initial closed reduction: (1) dorsal angulation >10°, (2) ulnar variance >3 mm, or (3) intra-articular step-off >2 mm. The primary outcome measure was the qDASH after 12 months. Secondary outcome measures were the PRWHE, EQ-5D-5L, ROM, grip strength, "satisfaction with wrist function" (score 0 to 10), and complications. In all, 89 women and 11 men were included. The mean age was 74 years (65–91 years). Nonoperative treatment was non-inferior to operation with a five-point difference in median qDASH score after 12 months (p = 0.206). After 3 and 6 months, the qDASH scores favored the operative group (p = 0.010 and 0.030, respectively). The median values for PRWHE were 19 in the operative group versus 10 in the nonoperative group at 3 months (p = 0.064), 9 versus 5 (p = 0.020) at 6 months, and 2 versus 0 (p = 0.019) after 12 months. ROM was similar between the groups. The EQ-5D-5L index score was better (mean difference 0.07) in the operative group at 3 and 12 months (p = 0.008 and 0.020, respectively). The complication rate was similar (p = 0.220). The operated patients were more satisfied with wrist function (median 8 vs 6) at 3 months (p = 0.002; 9 versus 8 at 6 months, p = 0.002; and 10 vs 8 at 12 months, $p < 0.001$). The conclusion was that nonoperative treatment was non-inferior to operative treatment based on the qDASH score after 1 year. Patients in the operative group had a faster recovery and were more satisfied with wrist function. Results from previous trials comparing operative and nonoperative treatment for displaced DRFs in the elderly vary between favoring the operative group and showing similar results between the treatments. This randomized trial suggested that most elderly patients may be treated nonoperatively [20].

14.6.6 Open Reduction and Volar Locking Plate Versus External Fixation with or Without Supplementary Pinning Versus Percutaneous Pinning

According to Chung et al., DRFs are common injuries among older adults and can result in substantial disability. Current evidence regarding long-term results in older adults is scarce. Chung et al. compared results across treatment groups at 24 months among adults with DRFs who participated in the WRIST trial [21]. The Wrist and Radius Injury Surgical Trial (WRIST) randomized, international, multicenter trial was conducted from April 1, 2012, through December 31, 2016 (trial registration, ClinicalTrials.gov; identifier, NCT01589692). Participants were adults aged 60 years or older with isolated, unstable DRFs at 24 health systems in the United States, Canada, and Singapore. Participants were randomized to open reduction and VLP, external fixation (EF) with or without supplementary pinning (EFP), and closed CR and percutaneous pinning (CRPP). The remaining participants chose closed reduction and casting. The primary outcome was the 24-month MHQ summary score. Secondary outcomes were scores on the MHQ subdomains hand strength and wrist motion. A total of 304 adults were recruited for the study, and 187 were randomized to undergo surgery, 65 to VLP, 64 to EFP, and 58 to CRPP; 117 participants opted for closed reduction and casting. Assessments were completed at 24 months for 182 participants (160 women [87.9%]; mean [SD] age, 70.1 [8.5] years). The mean MHQ summary scores at 24 months were 88 for VLP, 83 EFP, 85 for CRPP, and 85 for casting, with no clinically meaningful difference across groups after adjusting for covariates ($\chi 23 = 1.44$; $p = 0.70$). Pain scores also did not differ across groups at 24 months ($\chi 23 = 2.64$; $p = 0.45$). MHQ summary scores changed from 82 (95% CI, 80–85) to 85 (95% CI, 83–88) ($p = 0.12$) between 12 and 24 months across groups. The rate of malunion was higher in the casting group (26 participants [59.1%]) than in the other groups (4 participants [8.0%] for VLPS, 8 participants [17.0%] for EFP, and 4 participants [9.8%] for CRPP; $\chi 23 = 43.6$; $p < 0.001$), but malunion was not associated with the 24-month result difference across groups. This study did not find clinically meaningful patient-reported outcome differences 24 months after injury across treatment groups, with little change between 12 and 24 months. These findings suggested that long-term results need not necessarily be considered in deciding between treatment options. Patient needs and recovery goals that fit to relative risks and benefits of each treatment type will be more valuable in treatment decision-making [21].

14.6.7 Variable-Angle Volar Plate Versus Bridging External Fixator with K-Wire Augmentation in Comminuted Distal Radius Fractures

Mishra et al. compared the functional results between variable-angle volar plating and EF with K-wire augmentation in open reduction and internal fixation of DRFs [22]. A total of 62 adult patients with comminuted intra-articular DRFs were randomized into two groups: volar plate group and EF group. These patients aged between 18 and 60 years had unilateral fractures and agreed to be included in the study. Patients with a history of fracture, bilateral fracture, other associated injuries, delayed injury for more than 2 weeks, open fracture, preexisting arthrosis or disability, psychiatric illness, and pathological fracture were excluded. Patients were followed up at 6 weeks, 3 months, 6 months, and 1 year. The assessment of pain, functional activity, ROM, and grip strength was done at each stage of follow-up. The pain and functional activities were assessed by the PRWE and DASH scores. Patients in the volar plate group had superior PRWE and DASH scores at each stage of follow-up. At 1-year follow-up, the mean PRWE scores were 7.48 for the volar plate group and 7.35 for the EF group, while the mean DASH score was 4.65 for the volar plate group and 5.61 for the EF group, showing better flexion and extension ROM. They also had better pronation and supination ROM at initial follow-up; however, the difference was attenuated by 1 year. The volar plate group had significantly better grip strength than the EF group. Complication rates were higher in the EF group. The conclusion was that fixation with variable-angle volar plate resulted in early wrist mobilization, better ROM, less pain and disability, and early return of function [22].

14.6.8 Bilateral Distal Radius Fractures: External Fixation Versus Plate-Screw Treatment

Dagtas and Ünal compared the results of two surgical treatment options, EF or open reduction and internal fixation (ORIF), in patients with bilateral DRFs [23]. Twenty-one patients (11 males and 10 females; mean age, 40.0 years; range, 20–67 years) who underwent ORIF ($n = 10$) or EF ($n = 11$) due to bilateral DRF were retrospectively analyzed. The qDASH was used to calculate functional and symptomatic evaluation. The MWS was utilized to assess pain, functional status, ROM, and grip strength and the MHQ was used to measure hand performance in daily life. The operation time was statistically significantly longer in the ORIF group, compared to the EF group ($p < 0.001$). Radial shortening was statistically significantly greater in the EF group, compared to the ORIF group ($p < 0.001$). While the qDASH score was lower in the EF group on day 15 and at 1 and 2 months ($p < 0.001$, for each), it was similar between the groups at 1 year ($p = 0.507$). The MWS was higher in the EF group on day 15 and at 1 and 2 months and 1 year ($p < 0.05$, for each). While the MHOQ score was higher in the EF group on day 15 and at 1 and 2 months ($p < 0.001$, for each), it was similar between the groups at 1 year ($p = 0.557$). The conclusion was that in bilateral DRF cases, hand functions in the first 2 months after treatment were better in the EF group, compared to the ORIF group. This functional difference between the two groups gradually decreased in the first year and reached similar levels. This study demonstrated that EF can be a good alternative in the surgical treatment of bilateral DRFs owing to its acceptable outcomes, particularly in the short term [23].

14.7 Predictors of Management of Distal Radius Fractures in Patients Aged >65 Years

According to Walsh et al., treatment of DRFs in patients aged >65 years is controversial. They performed a study to identify what patient and fracture characteristics may influence the decision to pursue surgical versus nonsurgical treatment in patients aged >65 years sustaining a DRF. They queried their institutional DRF database for patients aged >65 years who presented to a single academic, tertiary center hand clinic over a 5-year period [24]. In all, 164 patients treated operatively were identified, and 162 patients treated nonoperatively during the same time period were selected for comparison (total $n = 326$). Demographic variables and fracture-specific variables were recorded. Patient and fracture characteristics between the groups were compared to determine which variables were associated with each treatment modality (operative or nonoperative). The average age in their cohort was 72 years, and 274 patients (67%) were women. The average Charlson Comorbidity Index (CCI) was 4.1. The CCI is a validated tool that predicts 1-year mortality based on patient age and a list of 22 weighted comorbidities. Factors associated with operative treatment in their population were largely related to the severity of the injury and included increasing dorsal tilt (odds ratio [OR], 1.09; 95% confidence interval [CI], 1.05–1.12; $p < 0.001$) and AO classification type C fractures (OR, 5.42; 95% CI, 2.35–11.61; $p < 0.001$). Increasing CCI was the only factor independently associated with nonoperative management (OR, 0.84; 95% CI, 0.72–0.997; $p = 0.046$) (Fig. 14.3). Fracture severity

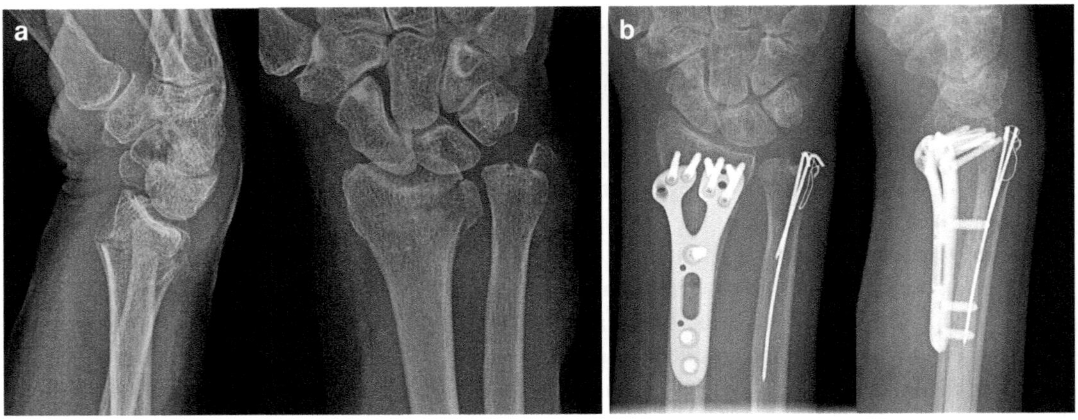

Fig. 14.3 (**a**, **b**) Distal radius and ulna fracture (**a**) treated with ORIF (open reduction and internal fixation)

was a strong driver in the decision to pursue operative management in patients aged >65 years, whereas increasing CCI predicted nonoperative treatment [24].

14.8 Conclusions

Distal radius fractures (DRFs) in the elderly population above 65 years of age represent 18% of all fractures and are therefore the second most common fracture in the elderly. The prevalence of DRFs is augmenting as life expectancy grows, leading to a larger population of patients who are at risk for these fractures. Most patients with minimally displaced DRFs can be treated nonoperatively with CR and 5-week cast immobilization, with satisfactory outcomes. However, DRFs in the elderly are often comminuted and intra-articular, therefore requiring surgical treatment. Three-dimensional preoperative planning for the osteosynthesis of DRFs has been proved to be reproducible with an error of about 2 mm for each reference point. It has been reported that Steinmann pin retractor-assisted CR combined with PP ameliorates fracture reduction and wrist function and can serve as an efficacious technique for A_2 (AO/OTA) and A_3 type of DRFs in the elderly with limited dorsal comminution, including intra-articular fractures with displacement less than 2 mm. DBP has been used most commonly in intra-articular, comminuted DRFs with overall functional wrist ROM, moderate patient-reported disability, and a 13% complication rate at follow-up. IlluminOss® System is a feasible alternative to treat DRFs with seemingly good clinical and functional result. However, one out of seven complications required surgical intervention. Fixation with VLP through the minimally invasive approach is a satisfactory and optional technique in the treatment of DRFs. This technique yields better early wrist function, shortens rehabilitation time, and obtains high psychological satisfaction. The plating method with a dual approach (dorsal and volar) may be an option for four-part intra-articular DRFs given its early mobility advantage and satisfactory functional and radiological results. It has been reported that prosthetic treatment of complex DRFs in elderly patients with the Cobra implant led to clinically and radiologically satisfactory midterm outcomes. However, the Cobra prosthesis still does not represent a gold standard but can be regarded as a feasible salvage option for complex DRFs when osteosynthesis may not be possible and nonoperative treatment will lead to further functional restrictions and wrist pain when performing activities of daily life in high functional demand patients. Restoration of anatomic and thus radiologic parameters of the radius may not be obligatory to achieve satisfactory functional result in patients with DRF aged 50 years or above. It has been reported that the patient is the most important "factor" in determining the adequate and successful treatment method for DRFs. A randomized clinical trial found no between-group differences in improvement in wrist pain or function at 12 months from VLP fixation over CR and cast immobilization for displaced DRFs in older people. Other randomized trial suggested that most elderly patients may be treated nonoperatively. A randomized study compared open reduction and VLP, external fixation with or without supplementary pinning, PP, and CR and casting. The study did not find clinically meaningful patient-reported outcome differences 24 months after injury across treatment groups, with little change between 12 and 24 months. Other reports compared a variable-angle volar plating and external fixator with K-wire augmentation in open reduction and internal fixation of DRFs. The conclusion was that the technique resulted in early wrist mobilization, better ROM, less pain and disability, and early return of function. It has been reported that factors associated with operative treatment in elderly patients are largely related to the severity of the injury and included increasing dorsal tilt and AO/OTA classification type C fractures. Increasing Charlson Comorbidity Index (CCI) was the only factor independently associated with nonoperative treatment. This study stated that fracture severity was a strong driver in the decision to pursue operative treatment in patients aged >65 years, whereas augmenting CCI predicted nonoperative treatment.

References

1. Thorninger R, Wæver D, Pedersen J, Tvedegaard-Christensen J, Tjørnild M, Lind M, Rölfing JD. Objective outcome measures continue to improve from 6 to 12 months after conservatively treated distal radius fractures in the elderly—a prospective evaluation of 50 patients. J Clin Med. 2021;10(9):1831.
2. Meena S, Sharma P, Sambharia AK, Dawar A. Fractures of distal radius: an overview. J Family Med Prim Care. 2014;3:325–32.
3. Corsino CB, Reeves RA, Sieg RN. Distal radius fractures. 2021 Aug 11. In: StatPearls [Internet]. Treasure Island (FL): StatPearls Publishing; 2021.
4. Vogt MT, Cauley JA, Tomaino MM, Stone K, Williams JR, Herndon JH. Distal radius fractures in older women: a 10-year follow-up study of descriptive characteristics and risk factors. The study of osteoporotic fractures. J Am Geriatr Soc. 2002;50:97–103.
5. Yoshii Y, Ogawa T, Shigi A, Oka K, Murase T, Ishii T. Three-dimensional evaluations of preoperative planning reproducibility for the osteosynthesis of distal radius fractures. J Orthop Surg Res. 2021;16(1):131.
6. Zhao B, Zhao W, Assan I, Li Z, Bi R. A novel retractor-assisted closed reduction combined with percutaneous pinning fixation for the treatment of elderly distal radius fractures: a retrospective cohort study. J Orthop Surg Res. 2021;16(1):409.
7. Fares AB, Childs BR, Polmear MM, Clark DM, Nesti LJ, Dunn JC. Dorsal bridge plate for distal radius fractures: a systematic review. J Hand Surg Am. 2021;46(7):627.e1–8.
8. Van Oijen GW, Vegt PA, Hagenaars T, Van Lieshout EMM, Verhofstad MHJ. Outcome after treatment of distal radius fractures in the elderly using the IlluminOss System. Eur J Trauma Emerg Surg. 2021;47:1129–36.
9. Fan J, Zhang X, Ji JQ, Yao Y, Li SZ, Yuan F, Cheng LM. Fixation of distal radius fracture with volar locking palmar plates while preserving pronator quadratus through the minimally invasive approach. Technol Health Care. 2021;29(1):167–74.
10. Uemura T, Yano K, Takamatsu K, Miyashima Y, Yasuda H, Konishi S, Nakamura H. Bone healing of distal radius nonunion treated with bridge plating with bone graft substitutes in combination with systemic romosozumab administration: a case report. Jt Dis Relat Surg. 2021;32:526–30.
11. Kibar B. Combined palmar and dorsal plating of four-part distal radius fractures: Our clinical and radiological results. Jt Dis Relat Surg. 2021;32:59–66.
12. Benedikt S, Kaiser P, Schmidle G, Kastenberger T, Stock K, Arora R. Lessons learned with the Cobra prosthesis in elderly patients with complex distal radius fractures-a retrospective follow-up study. Arch Orthop Trauma Surg 2021. https://doi.org/10.1007/s00402-021-04101-w. Online ahead of print.
13. Marchewka J, Szczechowicz J, Marchewka W, Golec E. Long-term outcomes and complications associated with operative and nonoperative treatment of distal radius fractures. Do we need to restore anatomy to have satisfactory clinical outcome? Folia Med Cracov. 2021;61:35–48.
14. Dobbe JGG, Peymani A, Roos HAL, Beerens M, Streekstra GJ, Strackee SD. Patient-specific plate for navigation and fixation of the distal radius: a case series. Int J Comput Assist Radiol Surg. 2021;16:515–24.
15. Belloti JC, Alves BVP, Faloppa F, Balbachevsky D, Netto NA, Tamaoki MJ. The malunion of distal radius fracture: Corrective osteotomy through planning with prototyping in 3D printing. Injury. 2021;52(Suppl 3):S44–8.
16. Zhang LY, Chi YJ, Liu FX, Gong WH, Yu C, Tang J, et al. Comparison of surgical effects between extension and flexion type of distal radius fracture. Zhongguo Gu Shang. 2021;34(2):101–7.

17. Fang C, Fang E, Yee DK, Kwan K, Leung G, Leung F. A comparison of six outcome measures across the recovery period after distal radius fixation-Which to use and when? J Orthop Surg (Hong Kong). 2021;29(1):2309499020971866.
18. Lawson A, Naylor JM, Buchbinder R, Ivers R, Balogh ZJ, Smith P, et al. Surgical plating vs closed reduction for fractures in the distal radius in older patients: a randomized clinical trial. JAMA Surg. 2021;156: 229–37.
19. Tahir M, Khan Zimri F, Ahmed N, Rakhio Jamali A, Mehboob G, Watson KR, Faraz A. Plaster immobilization versus anterior plating for dorsally displaced distal radial fractures in elderly patients in Pakistan. J Hand Surg Eur. 2021;46:647–53.
20. Hassellund SS, Williksen JH, Laane MM, Pripp A, Rosales CP, Karlsen Ø, et al. Cast immobilization is non-inferior to volar locking plates in relation to QuickDASH after one year in patients aged 65 years and older: a randomized controlled trial of displaced distal radius fractures. Bone Joint J. 2021;103-B: 247–55.
21. Chung KC, Kim HM, Malay S, Shauver MJ, WRIST Group. Comparison of 24-month outcomes after treatment for distal radius fracture: The WRIST randomized clinical trial. JAMA Netw Open. 2021;4(6):e2112710.
22. Mishra RK, Sharma BP, Kumar A, Sherawat R. A comparative study of variable angle volar plate and bridging external fixator with K-wire augmentation in comminuted distal radius fractures. Chin J Traumatol. 2021:S1008-1275(21)00078-X. https://doi.org/10.1016/j.cjtee.2021.04.005. Online ahead of print.
23. Dağtaş MZ, Ünal ÖK. The external fixation can be a good alternative to plate-screw treatment in the surgical treatment of bilateral distal radius fractures: a retrospective cohort study. Jt Dis Relat Surg. 2021;32:406–13.
24. Walsh A, Merchan N, Bernstein DN, Ingalls B, Harper CM, Rozental TD. Predictors of management of distal radius fractures in patients aged >65 Years. Hand (N Y). 2021:15589447211017217. https://doi.org/10.1177/15589447211017217. Online ahead of print.

15 Scapholunate Dissociation

Pablo Vadillo-Cardona, Alfonso Vaquero-Picado, and Fernando Corella

15.1 Introduction: Anatomy and Histology

The scapholunate interosseous ligament (SLIL) is an intrinsic, C-shaped ligament between the scaphoid and the lunate bones. The SLIL is anatomically divided in three portions: dorsal, proximal or membranous, and volar.

The dorsal SLIL is a taut structure composed of parallel collagen fibers and contributes to most of the tensile strength. Overstraeten et al. described the dorsal capsuloligamentous scapholunate septum (DCSS) [1]. It is an attachment between the dorsal wrist capsule, the dorsal part of the SLIL, and the dorsal intercarpal ligament. It inserts on to the scaphoid, the lunate, and the SLIL and it may play an important role in the stabilization of the scapholunate articulation.

The volar segment is similar in length and width but is approximately half as thick as the dorsal component and contains obliquely oriented fibers.

The proximal portion is histologically distinct because it is composed of fibrocartilage. It is difficult to identify the limits between the ligament and the scaphoid and lunate cartilage [2].

Hagert and Mataliotakis studied the histology of the SLIL. They described the different morphology of every portion of the ligament [3–5]. The dorsal portion is the strongest, rich in dense collagen fibers with few mechanoreceptors. The volar portion is well innervated and vascularized and there are fewer collagen fibers, but it is rich in mechanoreceptors. Finally, the proximal part is formed by conjunctive tissue centrally surrounded by fibrocartilage. There are some mechanoreceptors close to the palmar portion. According to these findings, the SLIL could be divided into a more mechanic dorsal portion and a more sensitive volar portion.

15.2 Pathomechanics

In a normal wrist there is an equilibrium between the flexion force applied over the scaphoid and the extension force applied over the triquetral. Both bones are stabilized to the lunate through the scapholunate and lunotriquetral ligaments. The scaphoid tends to flex the lunate and the triquetrum to extend it (Fig. 15.1).

The dorsal portion of the SLIL is the primary stabilizer of the scapholunate interval. The most important secondary stabilizers are the radioscaphocapitate (RSC), scaphocapitate (SC), and volar scaphotrapeziotrapezoid (STT) liga-

P. Vadillo-Cardona (✉) · A. Vaquero-Picado
Department of Orthopedic Surgery, "La Paz" University Hospital, Madrid, Spain
e-mail: pablo.vadillo@salud.madrid.org

F. Corella
Department of Orthopedic Surgery, "Infanta Leonor" Hospital, Madrid, Spain

E. C. Rodríguez-Merchán, A. Moreno-Garcìa (eds.), *Controversies in Orthopedic Surgery of The Upper Limb*, https://doi.org/10.1007/978-3-031-04907-1_15

ments. After complete lesion of the SLIL, there is no visible alteration in normal X-ray. However, under load, in stress X-rays, we can identify signs of scapholunate dissociation. Overstretching of secondary stabilizers with time may cause attenuation and rupture of these ligaments. In normal X-rays, we will identify scaphoid flexion and an increased scapholunate (SL) gap [6].

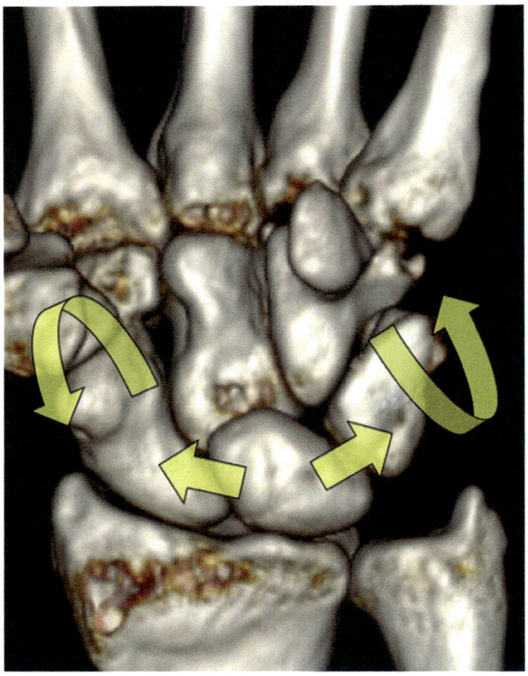

Fig. 15.1 The scaphoid tends to flex and the triquetrum to extend the lunate. The scapholunate and lunotriquetral ligaments stabilize the lunate in neutral position

In these cases, the scaphoid and lunate separate under the application of force, the lunate rotates into extension, and the scaphoid flexes, pronates, and moves dorsally and radially. The scaphoid proximal pole translates dorsoradially causing an alteration in the distribution of forces in the wrist. There is an increase of pressure in the dorsoradial area of the distal radius that may explain the frequent development of degenerative changes in the dorsolateral margin of the radioscaphoid fossa.

The extended lunate remains stable with the radius due to the fact that both articular surfaces have the same radius of curvature. Progression of the degenerative changes in the articulation with time may end in a predictable degenerative pattern termed scapholunate advanced collapse (SLAC) defined by Watson et al. [7]. Classically, it was thought that all SLIL lesions will progress to SLAC wrist. However, it is unclear which patients will end with an arthritic wrist. Some authors have described progressive deterioration of strength and mobility over time in an untreated SL lesion but the speed of progression in still unclear [8] (Fig. 15.2).

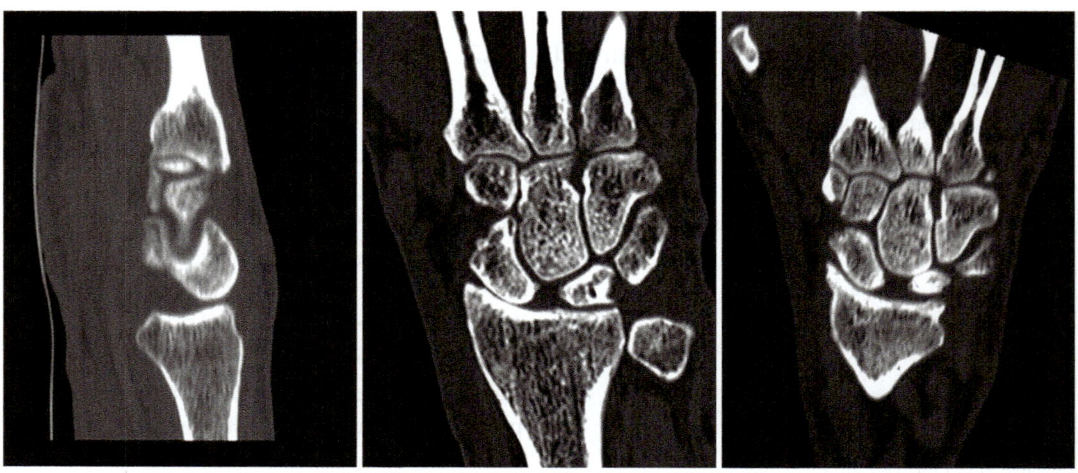

Fig. 15.2 Scapholunate advanced collapse (SLAC) classification. On the left: SLAC 1, degenerative changes limited to the dorsum of the scaphoid fossa. On the middle: SLAC 2, degenerative changes in the whole scaphoid fossa. On the right: SLAC 3, degenerative changes affecting the scaphoid and capitate

15.3 Diagnosis

The most common mechanism of injury of SLIL is a fall with the wrist in extension, ulnar deviation, and midcarpal supination. This mechanism can cause several lesions including concomitant fractures of the scaphoid or the distal radius.

Symptoms of SLIL injury may vary depending of the degree of disruption and the time from the lesion. A high index of suspicion is needed to avoid missing this injury. Most common complaints are poor grip strength, decreased mobility, and tenderness over the dorsal SLIL. Pain is variable and usually increased with activity. Sometimes the patients describe a "clunk" in the wrist after some movements due to the dislocation and reduction of the scaphoid.

15.3.1 Physical Exams

Scaphoid Shift Test or Watson Test: The examiner places four fingers in the dorsum of the radius and the thumb on the distal pole of the scaphoid. The other hand moves the wrist passively from ulnar to radial deviation. In SLIL lesions, pressure over the distal pole of the scaphoid during ulnar to radial deviation prevents flexion of the scaphoid. The scaphoid could be subluxated dorsally in complete lesions. When pressure is released, a painful "clunk" could be felt when the scaphoid reduces into the fossa. It is important to compare both wrists. Watson test could be positive in cases of hyperlaxity [9] (Fig. 15.3).

Scapholunate Ballottement Test: The lunate is stabilized with one hand and the scaphoid is displaced dorsally and volarly. The test is positive when there is pain, crepitus, or increased mobility (Fig. 15.4).

15.3.2 Radiological Examination

Radiological examination should include dorsopalmar, lateral, and stress views. AP fist with 30° ulnar deviation and clenched-fist views have the most consistent increase in scapholunate distance [10]. Contralateral views should be obtained for comparison (Fig. 15.5).

The radiographical signs of SLIL lesions are as follows:

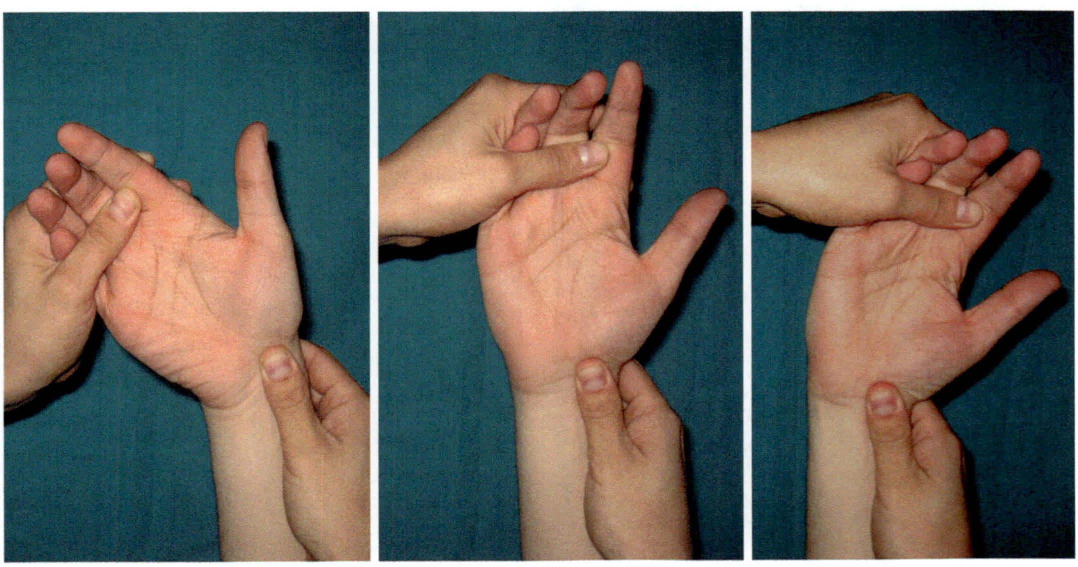

Fig. 15.3 Watson test

- Terry-Thomas sign, defined as a scapholunate distance >3 mm. Nevertheless, significant variability exists between patients.
- Signs of scaphoid flexion as the ring sign and shortening of the scaphoid in the PA view.
- Measurement of radiocarpal angles is difficult because of the irregular shape of the carpal bones. Small changes in wrist positioning can severely change measurements. High-quality views are needed for proper interpretation. Good-quality lateral views should show interposition of the scaphoid tubercle and pisiform and radius. Capitate and third metacarpals should be aligned.
  - Scapholunate angle >70° is considered a sign of abnormal flexion of the scaphoid; normal scapholunate angle ranges between 30° and 60°.
  - Radiolunate angle >15° is a defined sign of dorsal intercalated segment instability (Fig. 15.6).

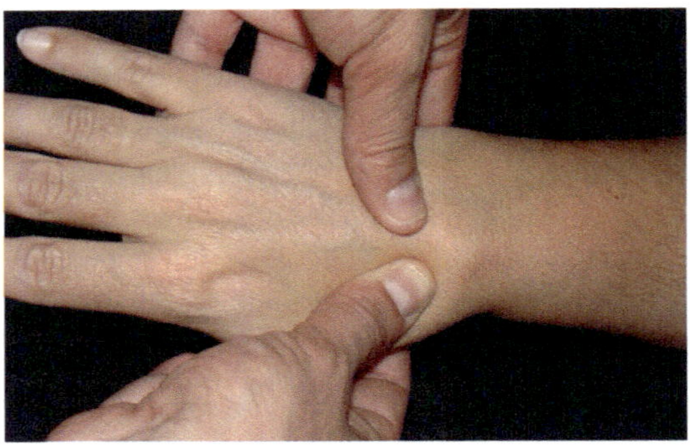

Fig. 15.4 Scapholunate ballottement test

SLIL injuries could be classified according to the radiological findings in four stages:

1. Pre-dynamic instability: standard and stress radiographs are normal. It corresponds to a partial SLIL rupture that can only be diagnosed by MRI or arthroscopy.
2. Dynamic instability: standard radiographs are normal and only stress views show signs of SLIL instability. It is associated with a complete SLIL rupture.
3. Static instability: there are radiographic signs of SLIL dissociation in standard and stress radiographs. It is associated with a complete rupture of the SLIL and attenuation of secondary stabilizers.

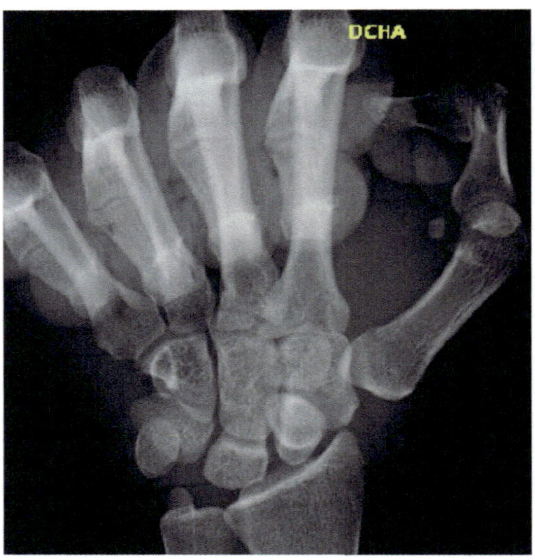

Fig. 15.5 Clenched-fist view showing and increased scapholunate (SL) gap

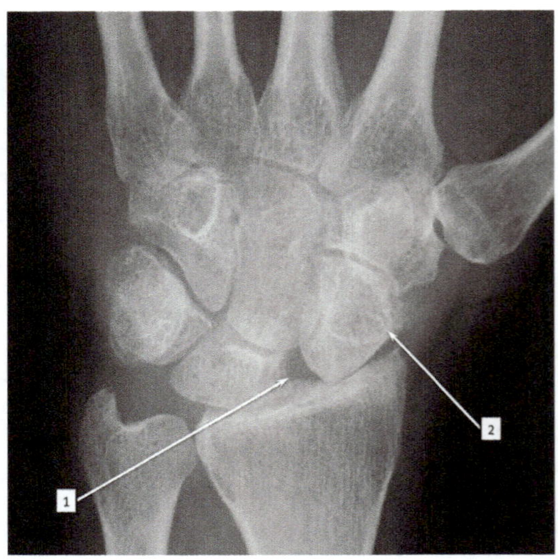

Fig. 15.6 A positive Terry-Thomas sign (marked as 1) and a ring sign (marked as 2)

4. Scapholunate advanced collapse (SLAC) wrist: Watson et al. described four different stages, which will be described later.

15.3.2.1 Advance Imaging

Magnetic resonance imaging (MRI) is not so accurate as in other joints due to the complex anatomy of the wrist ligaments [11]. According to a comparative study between magnetic resonance arthrography (MRA) and MRI, the sensitivity for detection of SLIL injury of 1.5 T MRI was 45% and 75.7% for 3 T. MRA sensitivity was higher but similar to 3 T MRI at 82.1% [12]. The use of 3 T MRI has improved the visualization of the ligaments of the wrist; however, SLIL lesions are still difficult to identify in MRI. Dietrich et al. published an interdisciplinary consensus on imaging of SL instability [13]. The consensus agreement suggested that radiographs, radiographic stress views, dynamic fluoroscopy, MRA, and CTA are currently the most useful and accurate imaging techniques for SL instability diagnosis.

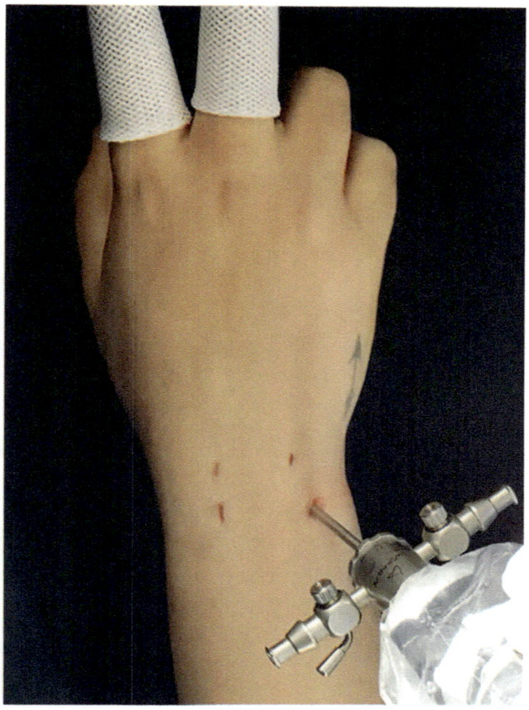

Fig. 15.7 Wrist arthroscopy. The scope is placed in the 6R portal

15.3.2.2 Arthroscopic Examination

Arthroscopy is considered the gold standard for the diagnosis of SLIL injuries. It allows the diagnosis and treatment of multiple pathologies. Initially, wrist arthroscopy was performed using constant saline flow irrigation [14]. The concept of dry wrist arthroscopy was developed by del Piñal et al. and it is very suitable for the diagnosis and treatment of SL lesions [15] (Fig. 15.7).

Geissler defined a treatment-oriented classification that evaluates the scapholunate interval. SLIL should be evaluated both through the radiocarpal and midcarpal joints [16]. When visualized from the radiocarpal joint, SLIL is best viewed through the 3–4 portal with a probe in the 6R portal. The normal scapholunate ligament is confluent between the scaphoid and the lunate and it is usually difficult to differentiate under direct visualization. On palpation, the scapholunate ligament is softer than the scaphoid and lunate. In the midcarpal joint, the SLIL is visualized through the midcarpal ulnar portal (MCU) and the probe in the midcarpal radial portal (MCR) (Table 15.1) (Fig. 15.8).

The European Wrist Arthroscopy Society (EWAS) modified in 2009 Geissler's classification [17] (Table 15.2):

The arthroscopic scaphoid 3D (dorsal, dynamic, displacement) test was described by Corella et al. to check the abnormal dorsal displacement of the scaphoid. To perform the test, traction should be released and the arthroscope set under the lunate (in the radiocarpal joint) or on the lunate (in the midcarpal joint). The scaphoid is manually pushed dorsally at the scaphoid tubercle. A negative test is defined when all the proximal row bones are minimally displaced, and

Table 15.1 Geissler classification of scapholunate ligament injuries

Stage	Radiocarpal view	Midcarpal view
I	Attenuation and hemorrhage of SL ligament	Tight SL interval. Probe cannot be inserted.
II	Attenuation and hemorrhage of SL ligament	Probe can be inserted but not rotated.
III	Radiocarpal step-off, SL tear	Probe enters SL interval and can be rotated.
IV	Radiocarpal step-off, SL tear	2.7-mm scope can be driven through the SL interval.

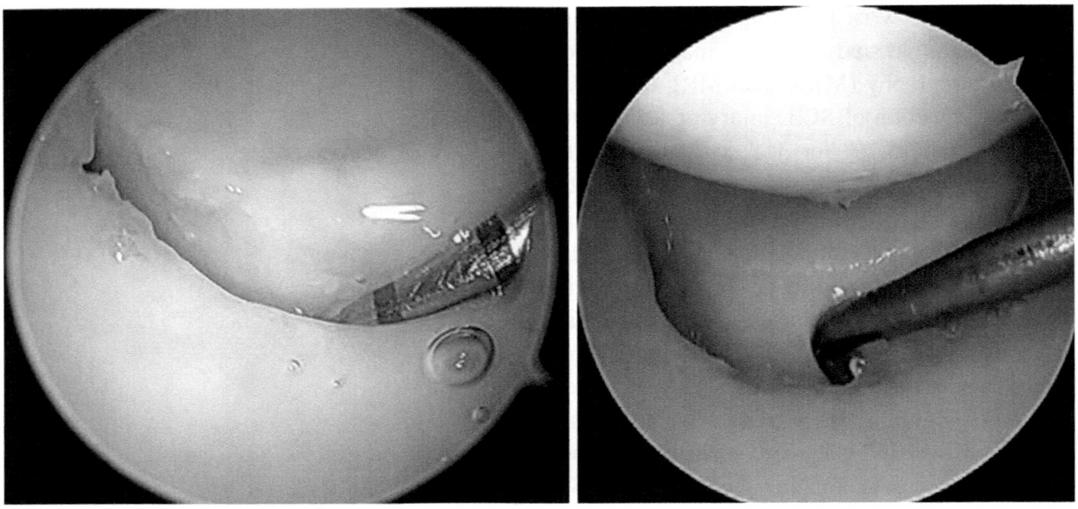

Fig. 15.8 On the left, Geissler grade III lesion; on the right, Geissler grade IV lesion

Table 15.2 European Wrist Arthroscopy Society (EWAS) classification of scapholunate ligament injuries

EWAS	Description	Arthroscopic test
I	As Geissler type I	Tight SL joint space; probe cannot be inserted.
II	As Geissler type II	Entry of the probe but not its rotation.
IIIA	Type II + volar SL ligament disruption	Volar laxity, no tension of the volar ligament when tested with the probe.
IIIB	Type II + dorsal SL ligament disruption	Dorsal laxity, no tension of the dorsal ligament when tested with the probe.
IIIC	Type II + volar and dorsal SL ligament disruption	Volar and dorsal laxity; probe can be rotated in SL interval.
IV	IIIC + SL gap, no misalignment or reducible	A 2.7 mm scope can be driven through the SL interval to the radiocarpal joint
V	IV + misalignment, not reducible	SL gap with radiographic abnormalities.

there is no scapholunate instability. A positive test is found when the scaphoid is displaced dorsally while the lunate remains static; this indicates scapholunate instability [18].

After evaluating SLIL lesions, it is important to check the rest of the joint for the presence of arthritis or other ligamentous injuries. These findings will help us to differentiate an acute lesion from a chronic rupture or a SLAC wrist.

Table 15.3 Garcia-Elias classification

	I	II	III	IV	V	VI
Is there a partial rupture with a normal dorsal SL ligament?	Yes	No	No	No	No	No
If ruptured, can the dorsal SL ligament be repaired?	Yes	Yes	No	No	No	No
Is the scaphoid normally aligned (RS <45°)?	Yes	Yes	Yes	No	No	No
Is the carpal malalignment easily reducible?	Yes	Yes	Yes	Yes	No	No
Is the articular cartilage normal?	Yes	Yes	Yes	Yes	Yes	No

15.4 Principles of Treatment

Treatment of SLIL lesions is controversial. There are numerous techniques described supported by limited evidence-based studies. Most treatment recommendations are based on expert opinions.

Garcia-Elias et al. proposed six questions to grade the scapholunate lesions in six stages, from a minor problem (stage I) to severe pathology (stage VI). Treatment recommendations were given for every stage [19] (Table 15.3).

15.4.1 Stage I: Partial SLIL Injury

The SLIL is only stretched or partially disrupted, and the dorsal portion of the ligament is intact. The degree of SLIL lesion varies from a distension (Geissler I) to a partial rupture (Geissler II). Wrist alignment is not altered but there is increased motion between the scaphoid and lunate causing cartilage loading and synovitis.

In standard and stress radiographs, there is no gap in the SL interval or malalignment. The SLIL lesion can only be diagnosed arthroscopically or by MRI. According to the radiographic findings, some authors defined this as occult or predynamic instability [20].

These patients, when symptomatic, could be treated by (1) arthroscopic debridement, (2) arthroscopic debridement and ligament shrinkage, or (3) reeducation of wrist proprioception.

15.4.1.1 Arthroscopic Debridement and Electrothermal Ligament Shrinkage

Synovectomy and debridement of torn and unstable ligament portions is performed in the radiocarpal and midcarpal joints. Electrothermal treatment is administered in short, non-ablative pulses over the SL ligament to produce a visible color and texture change. Specific focus is paid in the dorsal portion of the SLIL. The synovial fluid temperature should be monitored to avoid high temperatures that could cause chondrolysis.

Good clinical results, diminishing pain, and improving function are expectable with this technique, but the duration of the clinical relief is controversial. Lee et al. published good results in Geissler I and II lesions, reducing pain and improving grip strength in 14 patients with a mean follow-up of 53 months [21]. Burn et al. demonstrated excellent results in 9 patients with a follow-up of 5 years [22]. Patients had a mean grip strength equal to the contralateral extremity, near symmetric wrist motion, and a QuickDASH score improvement of 39 points.

15.4.1.2 Reeducation of Wrist Proprioception

Muscles act as carpal dynamic stabilizers; their contraction counteracts the displacement of the scaphoid in disrupted SLIL. Hagert et al. described the presence of mechanoreceptors in carpal ligaments that act as sensors to activate the contraction of the muscles to counteract the forces deforming the carpal bones [23]. Under axial load, the scaphoid tends to flex and pronate. Muscles that supinate the distal row compensate these forces. The abductor pollicis longus (APL) and extensor carpi radialis longus (ECRL) have demonstrated to supinate the carpal distal row, whereas the extensor carpi ulnaris (ECU) acts as a pronating muscle. The flexor carpi radialis (FCR) acts as a pronator muscle that supinates the scaphoid because of its relations to the scaphoid tuberosity [24]. Conservative management should focus on strengthening and proprioception reeducation of the supinator muscles (APL, ECRL, and FCR) while avoiding activation of the ECU. Certain orthosis could be modeled to place the wrist in slight extension, ulnar deviation, and supination to avoid contraction of the ECU [25, 26].

15.4.2 Stage II: Complete SLIL Injury, Repairable

In this stage, SLIL is completely disrupted but the dorsal portion is repairable. Arthroscopically, a complete Geissler grade III lesion is visualized. There is no malalignment and the secondary stabilizers are competent but tend to fail when loaded. There are only radiographic signs of instability in stress radiographs, SL gap or scaphoid flexion. This stage corresponds to a dynamic instability.

Anderson et al. described four types of dorsal SLIL ruptures: avulsion from the scaphoid (42%), avulsion from the lunate (18%), mid-substance rupture (20%), and partial rupture and elongation (22%) [27].

SLIL repairability depends on the quality of the ligament remnant. Mid-substance ruptures tend to degenerate very quickly and are often non-repairable. Bone avulsions are usually more favorable to repair. Lesions occurring after 3–4 months tend to degenerate and are usually not suitable for repair.

Treatment options for direct repair are (1) open reduction and dorsal ligament repair and (2) Arthroscopic repair.

15.4.2.1 Open Reduction and Dorsal SL Ligament Repair

A longitudinal, "Z-shaped," or transverse skin incision is made. The extensor retinaculum is open over the third extensor compartment, protecting the extensor pollicis longus tendon. Capsule incision varies depending of the posterior interosseous nerve. It could be excised, and a capsulotomy is made following the dorsal fiber-splitting approach described by Berger [28] or preserved using a nerve-sparing approach as described by Garcia-Elias. After exposing the SL interval, the ligament rupture is explored. According to the Anderson classification, the repair can be made by direct suture (mid-substance rupture) or by reinserting the ligament to the bone using an anchor. Usually, the repair is protected by transfixing the SL and SC joint with K-wires. Several authors recommend performing a dorsal capsulodesis during closure to reinforce the repair. Wires are removed after 8–10 weeks and a splint is maintained for a total of 12 weeks. A retrospective review of 82 patients showed acute repairs have better results than chronic ones [29]. Rosati et al. reported, in 18 patients with an average follow-up of 32 months, excellent or good functional outcomes in 88% of the patients [30]. Recently, Loisel et al. reported significant changes in carpal bone stability after performing the dorsal fiber-splitting approach in a cadaveric study [31]. They described a "window" approach that preserved the critical dorsal stabilizers and did not alter bone alignment (Fig. 15.9).

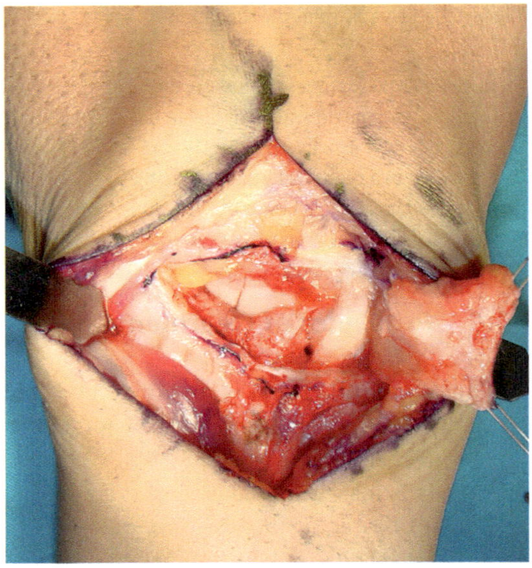

Fig. 15.9 Berger approach to reach the carpal bone

15.4.2.2 Arthroscopic Repair and Capsular Reinforcement

Arthroscopic repair and capsular reinforcement are performed through the four standard portals: 3–4, 6R, midcarpal radial (MCR), and midcarpal ulnar (MCU). The 6R portal is used for vision and the 3–4 as a working portal. Under direct vision, an anchor is introduced in the scaphoid or lunate upon the insertion of the SLIL, depending on where the SLIL has been detached. One side of the suture is passed through the remaining SLIL and both sutures are tied together. Depending on the lesion, sometimes more than one anchor is needed. The sutures of the implant are used for dorsal capsular plication. One side of the suture is passed to the midcarpal joint through the ligament and recovered to the radiocarpal joint between the capsule and the extensor tendons. Finally, both ends are tied together making a dorsal plication of the capsule. Carratala et al. reported good to excellent results in 79% of 19 patients with a follow-up of 1 year using this technique [32].

Mathoulin et al. described a capsuloligamentous repair performing a direct repair of the ligament and the dorsal capsule [33]. The indications were acute and chronic cases–Geissler 2, 3, and 4. K-wires were added in stage IV cases. Published results were good to excellent in most of cases (Fig. 15.10).

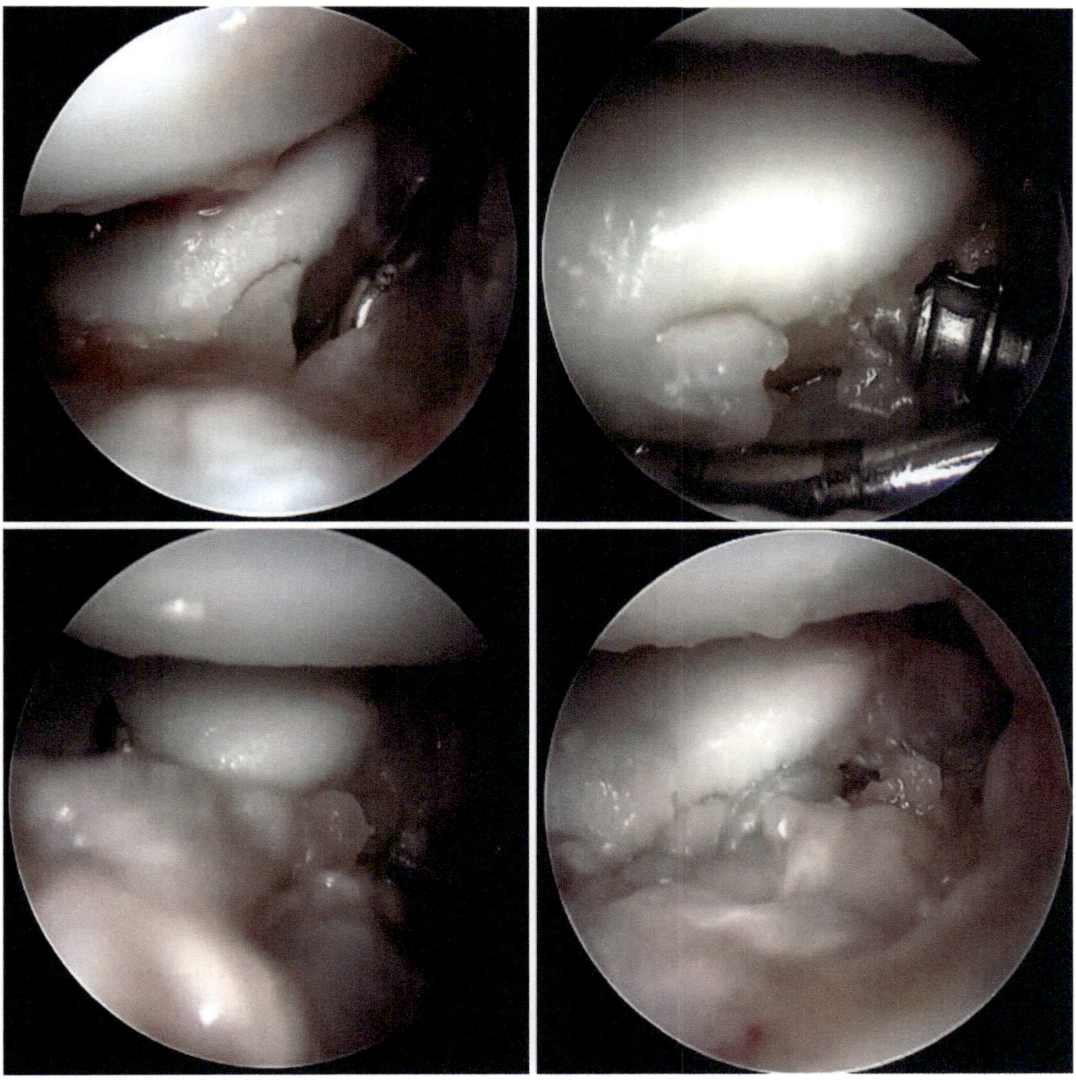

Fig. 15.10 Arthroscopic repair of a torn dorsal scapholunate (SL) ligament. Top left image: avulsion of the dorsal scapholunate interosseous ligament (SLIL). Top right image: anchor placement over the SLIL insertion. Down left image: suture passing through the SL remnant. Down right image: suture of the ligament

15.4.3 Stage III: Complete SLIL Lesion, Non-Repairable, No Malalignment

This is a complete lesion of the SLIL with poor healing potential, irreparable. There is still no malalignment because secondary stabilizers are still competent. This stage is radiographically defined as dynamic instability.

Most treatments for stage III utilize local tissues, like capsule, ligaments, or bone-ligament-bone autografts, to supplement local stabilizers. Treatment options are (1) dorsal capsulodesis, (2) bone-ligament-bone autografts, and (3) ligamentoplasties.

Dorsal Capsulodesis: It is carried out like the Blatt technique or Mayo Clinic scapholunate ligamentoplasty, using the capsule or the dorsal intercarpal ligament, respectively, to prevent scaphoid flexion. Both techniques showed improvement of symptoms but also significant reduction in range of motion and strength [34, 35].

Bone-Ligament-Bone Autografts: Grafts from the distal radius and dorsal retinaculum, or third metacarpal-capitate, have been used. There is still no long-term evidence of the results, but they have shown limited effect on preserving carpal alignment and preventing wrist arthritis.

Ligamentoplasties: Due poor results and decreased mobility of the aforementioned techniques, there is a trend to directly treat stage III lesions using scapholunate *ligamentoplasties*. These techniques will be described in the next section.

15.4.4 Stage IV: Complete, Irreparable SLIL Injury, Reducible Malalignment

In stage IV, there is a complete, irreparable SLIL lesion. Secondary stabilizers are stretched or disrupted. Plain radiographs show an increased SL gap in PA view and scaphoid flexion in lateral view. There is no cartilage damage. This stage is radiographically defined as static instability. The scaphoid will assume a flexed and pronated position and the lunate will be extended.

Three different treatment options have been described for this stage:

1. Reconstruction of the ruptured ligaments with tendon grafts:
   (a) Open reconstruction
   (b) Arthroscopic scapholunate ligamentoplasty
   (c) Arthroscopically assisted ligament reconstruction
2. Reduction-association of the SL joint (RASL) procedure

15.4.4.1 SLIL Ligamentoplasty Using a Tendon Graft

The "three-ligament tenodesis" uses the flexor carpi radialis (FCR) tendon to reconstruct the SLIL. The FCR is divided proximally, maintaining its insertion in the second metacarpal. A tunnel is made in the scaphoid from the insertion of the dorsal SLIL to the palmar tuberosity. The tendon strip is retrieved dorsally and fixed to the dorsum of the lunate using an anchor. The remainder of the tendon is pulled through the radiotriquetral ligament and sutured back in the lunate. K-wires are placed between the scaphoid and lunate and between the scaphoid and capitate to protect the reconstruction. Wrist immobilization is maintained for 6 weeks, and then a removable splint for additional 6 weeks. K-wires are removed at 8 weeks postoperatively. Garcia-Elias et al. published a series of 38 patients with an average follow-up of 46 months [36]. Pain relief at rest was obtained in 28 patients, 8 patients complained of mild discomfort during strenuous activity, and 2 had pain in most activities. Range of motion was 75% compared with the contralateral wrist and there was recurrence of malalignment in two wrists. Kakar et al. described a 360° reconstruction with tendon graft augmented with an internal brace [37]. The results in a cadaver study showed a significant superior biomechanical stability than tenodesis alone.

15.4.4.2 Arthroscopic Scapholunate Ligamentoplasty

Arthroscopic scapholunate ligamentoplasty combines the advantages of the arthroscopic and open techniques. Corella et al. described an arthroscopic ligamentoplasty that reconstructs the dorsal and volar SL ligament with a strip of the FCR [38]. To perform the technique, seven portals are used, and one more is needed to retrieve the FCR tendon: the four standard portals (3–4, 6R, MCR, and MCU), dorsal central (DC), volar central (VC), and radial distal (RD). A tunnel is created from the dorsal insertion of the SL ligament to the scaphoid tubercle. Another tunnel is drilled in the lunate parallel to the radiocarpal joint line. The tendon is retrieved through the scaphoid tunnel dorsally and then to the dorsum of the lunate intra-articularly. The tendon is then passed through the lunate tunnel volarly, passed extra-articularly to the scaphoid, and fixed to the scaphoid with an anchor. Interference screws are used to fix the tendon to the scaphoid and lunate. A removable splint is used for the first 6 weeks, and a dart-throwing motion is started at 2 weeks and progressive flexion-extension exercises at 4 weeks. At 6 weeks, progressive strength and proprioceptive exercises are started, and after 12 weeks, normal activity is resumed. They recently published the results in 46 patients showing a significant increase in grip strength and decrease in pain scales at 1 and 2 years postoperatively [39] (Fig. 15.11).

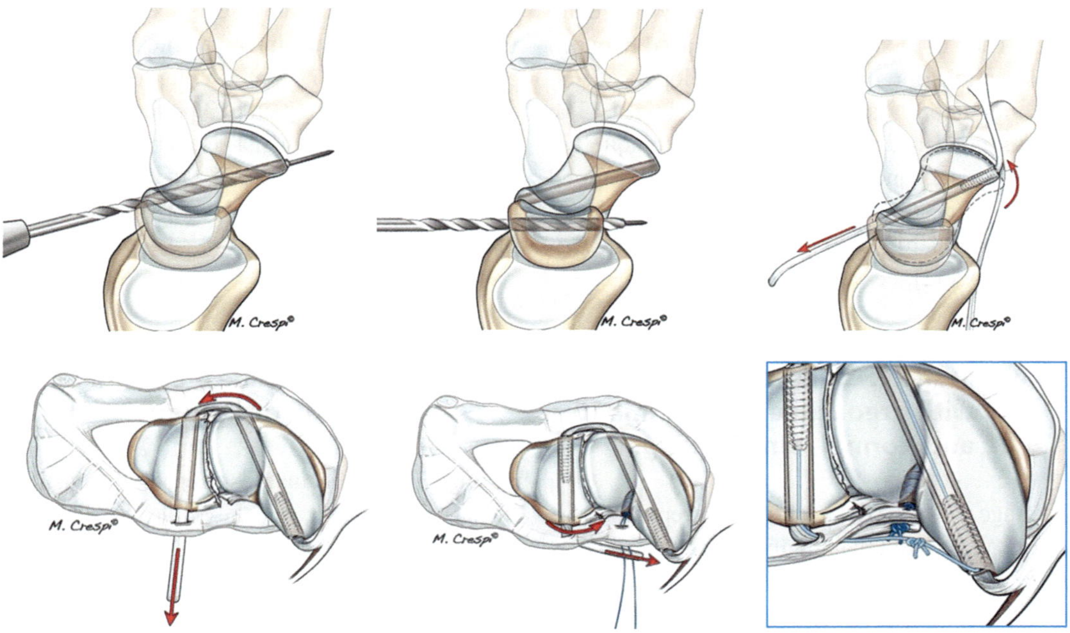

Fig. 15.11 Arthroscopic ligamentoplasty. Scaphoid tunnel is drilled from the dorsal insertion of the scapholunate ligament to the scaphoid tubercle. The second tunnel is drilled parallel to the joint surface of the lunate. A loop is passed from the dorsal to the 3–4 portal. Passage of the graft through the scaphoid tunnel and fixation using an interference screw. The graft is captured in the loop and recovered intra-articularly and dorsally on the lunate. The graft is passed through the lunate dorsal to volar and recovered through the volar central portal. The graft is fixed with a tenodesis screw. The graft is passed extra-articularly to the scaphoid and fixed with an anchor. Reprinted with permission from Corella F, Del Cerro M, Ocampos M, Simon de Blas C, Larrainzar-Garijo R. Arthroscopic scapholunate ligament reconstruction, volar and dorsal reconstruction. Hand Clin. 2017;33:687–707

15.4.4.3 Arthroscopically Assisted Ligament Reconstruction

Ho et al. described a combined limited open reconstruction with the assistance of arthroscopy [40]. They reconstructed the dorsal and volar portion of the SLIL using a palmaris longus tendon graft. The scaphocapitate joint was transfixed with Kirschner wires for 6–8 weeks after surgery. The authors published their results in 17 patients with a follow-up of 48.3 months. Eleven patients had no pain and 6 had some pain on maximum exertion or extreme motion. The mean grip was 120% of the preoperative status and motion improvement between 13% and 27%.

15.4.4.4 Reduction-Association of the SL Joint (RASL) Procedure

The reduction-association of the SL joint (RASL) procedure was initially described by White et al. [41]. They used a Herbert screw placed between the scaphoid and the lunate to develop a soft tissue nonunion that stabilized the bones. The results published with the RASL technique are controversial, and some authors endorse good results using this technique but there are cases describing hardware failure and recurrence of deformity [42].

15.4.5 Stage V: Chronic SL Injury with Irreducible Malalignment and Normal Joint Cartilage

In stage V, there is a chronic, irreparable SL lesion and a fixed malalignment. The cartilage is still preserved. Like stage IV, it is defined as a static instability. Treatment options are limited intercarpal arthrodesis. The goal of treatment is to reduce pain and preserve some range of motion at this stage [43].

15.4.5.1 Scapholunate Arthrodesis

Scapholunate arthrodesis has been attempted with little success, and published union rates are around 50%.

15.4.5.2 Scaphoid-Trapezium-Trapezoid Arthrodesis

Scaphoid-trapezium-trapezoid (STT) arthrodesis has a higher rate of union up to 86% (Stewart) with reduced range of motion and strength. There is a significant limited radial deviation and flexion of the scaphoid due to the arthrodesis. A radial styloidectomy has been described by some authors to increase mobility [44].

15.4.5.3 Radioscaphoid-Lunate Arthrodesis

Radioscaphoid-lunate fusion was developed to restore scaphoid position. Initially, wrist flexion was severely limited due to the scaphoid fixation. Garcia-Elias et al. described the excision of the distal pole of the scaphoid to allow more motion and decrease STT arthritis [45]. The midcarpal joint motion is preserved in the dart-thrower's plane when the distal pole is excised. Garcia-Elias et al. published, in 16 patients with an average follow-up of 37 months, complete pain relief in 10 patients, slight pain in 3 patients, and occasional pain in 3 patients. The average postoperative range of motion was 32° of flexion, 35° of extension, 14° of radial deviation, and 19° of ulnar deviation [45].

15.4.6 Stage VI: Chronic SL Injury with Irreducible Malalignment and Cartilage Damage

In stage VI, the ligament is irreparable, malalignment is not reducible, and the cartilage is damaged. Standard radiographs will show a static dissociation with osteoarthritis changes in the wrist. This stage corresponds to a scapholunate advance collapse (SLAC). SLAC wrist was divided in four stages as defined by Watson et al. [7].

1. Stage I is defined by limited osteoarthritis in the dorsum of the scaphoid fossa in the radius.
2. Stage II exhibits osteoarthritis and joint space narrowing in the whole scaphoid fossa in the radius.

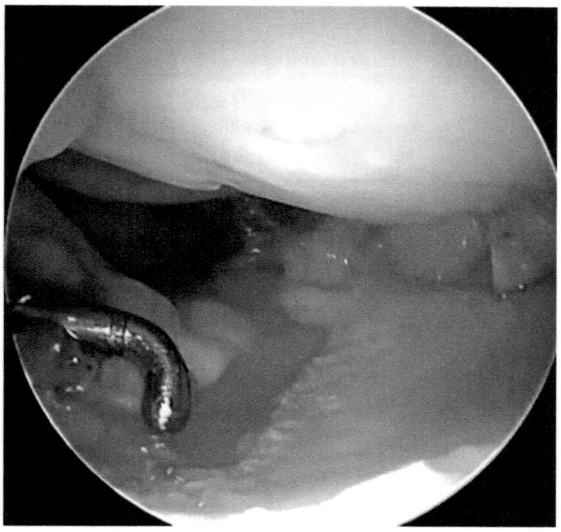

Fig. 15.12 Degenerative changes limited to the dorsum of the scaphoid fossa (scapholunate advanced collapse [SLAC] 1)

3. Stage III adds to stage 1 and 2 osteoarthritis between the lunate and capitate.
4. Stage IV is defined by the presence of osteoarthritis in the radiolunate fossa.

15.4.6.1 SLAC 1 Treatment

In stage I SLAC, the recommended treatment for symptomatic patients is a styloidectomy of the dorsum of the radioscaphoid fossa. It has been described as open or arthroscopically. In the arthroscopic technique, the 1 and 2 portals are commonly used to perform the styloidectomy [46] (Fig. 15.12).

15.4.6.2 SLAC 2 Treatment

Main options of treatment are a proximal row carpectomy (PRC) or the "four-corner arthrodesis."

PRC is performed by excising the scaphoid, lunate, and triquetrum bones. A new joint between the proximal pole of the capitate and the radius is created. Wall et al. published that in 16 patients, 35% required another surgery in a minimum follow-up of 20 years [47]. A 72% grip strength compared to contralateral wrist and an average flexion-extension arc of 68° was reported.

The four-corner arthrodesis (4CA) involves excision of the scaphoid and fusion of the capitate, hamate, lunate, and triquetrum. Arthrodesis could be performed open or arthroscopically using screws or specific plates. Traverso et al. followed 15 patients for an average of 18 years [48]. They reported a wrist flexion/extension arc of 68° and QuickDASH scores of 7.8 on average. Bain et al. reported significant pain relief and no reduction of grip strength in 31 patients at 1 and 10 years after surgery [49].

When comparing 4CA and PRC, there are no significant clinical differences between both techniques. In practice, although the decision is based on the etiology and extent of joint involvement, it is mostly influenced by the patient's functional demands and state of the wrist. PRC is contraindicated in stage III SLAC wrist due to the arthritic capitate that would become the focal point of wrist loading causing pain. PRC results are slightly better in terms of motion. Four-corner arthrodesis patients have higher grip strength with less mobility than PRC ones. Usually PRC is preferred in older patients who prefer mobility over strength and four-corner arthrodesis in younger patients who need a stronger wrist [50].

15.4.6.3 Stage III SLAC Treatment

Stage III SLAC wrist should not be treated by PRC. Four-corner arthrodesis is recommended.

15.4.6.4 Stage IV SLAC Treatment

Stage IV SLAC wrist has degenerative changes in the radiolunate joint. In cases of significant pain, a total wrist arthrodesis is frequently indicated. Published results show significant pain relief and functional grip strength [51]. Loss of wrist motion is well tolerated in selected patients. Wrist arthroplasty may be indicated in certain patients with SLAC IV wrist (Table 15.4).

Table 15.4 Scapholunate advanced collapse (SLAC) treatment

SLAC	Treatment
I	Dorsal styloidectomy
II	PRC or 4CA
III	4CA
IV	Total wrist arthrodesis

Table 15.5 Author-preferred treatment summary

Instability	Garcia-Elias	EWAS	Geissler	Treatment
Pre-dynamic	1	I, II, or IIIa	I or II	Synovectomy
Dynamic	2	IIIb or IIIc	III	Suture and capsular plicature
Dynamic	3	IV	IV	Ligamentoplasty
Static	4			Ligamentoplasty
Static	5	V		Limited arthrodesis
SLAC	6			Salvage procedure

15.5 Authors' Preferred Treatment

Wrist arthroscopy has improved the knowledge of SLIL lesions, allowing a precise diagnosis. In addition, it permits to repair carpal lesions without extensive approaches that may damage secondary stabilizers, blood vessels, and wrist proprioception. We systematically performed wrist arthroscopy in cases of suspected SL lesions.

Stage I: In cases of symptomatic partial lesions, we usually perform a synovectomy and limited debridement of the torn ligament.

Stage II: Cases of complete reparable disruption are treated by direct repair. Suture and dorsal capsule plicature are used as described by Carratala et al. or Mathoulin.

Stages III and IV: In cases of complete, irreparable rupture or reducible malalignment, we performed a ligamentoplasty as described by Corella et al.

Stage V: We usually recommend observation and perform a radiolunate-scaphoid partial arthrodesis in cases of intolerable pain.

Stage VI: In SLAC wrists, we do salvage procedures according to the stage of SLAC. In stage I arthroscopic dorsal styloidectomy, stage II arthroscopic proximal row carpectomy or four-corner fusion, stage III arthroscopic four-corner fusion, and stage IV total wrist arthrodesis (Table 15.5).

15.6 Conclusions

Injury to the scapholunate interosseous ligament (SLIL) is the most common cause of carpal instability and can cause important functional impairment to the patient. Initially, SLIL lesions are well tolerated due to the function of the secondary stabilizers. Nevertheless, chronic lesions may cause instability and osteoarthritis, as evidenced by clinical conditions such as dorsal intercalated segment instability (DISI) and scapholunate advanced collapse (SLAC).

References

1. Overstraeten LV, Camus EJ, Wahegaonkar A, Messina J, Tandara AA, Binder AC, et al. Anatomical description of the dorsal capsulo-scapholunate septum (DCSS)-arthroscopic staging of scapholunate instability after DCSS sectioning. J Wrist Surg. 2013;2:149–54.
2. Rajan PV, Day CS. Scapholunate interosseous ligament anatomy and biomechanics. J Hand Surg Am. 2015;40:1692–702.
3. Hagert E, Forsgren S, Ljung BO. Differences in the presence of mechanoreceptors and nerve structures between wrist ligaments may imply differential roles in wrist stabilization. J Orthop Res. 2005;23:757–63.
4. Hagert E, Garcia-Elias M, Forsgren S, Ljung BO. Immunohistochemical analysis of wrist ligament innervation in relation to their structural composition. J Hand Surg Am. 2007;32:30–6.
5. Mataliotakis G, Doukas M, Kostas I, Lykissas M, Batistatou A, Beris A. Sensory innervation of the subregions of the scapholunate interosseous ligament in relation to their structural composition. J Hand Surg Am. 2009;34:1413–21.
6. Short WH, Werner FW, Green JK, Masaoka S. Biomechanical evaluation of ligamentous stabilizers of the scaphoid and lunate. J Hand Surg Am. 2002;27:991–1002.
7. Watson HK, Ballet FL. The SLAC wrist: scapholunate advanced collapse pattern of degenerative arthritis. J Hand Surg Am. 1984;9:358–65.
8. O'Meeghan CJ, Stuart W, Mamo V, Stanley JK, Trail IA. The natural history of an untreated isolated scapholunate interosseous ligament injury. J Hand Surg Br. 2003;28:307–10.
9. Watson HK, Ashmead D IV, Makhlouf MV. Examination of the scaphoid. J Hand Surg Am. 1988;13:657–60.

10. Lee SK, Desai H, Silver B, Dhaliwal G, Paksima N. Comparison of radiographic stress views for scapholunate dynamic instability in a cadaver model. J Hand Surg Am. 2011;36:1149–57.
11. Daunt N. Magnetic resonance imaging of the wrist: anatomy and pathology of interosseous ligaments and the triangular fibrocartilage complex. Curr Probl Diagn Radiol. 2002;31:158–76.
12. Hafezi-Nejad N, Carrino JA, Eng J, Blackmore C, Shores J, Lifchez SD, et al. Scapholunate interosseous ligament tears: diagnostic performance of 1.5 T, 3 T MRI, and MR arthrography-a systematic review and meta-analysis. Acad Radiol. 2016;23:1091–103.
13. Dietrich TJ, Toms AP, Cerezal L, Omoumi P, Boutin RD, Fritz J, et al. Interdisciplinary consensus statements on imaging of scapholunate joint instability. Eur Radiol. 2021:10.1007/s00330-021-08073-8. Online ahead of print.
14. Palmer AK. Triangular fibrocartilage disorders: injury patterns and treatment. Arthroscopy. 1990;6:125–32.
15. del Piñal F, García-Bernal FJ, Pisani D, Regalado J, Ayala H, Studer A. Dry arthroscopy of the wrist: surgical technique. J Hand Surg Am. 2007;32: 119–23.
16. Geissler WB, Freeland AE, Savoie FH, McIntyre LW, Whipple TL. Intracarpal soft-tissue lesions associated with an intra- articular fracture of the distal end of the radius. J Bone Joint Surg Am. 1996;78:357–65.
17. Messina JC, van Overstraeten L, Luchetti R, Fairplay T, Mathoulin CL. The EWAS classification of scapholunate tears: an anatomical arthroscopy study. J Wrist Surg. 2013;2:105–9.
18. Corella F, Ocampos M, Cerro MD. Arthroscopic scaphoid 3D test for scapholunate instability. J Wrist Surg. 2018;7:89–92.
19. Garcia-Elias M, Lluch AL, Stanley JK. Three-ligament tenodesis for the treatment of SL dissociation: indications and surgical technique. J Hand Surg Am. 2006;31:125–34.
20. Watson HK, Weinzweig J, Zeppieri J: The natural progression of scaphoid instability. Hand Clin 1997;13:39–49.
21. Lee JI, Nha KW, Lee GY, Kim BH, Kim JW, Park JW. Long-term outcomes of arthroscopic debridement and thermal shrinkage for isolated partial intercarpal ligament tears. Orthopedics. 2012;35:e1204–9.
22. Burn MB, Sarkissian EJ, Yao J. Long-term outcomes for arthroscopic thermal treatment for scapholunate ligament injuries. J Wrist Surg. 2020;9:22–8.
23. Hagert E. Proprioception of the wrist joint: a review of current concepts and possible implications on the rehabilitation of the wrist. J Hand Ther. 2010;23:2–17.
24. Esplugas M, Garcia-Elias M, Lluch A, Llusá PM. Role of muscles in the stabilization of ligament-deficient wrists. J Hand Ther. 2016;29:166–74.
25. Lluch A, Salvà G, Esplugas M, Llusá M, Hagert E, Garcia-Elias M. El papel de la propiocepción y el control neuromuscular en las inestabilidades del carpo. Revista Iberoamericana de Cirugía de la Mano. 2015;43:70–8.
26. Salvà-Coll G, Garcia-Elias M, Leon-Lopez MT, Llusa-Perez M, Rodríguez-Baeza A. Effects of forearm muscles on carpal stability. J Hand Surg Eur. 2011;36:553–9.
27. Andersson JK, Garcia-Elias M. Dorsal scapholunate ligament injury: a classification of clinical forms. J Hand Surg Eur. 2013;38:165–9.
28. Berger RA. The ligaments of the wrist: a current overview of anatomy with considerations of their potential functions. Hand Clin 1997;13:63–82.
29. Rohman EM, Agel J, Putnam MD, Adams JE. Scapholunate interosseous ligament injuries: a retrospective review of treatment and outcomes in 82 wrists. J Hand Surg. 2014;39:2020–6.
30. Rosati M, Parchi P, Cacianti M, Poggetti A, Lisanti M. Treatment of acute scapholunate ligament injuries with bone anchor. Musculoskelet Surg. 2010;94:25–32.
31. Loisel F, Wessel LE, Morse KW, Victoria C, Meyers KN, Wolfe SW. Is the dorsal fiber-splitting approach to the wrist safe? A kinematic analysis and introduction of the "window" approach. J Hand Surg Am. 2021:S0363-5023(21)00368-3.
32. Carratalá V, Lucas FJ, Miranda I, Prada A, Guisasola E, Miranda FJ. Arthroscopic reinsertion of acute injuries of the scapholunate ligament technique and results. J Wrist Surg. 2020;9:328–37.
33. Mathoulin CL, Dauphin N, Wahegaonkar AL. Arthroscopic dorsal capsuloligamentous repair in chronic scapholunate ligament tears. Hand Clin. 2011;27:563–72.
34. Moran SL, Cooney WP, Berger RA, Strickland J. Capsulodesis for the treatment of chronic scapholunate instability. J Hand Surg. 2005;30:16–23.
35. Megerle K, Bertel D, Lehnhardt M, Guenter P, Hellmich S. Long-term follow-up of modified Blatt's capsulodesis for the treatment of scapholunate ligament injuries. J Hand Surg Am. 2011;36(8):52.
36. Garcia-Elias M, Lluch AL, Stanley JK. Three-ligament tenodesis for the treatment of scapholunate dissociation: indications and surgical technique. J Hand Surg Am. 2006;31:125–34.
37. Kakar S, Greene RM, Denbeigh J, Van Wijnen A. Scapholunate ligament internal brace 360 tenodesis (SLITT) procedure: a biomechanical study. J Wrist Surg. 2019;8:250–4.
38. Corella F, Del Cerro M, Ocampos M, Simon de Blas C, Larrainzar-Garijo R. Arthroscopic scapholunate ligament reconstruction, volar and dorsal reconstruction. Hand Clin. 2017;33:687–707.
39. Nakamura T, Cheong Ho P, Atzei A, Corella F, Haugstvedt JR. Revolutions in arthroscopic wrist surgeries. J Hand Surg Eur. 2022;47:52–64.
40. Ho PC, Wong CW, Tse WL. Arthroscopic-assisted combined dorsal and volar scapholunate ligament reconstruction with tendon graft for chronic SL instability. J Wrist Surg. 2015;4:252–63.
41. White NJ, Raskolnikov D, Crow SA, Swart E, Rosenwasser MP. Reduction and association of the scaphoid and lunate (RASL): long-term follow-up of

a reconstruction technique for chronic scapholunate dissociation. J Hand Surg Am. 2017;35:16–7.
42. Larson TB, Stern PJ. Reduction and association of the scaphoid and lunate procedure: short-term clinical and radiographic outcomes. J Hand Surg. 2014;39:2168–74.
43. Stewart DT, Froelich JM, Shin AY. Intercarpal arthrodeses. J Hand Surg. 2014;39:373–7.
44. Bain GI, McGuire DT. Decision making for partial carpal fusions. J Wrist Surg. 2012;1:103–14.
45. Garcia-Elias M, Lluch A, Ferreres A, Papini-Zorli I, Rahimtoola ZO. Treatment of radiocarpal degenerative osteoarthritis by radioscapholunate arthrodesis and distal scaphoidectomy. J Hand Surg Am. 2005;30:8–15.
46. Yao J, Osterman AL. Arthroscopic techniques for wrist arthritis (radial styloidectomy and proximal pole hamate excisions). Hand Clin. 2005;21:519–26.
47. Wall LB, Didonna ML, Kiefhaber TR, Stern PJ. Proximal row carpectomy: minimum 20-year follow-up. J Hand Surg. 2013;38:1498–04.
48. Traverso P, Wong A, Wollstein R, Carlson L, Ashmead D, Watson HK. Ten-year minimum follow-up of 4-corner fusion for SLAC and SNAC wrist. Hand (N Y). 2017;12:568–72.
49. Bain GI, Watts AC. The outcome of scaphoid excision and four-corner arthrodesis for advanced carpal collapse at a minimum of ten years. J Hand Surg Am. 2010;35:719–25.
50. Laulan J, Bacle G, de Bodman C, Najihi N, Richou J, Simon E, et al. The arthritic wrist. II--the degenerative wrist: indications for different surgical treatments. Orthop Traumatol Surg Res. 2011;97(4 Suppl):S37–41.
51. Rauhaniemi J, Tiusanen H, Sipola E. Total wrist fusion: a study of 115 patients. J Hand Surg Br. 2005;30:217–9.

Wrist Arthritis: Total Versus Limited Fusion Versus Arthroplasty

16

Emmet Thompson and Olivia Flannery

16.1 Introduction

Wrist arthritis is a progressive, destructive, deforming and debilitating disease (Fig. 16.1) that results in severe loss of hand function for those affected. This broad term is often used to describe degenerative changes seen in the radiocarpal joint, the intercarpal joints or, in some conditions, both. It can affect the younger, higher-demand patient population as the end stage of Kienböck disease or more commonly in the post-traumatic setting of a SNAC (scaphoid non-union advanced collapse) or SLAC (scapholunate advanced collapse) wrist, post-traumatic arthritis following distal radius fracture or fracture malunion. In older patients it may also present as a post-traumatic condition or as a sequelae of inflammatory arthropathy such as rheumatoid or psoriatic arthritis or as primary osteoarthritis. The diversity of the underlying aetiologies and functional demands of those affected has led to considerable debate and controversy on the optimal management of this condition, namely, motion-sacrificing versus motion-sparing techniques. A significant volume of work has been published on the surgical management of wrist

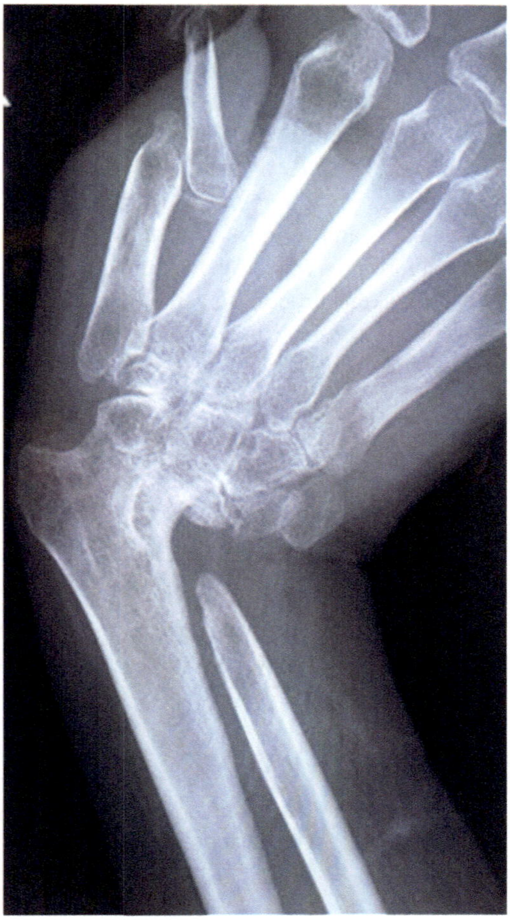

Fig. 16.1 Radiograph of end-stage degenerative change in the wrist of a patient suffering from rheumatoid arthritis. Note the apparent partial auto-fusion at the radiocarpal joint, the destructive change and subsequent instability at the thumb metacarpal phalangeal joint and previous distal ulnar resection arthroplasty

E. Thompson · O. Flannery (✉)
Connolly Hospital Blanchardstown, Dublin, Ireland

National Orthopaedic Hospital Cappagh,
Dublin, Ireland
e-mail: oliviaflannery@hermitageclinic.ie

E. C. Rodríguez-Merchán, A. Moreno-Garcìa (eds.), *Controversies in Orthopedic Surgery of The Upper Limb*, https://doi.org/10.1007/978-3-031-04907-1_16

arthritis and the authors aim to highlight the evolution and changing trends in this field focusing on total wrist fusion, limited or partial wrist fusion and wrist arthroplasty and the related areas of controversy and debate. It is by no means a treatise on surgical technique or an exhaustive review, the likes of which have already been published and can be easily found through any scholastic online search engine. However, we hope these discussion points might better inform the reader of the surgical options available, evidence behind these options and potential future developments while also drawing attention to several key questions which remain to be answered.

16.2 Treatment Algorithm for the Surgical Management of Wrist Arthritis

Many authors and surgeons have their own treatment algorithm which they employ in the decision-making process to tailor their surgical interventions for each individual patient. These are often based on training, experience and personal preference. Below is an example of the senior author treatment algorithm for the surgical management of wrist arthritis based on the location and extent of the degenerative process (Fig. 16.2). We advocate the use of a detailed, but focused history and examination, as well as appropriate radiographs and higher-order imaging including computed tomography (CT), single-photon emission computed tomography (SPECT) and magnetic resonance imaging (MRI) to fully evaluate each patient. We also advocate the use of diagnostic wrist arthroscopy (Fig. 16.3), particularly in cases where the extent of degenerative change is uncertain, where there is ambiguity between the clinical and radiographic findings and in cases where there is the potential to perform and limited fusion procedure. It should be noted that this algorithm does not include the many patient demographics such as age, aetiology, hand dominance, previous and current hand function, occupation and post-treatment expectations of the patient. Each of these factors should be taken into account when developing a treatment plan in tandem with patient wishes, with reason.

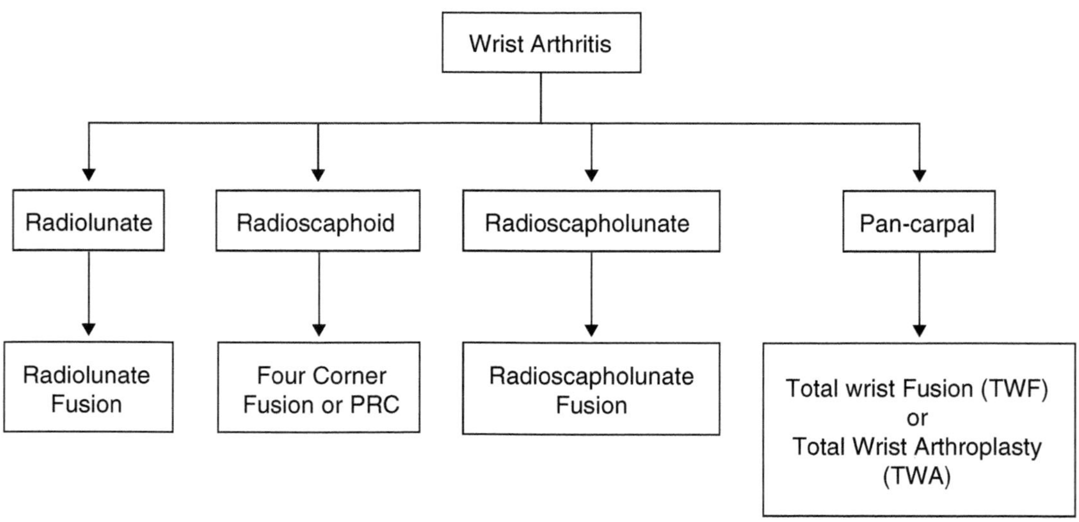

Fig. 16.2 Treatment algorithm for the surgical management of wrist arthritis based on the confirmed location and extent of the degenerative changes within the wrist

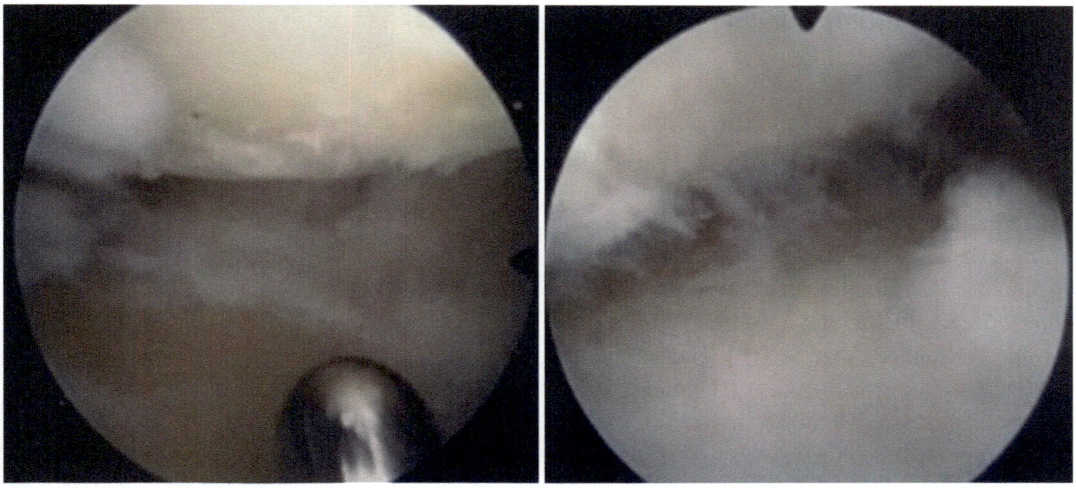

Fig. 16.3 Intraoperative photo taken during diagnostic wrist arthroscopy showing severe articular cartilage loss with bone-on-bone arthritis at the radioscaphoid articulation (left) and severe degenerative change at the radiolunate articulation. The remaining intercarpal articulations were well preserved and this patient went onto radioscapholunate (RSL) fusion

16.3 Normal Wrist Motion and Biomechanics and Its Importance in the Surgical Management of Wrist Arthritis

The importance of dart thrower's motion (DTM) has been emphasized in the literature [1–3]. This describes one of the most frequently used planes of wrist motion, bringing the wrist from a radially deviated extended position (radial extension) to an ulnarly deviated flexed position (ulnar flexion), occurring mainly in the midcarpal joint [4]. This is not aligned with the anatomic sagittal or coronal axes of the wrist [5]. Mapping of all possible wrist positions results in an ellipsoidal shape oriented obliquely to the sagittal plane of motion. It is now believed that DTM actually consists of several different paths that cumulatively contribute to a wide variety of functional activities [6]. Previous total wrist arthroplasty designs have tried to recreate the contour and kinematics of the radiocarpal joint with little attention paid to the midcarpal joint which is either defunct due to PRC or fused. Thus, many total wrist arthroplasties (TWAs) restrict motion to the anatomical directions and minimizing the important dart thrower's arc. Fourth-generation TWA using ellipsoidal polyethylene articular surfaces may improve the general range of motion possible but do not allow for the true replication of the DTM and its functional benefits.

In terms of fusion procedures, total wrist fusion (TWF) abolishes any DTM. Partial wrist fusions such as radioscapholunate (RSL) fusion preserves critical midcarpal motion and carpal height, thus retaining possible DTM. However, RSL fusion may reduce total wrist movement by 40% [7] but has the potential to maintain a greater degree of midcarpal motion and DTM.

16.4 Partial/Limited Wrist Fusion

Partial/limited wrist fusions are most commonly performed for debilitating painful arthritis. The goal of a partial wrist fusion is to fuse the painful, diseased joints while preserving movement of the healthy joints. There are various options of partial wrist fusions, depending on the extent of the disease process. The most common fusions performed include radiolunate, radioscapholunate and four-corner fusions.

16.4.1 Radiolunate Fusion (Chamay Fusion)

Indications for radiolunate (RL) fusion include post-traumatic osteoarthritis of the radiolunate joint typically following die-punch distal radial fractures, rheumatoid arthritis with ulnar and volar translocation of the carpus and complex ligament instabilities deemed unreconstructable [8, 9]. An RL fusion may also be considered for advanced Kienböck disease [10]. The neighbouring radioscaphoid and midcarpal joints need to be free of disease. Methods for fixation include headless compression screws, staples, plate and screws and Kirschner wires.

The lunate is fused in neutral alignment relative to the radius. Radiolunate fusions appear to be associated with low rates of non-union and low rates of progression to total wrist arthrodesis [11].

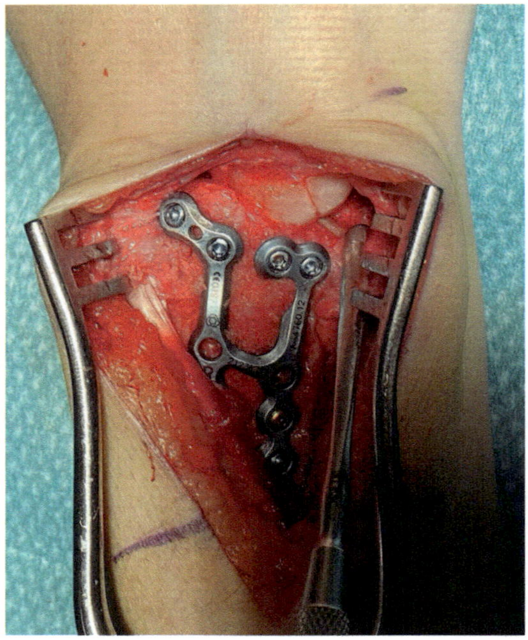

Fig. 16.4 Intraoperative photo taken during radioscapholunate (RSL) fusion for the treatment of end-stage radioscapholunate arthritis using a purpose-specific plate. Note the obvious defect created by the excision of the triquetrum being pointed out by the Freer elevator. This patient also had a distal pole scaphoidectomy

16.4.2 Radioscapholunate (RSL) Fusion

It is more common to have RSL osteoarthritis than RL osteoarthritis in isolation. The midcarpal joint must be intact to proceed with an RSL fusion. However, there is concern regarding the high rates of non-union and progression to midcarpal arthritis [12]. Change from the use of k-wires to memory staples, compression screws, plate and screw fixation and modification of the surgical technique have improved union rates. Wrist motion is significantly affected as the immobile scaphoid bridges the remaining midcarpal joint. Distal scaphoid excision has been shown to release the midcarpal joint. This results in a significantly greater wrist motion as well as reduces the risk of scaphotrapeziotrapezoid (STT) joint and midcarpal joint osteoarthritis and improves union rates [13]. Given the preservation of the midcarpal joint, wrist motion at or above the level of functional wrist motion required to perform most activities of daily living is maintained [11]. The addition of triquetrum excision has been shown to improve range of movement while providing extra bone for grafting [14, 15]. The senior author's preference is distal pole scaphoidectomy, excision of triquetrum and RSL fusion using the purpose-designed RSL fusion plate (Fig. 16.4).

16.4.3 Four-Corner Fusion

Four-corner fusions are widely used to treat symptomatic arthritis seen in scaphoid non-union advance collapse (SNAC) and scapholunate advanced collapse (SLAC). It is typically used when there is involvement of the capitolunate joint but can also be used if the capitolunate joint is preserved and if a fusion is preferred over a proximal row carpectomy. Various methods of fixation include K-wire, screws, staples and more commonly a circular plate and screws, which is the senior author's preference (Fig. 16.5).

Moreover, 40% to 50% of movement and grip strength can be expected post-operatively and overall good long-term outcome is achieved [16]. Non-union remains a concern, particularly at the

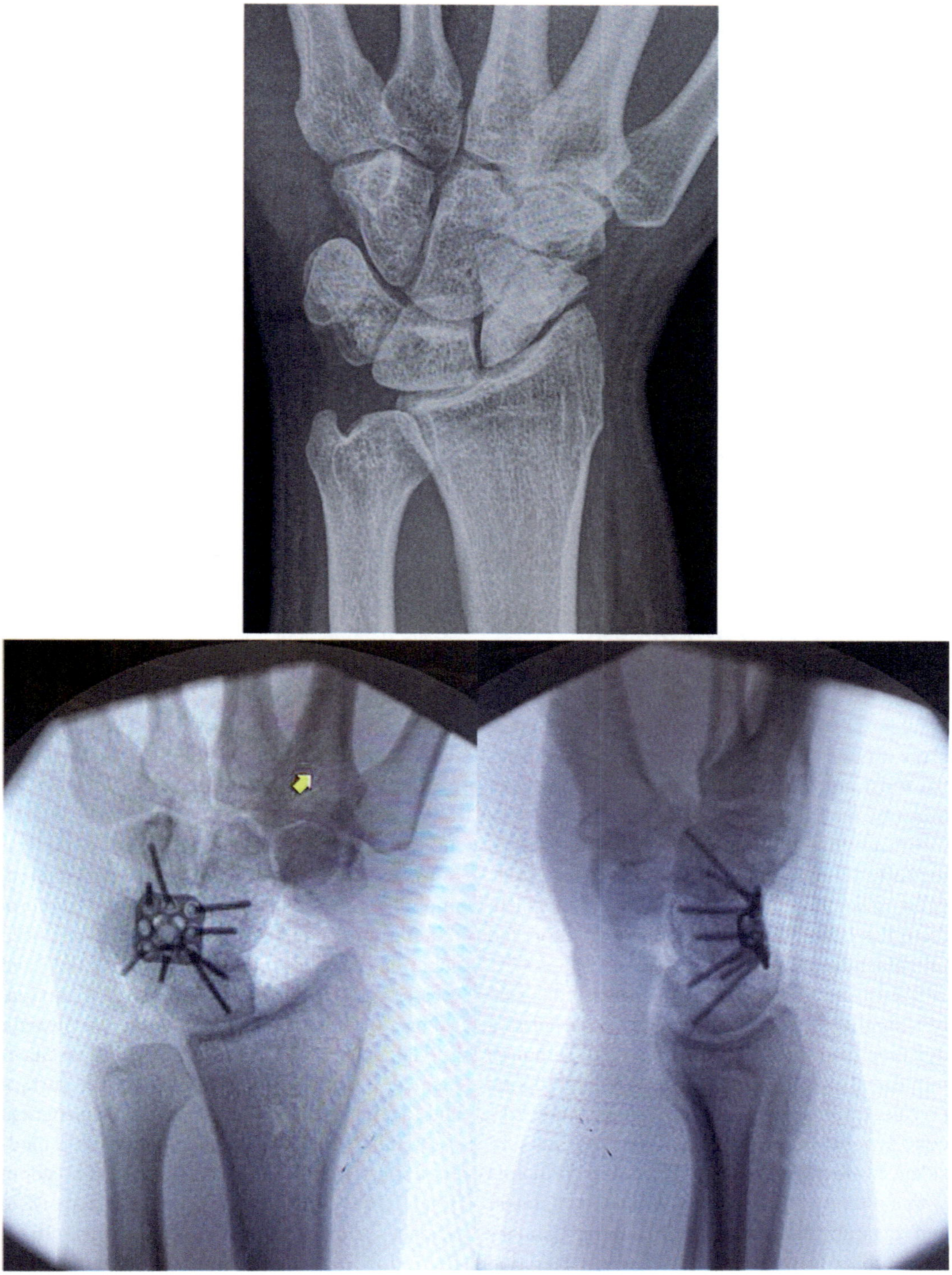

Fig. 16.5 Preoperative and intraoperative images of a patient with localized degenerative at the radioscaphoid articulation treated with a limited intercarpal/four-corner fusion. Note the multiple screw options to ensure appropriate fixation and compression of the fusion mass. Note also how this system allows recession of the plate to limit impingement of the plate against the dorsal lip of the distal radius during wrist extension and to reduce the risk of extensor tendon irritation. Images courtesy of Ms. E. Conroy, University Hospital Kerry

triquetrum. However, union is typically achieved following regrafting and fusion.

More recently, a three-corner fusion has been described, where the triquetrum is excised in addition to the scaphoid. This gives extra bone for grafting and improves ulnar deviation. Higher union rates have also been reported [17]. At the time of writing, the PARTE (PARtial wrist fusion with or without Triquetral Excision) trial is currently underway [18]. This multi-centre double-blind prospective randomized clinical trial will assess the impact of four-corner arthrodesis (without triquetral excision) or three-corner/capitolunate arthrodeses with triquetral excision on grip strength and range of motion in eligible participants with SNAC or SLAC wrist arthritis who have been deemed operative candidates. The results of this study may help to conclude which salvage procedure is best for this cohort.

16.5 Total Wrist Arthroplasty

Total wrist arthroplasty (TWA) has the potential to alleviate pain, improve wrist function and preserve motion for patients with end-stage pancarpal wrist arthritis. These benefits are somewhat offset by their higher complication rates.

Since wrist arthroplasty was first reported in the early 1890s by the German physician and surgeon, Themistocles Gluck (1853–1942) [19], there has been a slow but gradual evolution and refinement in implant design.

First-generation wrist arthroplasties consisted of a single-piece silicone implant that acted as a dynamic spacer at the radiocarpal joint. Although initial studies were encouraging [20], later reports revealed problems such as implant fracture, silicone synovitis [21], osteolysis and implant subsidence. However, the general design principle with a proximal intramedullary radial component and transcapitate/third metacarpal intramedullary distal component is used in fourth-generation implants such as the Motec® (Swemac Orthopaedics, Linkoping, Sweden) prosthesis.

Second-generation designs such as the Meuli (Sulzer Orthopaedics Ltd., Winterthur, Switzerland, and later revised to the MWP III Total Wrist Prosthesis, Zimmer, Warsaw, IN, USA) and Volz (Howmedica Company, Rutherford, NJ, USA) type implants sought to improve durability by using titanium (Meuli) or cobalt chrome (Volz), which were unconstrained ball and socket (Meuli) or semi-constrained hemispherical (Volz) designs with separate radial and carpal components that relied on proximal and distal cement fixation. Unfortunately, distal implant loosening and difficulties in centring the implants in the distal radius and metacarpals due to design constraints made balancing the wrist technically challenging.

Third-generation implants such as the tri-spherical implants, Biax total wrist prosthesis (DePuy Orthopaedics, Warsaw, IN, USA) and the Universal total wrist implant (Kinetikos Medical, Carlsbad, CA, USA) incorporated features including an axle constraint to lock the radial and carpal components, ellipsoidal (Biax) or toroidal (Universal) polyethylene articulating surface, screw fixation and reduced bone resection to restore soft tissue balance and stability [22–24]. These improvements lead to enhanced patient outcomes but were still hampered with complications including loss of fixation, periprosthetic fracture due to stem breakout and dislocation.

Current fourth-generation designs aim to reduce design-related difficulties and complications, improve biomechanics of the articulation, minimize instability and maximize long-term fixation and bone stock [25]. This has been achieved through improved centralization and greater contact during the total arc of motion, using an ellipsoidal ultrahigh-molecular-weight polyethylene articular surface [26] and uncemented fixation using porous textured surface and locking and fixed-angle screws to encourage osseointegration. The most commonly used modern implants include the Universal 2 and Freedom Total Wrist Implant Systems (Integra Life Sciences, Plainsboro, NJ, USA; Fig. 16.6), ReMotion Total Wrist (Small Bone Innovations, Morrisville, PA, USA) and Maestro Total Wrist System (Biomet, Warsaw, IN, USA), although the latter was voluntarily withdrawn from the marketplace in 2018 despite excellent results. Single-component interposition pyrocarbon

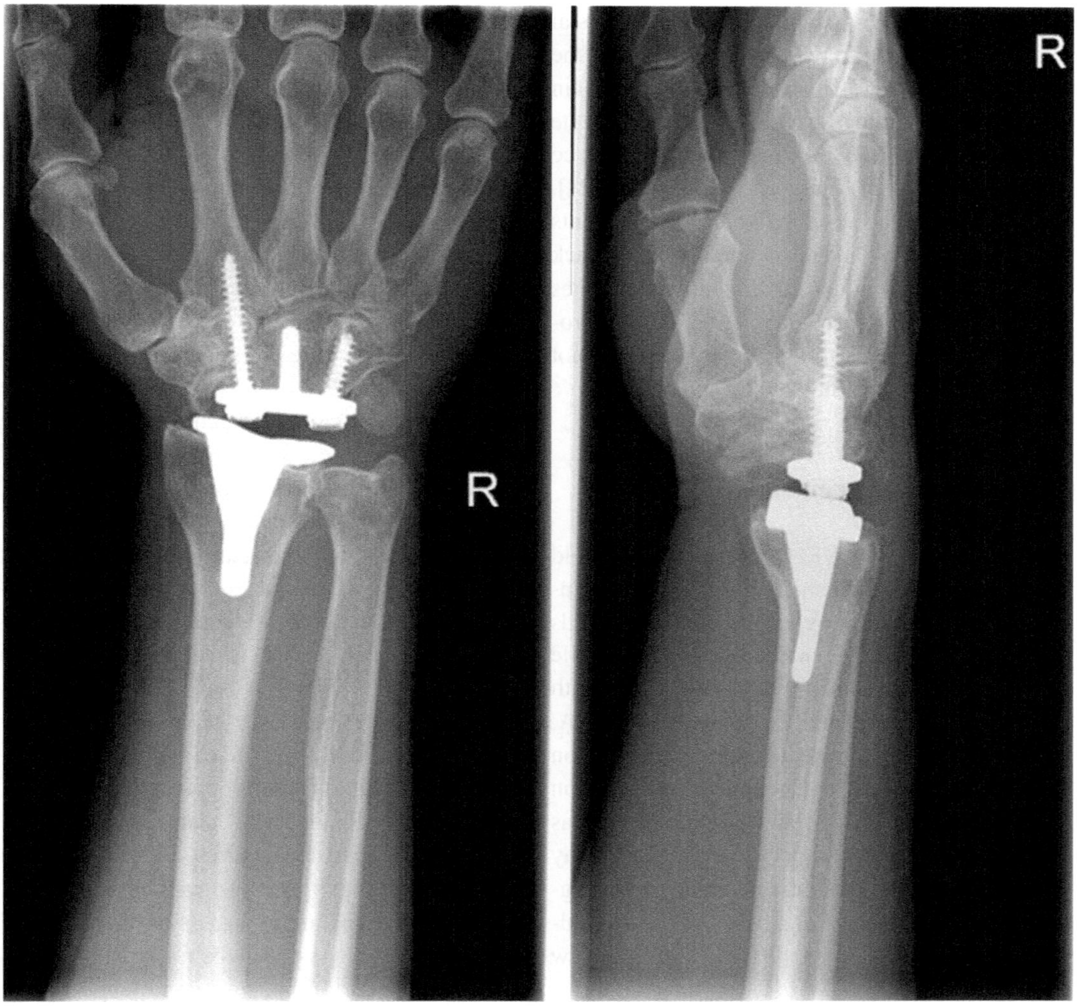

Fig. 16.6 Radiograph of a total wrist arthroplasty using the Freedom Total Wrist Implant System. Images courtesy of Mr. K. O'Shea, National Orthopaedic Hospital, Cappagh, Dublin

arthroplasty such as the Amandys (Tornier SAS–Bioprofile, St. Martin, France) has been recently introduced with encouraging PROMs results. This very different concept uses a quadric elliptical component that acts like a mobile spacer and potentially allows for a ligament-sparring approach to the wrist. However, like the other fourth-generation implants for TWA, only short-term data on their performance is currently available.

Hemiarthroplasty should also be mentioned. As there is less bone and soft tissue resection and dissection, this procedure has been advocated for use in managing younger patients and those with post-traumatic causes including SNAC and SLAC wrist and even in distal radius fractures [27–29]. Depending on the underlying aetiology, a proximal row carpectomy may be undertaken followed by either replacement of the distal radius articular surface alone [27] or in combination with midcarpal resection hemiarthroplasty [28] with maintenance of the distal carpal row or with replacement of the distal carpal row articular surface and maintenance of the distal radius articular surface [29]. Replacement of the distal radius articular surface in isolation has been reported in several centres in Europe for the management of acute distal radius fractures. Midcarpal resection involves using a monoblock prosthesis implanted into the distal radius and designed to recreate the contour of the proximal carpal row. This is believed to maintain the centre of rotation of the wrist and allow for the dart thrower's motion to occur and hence produce a better functional range of movement [28]. However, due to the very small number of patients treated in specialist and designer centres, the lack of long-term follow-up, significant failure rates reported and availability of reliable, proven procedures, wrist hemiarthroplasty is currently not recommended at this time by the authors.

16.6 Total Wrist Fusion

Total wrist fusion (TWF) is considered the gold standard for the management of end-stage symptomatic wrist arthritis by any surgeon. It affords the ability to correct significant deformity while providing stability and reliable pain relief with lower rates of complications compared to TWA, with high levels of patient-reported satisfaction and function [30] despite the loss of wrist motion requiring adaptation of functional tasks such as perineal hygiene. Failed wrist arthroplasty may be used to salvage wrist fusion, although managing bone loss and achieving bone union are challenging in this setting [30]. There are few contraindications to TWF. These include active infection at the wrist joint or lack of an adequate soft tissue envelope. Poor bone stock in patients with rheumatoid arthritis or after failed wrist arthroplasty has been considered a relative contraindication but modern-day locking plates and refinement in surgical technique have generally overcome this.

During wrist fusion the radiocarpal, intercarpal and midcarpal joints are denuded of articular to expose the preferably bleeding subchondral bone to create the fusion bed. At this time additional procedures involving the extensor tendons or the distal radioulnar joint (DRUJ) can be performed if required depending on the pre-existing pathology and as functional deficits. In the case of patients with severe deformity, proximal row carpectomy (PRC) can be included to de-tension soft tissue structures and help in reducing the hand onto the distal radius. The secondary benefit of this is a ready supply of autologous bone graft from the resected carpal bones. Alternatively, the triquetrum, radial styloid or distal scaphoid can be excised in isolation or in combination to avoid impingement or ulnocarpal impaction.

Historically, fusion constructs consisted of retrograde trans-carpal intramedullary pins (Rush or Steinman, either single or multiple) traversing from the second or third metacarpal to the distal radius. This provided compression and some rotational control, with the use of one or more staples used in modified techniques to provide complimentary fixation. Although largely superseded by plate-assisted fusion (discussed below), this procedure is still advocated in patients requiring concomitant metacarpophalangeal joint implant arthroplasties or in those in whom forearm dissection can be problematic. In such situations, rotational control is achieved using two Steinmann pins [31].

The growing use of the AO (Arbeitsgemeinschaft für Osteosynthesefragen) plating philosophy in the 1970s and 1980s heralded the advent of plate-assisted fusion with plates spanning the metacarpals to the distal radius. Subsequent iterations resulted in purpose-designed pre-contoured, low-contact, dynamic compression titanium and stainless-steel plating systems for wrist arthrodesis, with modern implants employing locking screw holes. Such systems allow compression of the fusion mass by the plate itself and can provide rigid fixation, even in patients with poor bone stock (Fig. 16.7a, b).

From a technical standpoint, ideal wrist fusion position and the joints that should be included in the fusion are still hotly debated in the literature, with no consensus regarding optimal positioning, particularly if arthrodesis is to be performed on both wrists.

Classical techniques are somewhat limited in the position the wrist could be placed because the pin was straight, and the wrist was fused in a neutral flexion-extension position. Some ulnar deviation could be built into the fusion by placing the pin in the second metacarpal, hence offsetting the longitudinal axis of the wrist. In plate-assisted fusion, the position is set by the contour of the

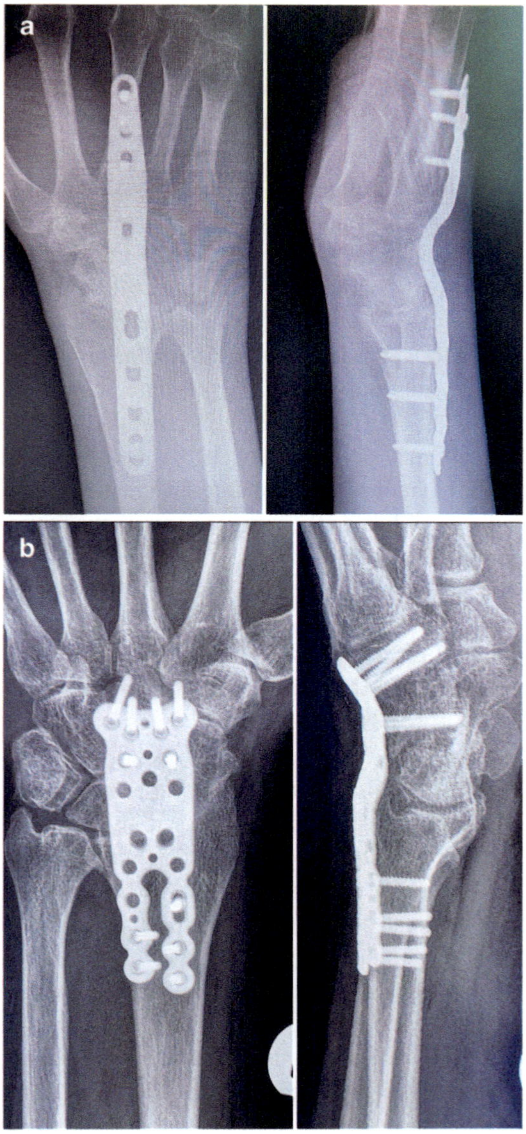

Fig. 16.7 (**a**) Radiograph of a total wrist fusion using a purpose-specific pre-contoured wrist fusion plate spanning from the distal radius to the third metacarpal. (**b**) Radiograph of a total wrist fusion using a modern, low-profile pre-contoured locking wrist fusion plate. Note how the plate extends only as far as the distal carpal row, thus preserving the carpometacarpal (CMC) articulations and also preserving the intramedullary canal of the metacarpal allowing for concomitant metacarpophalangeal (MCP) joint arthroplasty if necessary

plate itself with some minor customization possible. Most modern plates lend themselves to fusing the wrist in some extension and ulnar deviation to maximize post-operative power grip.

The few contraindications to total wrist arthrodesis include an active wrist infection or lack of an adequate soft tissue envelope. Although inadequate bone stock for fusion in patients with rheumatoid arthritis or after failed wrist arthroplasty was historically considered a relative contraindication to plate fixation, the advent of locking plate technology has largely overcome this issue. Major complications include nonunion, ulnocarpal impaction syndrome and implant-related problems, such as plate prominence requiring plate removal due to tenderness and/or extensor tendon irritation and periprosthetic fractures around the plate, mostly metacarpal fractures.

16.7 TWA Versus TWF

Despite the growing body of publication regarding TWA in general, there is a limited volume of level 1 evidence comparing total wrist arthroplasty versus total wrist fusion, the popularly accepted current gold standard. Furthermore, much of this literature deals specifically with rheumatoid arthritis patients [32–34] and hence may not be applicable to other conditions, although this concept is being challenged. There have been several systematic reviews that have tried to address and answer the questions of who the appropriate patients for TWA are and what are the functional benefits for the recipients [30, 32–35].

16.7.1 Indications and Patient Selection

Perhaps the most controversial topic regarding wrist replacement versus fusion is the debate surrounding indications and patient selection with many experts predominantly polarized between the rheumatoid wrist and idiopathic or post-traumatic arthritis. Life expectancy, bone stock and functional demands are frequently cited as determining factors.

TWA may be ideal for frail, low-demand patients with rheumatoid arthritis (RA) or osteoarthritis, looking for pain relief and maintenance of wrist motion. It is a more functionally acceptable option for patients with a contralateral wrist fusion who wish to maintain wrist motion in one wrist, or in patients with arthritis affecting another ipsilateral upper extremity joint, such as the shoulder, elbow and hand [22], which limits the ability to compensate for a stiff wrist. Ironically, patients with a better soft tissue envelope and bone stock are more likely to achieve better outcomes from TWA [23], which is seldom the case in patients with end-stage inflammatory arthritis.

Whereas wrist arthrodesis may be better suited in younger patients, manual labourers, where there is a history of infection or those requiring the use of a walking aid, or have a pre-existing lack active wrist motion [36]. A wrist arthrodesis is more appropriate in patients whose function will not be improved by a motion-saving procedure such as those suffering from nerve palsy; cervical spinal cord or brachial plexus injury; paralytic, spastic or connective tissue disorders; and bone loss due to underlying inflammatory conditions, trauma or following tumour resection. Wrist fusion can also be considered the treatment of choice in complex carpal instability and salvage for failed total wrist replacement, proximal row carpectomy or limited intercarpal arthrodesis [37].

As the reported functional benefits and survival of TWA improve with fourth-generation implants and modern surgical techniques, including perioperative management, so too have the indications expanded for its use as a treatment method for an increasing number of conditions. In keeping with the management of hip, proximal (and to a lesser extent distal) humeral fractures, TWA has been reported in the primary treatment of acute irreparable distal radius fractures in the elderly [38]. This is still very much experimental, and although good objective and subjective function at 1-year follow-up is reported, its long-term benefit and survival are currently unknown. This, along with other proposed expanded indications for TWA such as SLAC and SNAC wrist, malunited intra-articular distal radius fractures and Kienbock disease, lacks the robust weight of evidence published relating to its use in rheumatoid arthritis, and as such, the authors are reluctant to promote TWA in these conditions currently. However, the Norwegian Registry has reported no difference in revision rates comparing RA with other aetiologies [39] and there is some evidence of equivalent results in rheumatoid and non-rheumatoid patients [36, 40]. In addition, medical advances in the treatment of RA through the use of disease-modifying antirheumatic drugs (DMARDs) has led to the reduction in severe RA progression and subsequent need for hand surgery [41–43]. Therefore, with careful selection, patients may do equally well but there is still a lack of evidence to help surgeons identify which indications lead to the best results with the fewest complications.

16.7.2 Quality Assessment of Studies and Outcomes Reporting Tools

The surgical management of wrist arthritis is by its nature a subspecialist field within hand surgery and does not lend itself to large multi-centre prospective or randomized control trials. Bearing that in mind, it is clear from the literature that most data relate to retrospective observational studies from single surgeons or implant designers, with no blinding, often missing data or high numbers of patients lost to follow-up. Furthermore, significant heterogeneity is commonly observed in terms of the underlying pathology, interventions and procedures undertaken, implants used and outcome measures along with small sample sizes [33, 40]. The nature of the reported data is not amenable to robust statistical testing, so much so that authors have had to choose to do systematic reviews of the topic rather than a meta-analysis [32]. Finally, generic non-validated assessment tools lacking specificity and sensitivity may not be designed to measure specific impairment in this patient cohort and thus fail to recognize if any true functional advantages exist. For example, the DASH (Disabilities of the Arm, Shoulder and Hand) score is frequently used in assessment after TWA or TWF. This tool is potentially subject to misinterpretation in patients with multiple-joint involvement such as in the case of RA as their scores may be affected by concurrent impairment in other joints of the same upper limb [44]. Generally, it is felt that the GRADE (Grading of Recommendations, Assessment, Development and Evaluations) quality assessment in this field is low, at best.

16.7.3 Motion, Function and Satisfaction After TWA and TWF

As discussed above, wrist biomechanics and kinematics are a complex interplay of radiocarpal and midcarpal movements in several plains occurring simultaneously. Despite advances in component design, current generations of implants simplify normal wrist kinematics to create a stable platform with a functional range of motion. TWA has been shown to improve range of motion (ROM) in absolute terms in all planes with mean post-operative increases of 9o in flexion/extension, 12o in radial/ulnar deviation and 31o in pronation/supination [33]. Although an increase from baseline can be seen, the average total wrist arthroplasty patient fails to achieve a functional active arc of motion as described by Palmer et al. [1]. Moreover, there is little evidence to assess the impact of TWA on improving the dart thrower's motion (DTM), arguably the most important functional wrist movement. Some newly licenced total wrist arthroplasties (KinematX total wrist arthroplasty, Extremity Medical, Parsippany, NJ, USA, and WristMotion Total Wrist Arthroplasty, Anika Therapeutics, Bedford, MA, USA) claim to reproduce the DTM, but long-term, large sample studies in non-designer centres have not been performed to corroborate these claims.

Arthroplasty may improve wrist motion, but for many patients, it offers the potential to preserve their current level of movement. Despite this perceived advantage, it does not appear to reflect an obvious benefit on objective assessment of function, pain relief or complications. That being said, several studies have reported improved function and patient preference towards replacement in those initially treated with TWF and who subsequently received a TWA on the contralateral wrist [45–47]. In contrast, the restricted ROM caused by arthrodesis does not necessarily translate into dissatisfaction or poor function as there are multiple reported retrospective reviews which have found that patients are overall happy with their function after bilateral wrist fusions and have adapted well and the overwhelming majority would repeat the surgery [48]. Greater increases in grip strength for arthrodesis (76% increase from pre-op) compared to arthroplasty (31%) have been reported [33]. Despite these data relating to a group of rheumatoid patients, this raises the possibility that arthrodesis may be a better option for those requiring enhanced grip strength. Satisfaction rates have been found to be high for both interventions (arthroplasty 91% vs. arthrodesis 93%), but TWF provided more reliable pain relief, a lower rate of complications and less frequent need for revision than TWA [31].

16.7.4 Financial Factors Influencing the Choice Between TWA and TWF

TWA is more costly than wrist fusion due to the cost of the implants themselves as well as those associated with complications and revisions should they arise. Counterintuitively, when quality-adjusted life years (QALYs) are taken into account, the incremental cost per QALY accrued for TWA relative to TWF is substantially less ($2328) than the national standard of $50,000/QALY deemed acceptable for adoption in the USA [49] or the £20,000–£30,000/QALY threshold range for adopting new treatment recommended by the National Institute for Health and Care Excellence (NICE) in the UK [50]. Both TWA and total wrist arthrodesis can be considered as very cost effective, and the price of a TWA seems to be within the reasonable cost range. Be that as it may, we believe that total wrist arthroplasty outcomes should be markedly better than those of TWF to justify the additional costs and risks of the procedure, and the evidence currently available does not support this viewpoint.

16.7.5 Changing Complication Rates Between TWA and TWF

Historically, TWA for end-stage rheumatoid disease of the wrist has been hampered by high rates of complications post-operatively compared to TWF. In counterpoint to this, recent systematic reviews now suggest similar complication rates between TWA and TWF [33, 40]. Complications in TWA are primarily related to prosthetic loosening and dislocation, which in time may be overcome by better prosthetic designs. Indeed, the complication profile of newer fourth-generation prosthesis appears to be improved relative to earlier generations, at least in the short to medium term [33, 40]. However, the complications related to TWF are primarily related to carpal tunnel syndrome, metal work prominence and extensor tendon issues, which may be inherent to the procedure itself and may be less amenable to remedy despite procedural refinement. As the perceived high rate of complications may deter surgeons from offering TWA on a more generous basis, this levelling of the risk profile for TWA could be interpreted as an argument for more widespread, liberal use of TWA. To accurately capture complication rates, as well as long-term clinical outcomes, implant survival and revision data, national joint registries with compulsory reporting for wrist arthroplasty, like those widely seen in hip, knee, shoulder, elbow and ankle arthroplasty, should be established. Such registries are few and far between but may help to address publication bias and portray real-life practices outside of subspecialist and designer centres.

16.8 Conclusions

Multiple surgical options are available for the management of symptomatic wrist arthritis. Partial wrist fusions can be tailored to the specific wear patterns and demographics of the patient, providing good pain relief while still maintaining wrist motion. Total wrist fusion sacrifices effectively all wrist movement but is still considered the gold standard by many because of its reliable outcomes. Total wrist arthroplasty is an attractive option for patients with diffuse symptomatic wrist arthritis. However, due to its complexity, cost implications, high rate of complications (although this may be less problematic with modern implants and arthroplasty techniques) and the existence of reliable alternatives [51], it is best reserved for a select cohort of patients.

Similar to the utility of total hip and knee national joint registries, total wrist arthroplasty registries in conjunction with prospective, randomized controlled trials comparing total wrist arthroplasty with wrist fusion are needed to draw meaningful conclusions on which treatment pathways are likely to provide superior clinical outcomes for patients with wrist arthritis. Standardized pre- and post-operative functional evaluations, quality of life assessments, patient-reported satisfaction and long-term follow-up will be essential to determine the true benefit of these interventions. These robust data will help to inform both patients and surgeons during the decision-making process to identify which patients are likely to gain the greatest benefit from either procedure [4] and will foster discussion and debate to definitively settle the areas of controversy that still remain.

References

1. Palmer AK, Werner FW, Murphy D, Glisson R. Functional wrist motion: a biomechanical study. J Hand Surg Am. 1985;10:39–46.
2. Saffar P, Semaan I. The study of the biomechanics of wrist movements in an oblique plane—a preliminary report. In: Schuind F, An KN, Cooney III WP, Garcia-Elias M, editors. Advances in the biomechanics of the hand and wrist. Springer; 1994. p. 305–11. ISBN: 978-1-4757-9109-9.
3. Wolfe SW, Crisco JJ, Orr CM, Marzke MW. The dart-throwing motion of the wrist: is it unique to humans? J Hand Surg Am. 2006;31:1429–37.
4. Moritomo H, Apergis EP, Herzberg G, Werner FW, Wolfe SW, Garcia-Elias M. 2007 IFSSH committee report of wrist biomechanics committee: biomechan-

ics of the so-called dart-throwing motion of the wrist. J Hand Surg Am. 2007;32:1447–53.
5. Crisco JJ, Heard WM, Rich RR, Paller DJ, Wolfe SW. The mechanical axes of the wrist are oriented obliquely to the anatomical axes. J Bone Joint Surg Am. 2011;93:169–77.
6. Apergis EP, Garcia-Elias M, Werner F, Wolfe S. IFSSH Scientific Committee on Anatomy and Biomechanics 2013.
7. Leventhal EL, Moore DC, Akelman E, Wolfe SW, Crisco JJ. Carpal and forearm kinematics during a simulated hammering task. J Hand Surg Am. 2010;35:1097–104.
8. Linscheid RL, Dobyns JH. Radiolunate arthrodesis. J Hand Surg Am. 1985;10(6 Pt 1):821–9.
9. Garcia-Elias M, Lluch AL, Ferreres A, Papini-Zorli I, Rahimtoola ZO. Treatment of radiocarpal degenerative osteoarthritis by radioscapholunate arthrodesis and distal scaphoidectomy. J Hand Surg Am. 2005;30:8–15.
10. Tambe A, Ali F, Trail I, Stanley J. Is radiolunate fusion a viable option in advanced Kienböck disease? Acta Orthop Belgica. 2007;73(5):598.
11. Fakunle OP, EL DM, Spencer CC, Kumar AD, Gottschalk MB, Wagner ER. Two sides of the same coin: a systematic review of radiolunate and radioscapholunate arthrodesis. J Hand Surg Global Online. 2021;3:81–7.
12. Montoya-Faivre D, Pomares G, Calafat V, Dap F, Dautel G. Clinical and radiological outcomes following radioscapholunate fusion. Orthop Traumatol Surg Res. 2017;103:1093–8.
13. McCombe D, Ireland DC, McNab I. Distal scaphoid excision after radioscaphoid arthrodesis. J Hand Surg. 2001;26:877–82.
14. McNary SM, Heyrani N, Volk I, Szabo RM, Bayne CO. The effect of radioscapholunate fusion with and without distal scaphoid and triquetrum excision on capitolunate contact pressures. J Hand Surg. 2019;44:420.e1–7.
15. Pervaiz K, Bowers WH, Isaacs JE, Owen JR, Wayne JS. Range of motion effects of distal pole scaphoid excision and triquetral excision after radioscapholunate fusion: a cadaver study. J Hand Surg. 2009;34:832–7.
16. Trail IA, Murali R, Stanley JK, Hayton MJ, Talwalkar S, Sreekumar R, et al. The long-term outcome of four-corner fusion. J Wrist Surg. 2015;4:128–33.
17. Delattre O, Goulon G, Vogels J, Wavreille G, Lasnier A. Three-corner arthrodesis with scaphoid and triquetrum excision for wrist arthritis. J Hand Surg. 2015;40:2176–82.
18. Alberta Uo. Randomized comparison of partial wrist fusion with or without triquetral excision (PARTE) 2020. https://clinicaltrials.gov/ct2/show/NCT04580225.
19. Ritt M, Stuart P, Naggar L, Beckenbaugh R. The early history of arthroplasty of the wrist from amputation to total wrist implant. J Hand Surg Br Eur. 1994;19:778–82.
20. Swanson AB, de Groot SG, Maupin BK. Flexible implant arthroplasty of the radiocarpal joint. Surgical technique and long-term study. Clin Orthop Related Res. 1984;187:94–106.
21. Chakrabarti I. Total wrist arthroplasty: a review. J Hand Microsurg. 2009;1:72–5.
22. Kennedy CD, Huang JI. Prosthetic design in total wrist arthroplasty. Orthop Clin. 2016;47:207–18.
23. Nair R. Past, present, and future in total wrist arthroplasty: a perspective. Curr Orthop Pract. 2015;26:318–9.
24. Shepherd DE, Johnstone AJ. Design considerations for a wrist implant. Med Eng Phys. 2002;24:641–50.
25. Srnec JJ, Wagner ER, Rizzo M. Total wrist arthroplasty. JBJS Rev. 2018;6(6):e9.
26. Grosland N, Rogge R, Adams B. Influence of articular geometry on prosthetic wrist stability. Clin Orthop Relat Res. 2004;421:134–42.
27. Morrell NT, Weiss A-PC. Total wrist arthroplasty for treatment of distal radius fractures. In: Arthroplasty for the treatment of fractures in the older patient: indications and current techniques. Borrelli Jr J, Anglen JO, eds. Springer; 2018. pp. 81–90. ISBN: 978-3-030-06812-7.
28. Vance MC, Packer G, Tan D, Crisco JT, Wolfe SW. Midcarpal hemiarthroplasty for wrist arthritis: rationale and early results. J Wrist Surg. 2012;1:61–8.
29. Huish EG Jr, Lum Z, Bamberger HB, Trzeciak MA. Failure of wrist hemiarthroplasty. Hand (NY). 2017;12:369–75.
30. Berber O, Gidwani S, Garagnani L, Spiteri M, Riley N, McNab I, et al. Salvage of the failed total wrist arthroplasty: a systematic review. J Wrist Surg. 2020;9:446–56.
31. Wei DH, Feldon P. Total wrist arthrodesis: indications and clinical outcomes. J Am Acad Orthop Surg. 2017;25:3–11.
32. Cavaliere CM, Chung KC. A systematic review of total wrist arthroplasty compared with total wrist arthrodesis for rheumatoid arthritis. Plast Reconstr Surg. 2008;122:813–25.
33. Hussein A, Sallam A, Elnahas W, Mallina R, Briffa N, Imam M. Wrist arthroplasty leads to better outcomes than arthrodesis for treatment of patients with advanced rheumatoid arthritis of the wrist: a review of literature. Austin Orthop. 2017;2(1):1003.
34. Zhu XM, Perera E, Gohal C, Dennis B, Khan M, Alolabi B. A systematic review of outcomes of wrist arthrodesis and wrist arthroplasty in patients with rheumatoid arthritis. J Hand Surg Eur. 2021;46:297–303.
35. Berber O, Garagnani L, Gidwani S. Systematic review of total wrist arthroplasty and arthrodesis in wrist arthritis. J Wrist Surg. 2018;7:424–40.
36. Nydick JA, Watt JF, Garcia MJ, Williams BD, Hess AV. Clinical outcomes of arthrodesis and arthroplasty for the treatment of posttraumatic wrist arthritis. J Hand Surg. 2013;38:899–903.

37. Jebson PJ, Adams BD. Wrist arthrodesis: review of current techniques. J Am Acad Orthop Surg. 2001;9:53–60.
38. Schmidt I. Can total wrist arthroplasty be an option for treatment of highly comminuted distal radius fracture in selected patients? Preliminary experience with two cases. Case Rep Orthop. 2015;2015:380935.
39. Krukhaug Y, Lie SA, Havelin LI, Furnes O, Hove LM. Results of 189 wrist replacements: a report from the Norwegian Arthroplasty Register. Acta Orthop. 2011;82:405–9.
40. Yeoh D, Tourret L. Total wrist arthroplasty: a systematic review of the evidence from the last 5 years. J Hand Surg Eur. 2015;40:458–68.
41. Gogna R, Cheung G, Arundell M, Deighton C, Lindau TR. Rheumatoid hand surgery: is there a decline? A 22-year population-based study. Hand. 2015;10:272–8.
42. Dafydd M, Whitaker I, Murison M, Boyce D. Change in operative workload for rheumatoid disease of the hand: 1,109 procedures over 13 years. J Plast Reconstr Aesthet Surg. 2012;65:800–3.
43. Aletaha D, Smolen JS. Diagnosis and management of rheumatoid arthritis: a review. JAMA. 2018;320:1360–72.
44. Murphy DM, Khoury JG, Imbriglia JE, Adams BD. Comparison of arthroplasty and arthrodesis for the rheumatoid wrist. J Hand Surg. 2003;28:570–6.
45. Ferreres A, Lluch A, Del Valle M. Universal total wrist arthroplasty: midterm follow-up study. J Hand Surg Am. 2011;36:967–73.
46. Vicar AJ, Burton RI. Surgical management of the rheumatoid wrist—fusion or arthroplasty. J Hand Surg Am. 1986;11:790–7.
47. Goodman MJ, Millender LH, Nalebuff ED, Phillips CA. Arthroplasty of the rheumatoid wrist with silicone rubber: an early evaluation. J Hand Surg Am. 1980;5:114–21.
48. Wagner ER, Elhassan BT, Kakar S. Long-term functional outcomes after bilateral total wrist arthrodesis. J Hand Surg Am. 2015;40:224–8 e1.
49. Cavaliere CM, Chung KC. A cost-utility analysis of nonsurgical management, total wrist arthroplasty, and total wrist arthrodesis in rheumatoid arthritis. J Hand Surg Am. 2010;35(379–91):e2.
50. Gandjour A. Willingness to pay for new medicines: a step towards narrowing the gap between NICE and IQWiG. BMC Health Serv Res. 2020;20(1):343.
51. Rosenfeld JF, Nicholson JJ. History and design considerations for arthroplasty around the wrist. Hand Clin. 2013;29:1–13.

Controversies in Carpal Tunnel Syndrome in Adults: Endoscopic Versus Open Carpal Tunnel Release

17

Juan Ameztoy-Gallego, Alfonso Vaquero-Picado, and Pablo Vadillo-Cardona

17.1 Introduction

Carpal tunnel syndrome is the most common compression neuropathy in the human body, arising from increased pressure in the carpal tunnel. Trauma, systemic conditions such as diabetes, or hypothyroidism amongst other clinical conditions may lead to carpal tunnel syndrome. However, the idiopathic condition is the most frequent. If conservative treatment fails, a procedure to release carpal tunnel is usually indicated [1].

Surgical treatment for carpal tunnel syndrome involves cutting the transverse carpal tunnel ligament to release pressure on the median nerve. Traditional open surgery requires a wide incision from the wrist creases to the middle of the palm to fully visualize the ligament and surrounding structures.

The development of endoscopic techniques in orthopedic surgeries drove a new horizon for carpal tunnel release. Over the last decades, orthopedic surgeons realized potential advantages of applying an endoscopic, minimally invasive, technique to treat carpal tunnel syndrome symptoms. Endoscopic carpal tunnel release is expected theoretically to yield better outcomes in terms of pain, speed of healing, and return to normal activities because it is minimally invasive and leave structures overlying the transverse carpal tunnel ligament intact.

Endoscopic procedure was first described by Okutso [2]; he described a one-portal endoscopic approach. Local anesthesia was used, without tourniquet. A transverse incision was made including skin and fascia approximately 3 cm proximal to the proximal carpal crease through which the endoscope was introduced into the carpal tunnel. The transverse carpal ligament was examined under the endoscope, paying special attention to the location of the superficial palmar arch and possible anatomic variations of the motor branch of the median nerve. The transverse carpal ligament was incised in its ulnar side using a knife under complete endoscopic vision.

Hereafter, Chow [3] developed a two-portal endoscopic technique. Using the same proximal incision, a trocar is introduced and advanced distally with the wrist in hyperextension under the carpal tunnel ligament and then subcutaneously and pushed through a second small incision. A hook knife is inserted, and the carpal tunnel ligament is released completely from proximal to distal. Here the ligament can be inspected both distally and proximally. The ligament is separated distally and proximally in two steps, each one within view of the endoscope from the opposite end.

J. Ameztoy-Gallego · A. Vaquero-Picado
P. Vadillo-Cardona (✉)
Department of Orthopedic Surgery, La Paz University Hospital, Madrid, Spain
e-mail: pablo.vadillo@salud.madrid.org

E. C. Rodríguez-Merchán, A. Moreno-Garcìa (eds.), *Controversies in Orthopedic Surgery of The Upper Limb*, https://doi.org/10.1007/978-3-031-04907-1_17

17.2 Clinical Results

Endoscopic carpal tunnel release and open carpal tunnel release are two procedures which provide satisfactory results in terms of symptom relief, with a relatively short recovery time [4]. Both procedures have been compared in multiple studies without evidence of significant difference in terms of clinical results [5]. Open release efficacy is well proven, but since the irruption of the endoscopic technique, multiple studies have compared both techniques.

Parajdi et al. [6] analyzed 14,871 patients that had an endoscopic carpal tunnel release scattered in 15 years. They obtained an 88% pain and symptom relief in the first 10 days after surgery, which raised to a 100% at 2 months after surgery. They also described an 88% recovery in grip strength in 40 days which raised to a 93% in 6 months.

When comparing the open traditional approach versus the endoscopic technique, several authors like Sayegh et al. [5] described an overall improvement of carpal tunnel syndrome symptoms having equal likelihood after endoscopic and open release, with no differences between both groups in the rate of persistent symptoms, including pain, numbness, paresthesia, subjective weakness, or night symptoms. Also, the digital sensibility testing showed no differences between the open and endoscopic technique according to the Semmes-Weinstein monofilament test score, static two-point discrimination, or static two-point sensory threshold. Both strategies showed similar improvement in the components of the Boston Carpal Tunnel Syndrome Questionnaire (BCTQ) score including symptom severity and functional status scores. The findings of this meta-analysis suggest that symptom relief and clinical outcomes, according to the validated BCTQ symptom severity and functional status indices, were no different for patients treated with endoscopic versus open surgery. Table 17.1 shows the advantages and disadvantages of endoscopic carpal tunnel release.

Table 17.1 Advantages and disadvantages of endoscopic carpal tunnel release

Advantages	Disadvantages
Earlier return to work	Costs
Reduced postoperative pain	"Blind" technique
Earlier mobility	Higher risk of neurapraxia
Reduced scar complications	Higher skills/training
Minimal incision	
Earlier recovery of grip strength	

17.3 Recurrence/Reoperation

Theoretically, endoscopic release carries the disadvantage of not directly identifying the distal edge of the carpal tunnel ligament which potentially can lead to incomplete release and recurrence of symptoms (recurrence defined as documented carpal tunnel syndrome after resolution from prior surgical technique). Incomplete carpal tunnel release has been identified as a cause for recurrence and reoperation.

The distal border of the retinaculum is embedded in a 3-mm average layer of palmar fat and is therefore not directly endoscopically visible. Findings from cadaver studies using the Agee or Chow endoscopic technique report incomplete retinaculum transection rates, ranging from 0% to 56% [7–12]. In this context, Shinya et al. [13] recommended to first separate the distal third of the retinaculum and then to advance the endoscope distally to confirm complete transection. Following the complete carpal tunnel release, the palmar fat prolapses into the carpal tunnel; the view is therefore inhibited especially distally, and remaining fibers may thus be overlooked. However, there is still controversy regarding the importance of the division of the distal end of the carpal tunnel ligament. Research made by Cobb and Cooney [14] showed that dividing the distal 4 mm of the carpal tunnel ligament had no impact on carpal arch widening when compared to incomplete division. Several studies suggest that endoscopic release is equally effective clinically, presumably resulting in a complete release of the carpal tunnel, although it is unclear if this is correlated to a complete division of the carpal tunnel ligament. Langloh et al. [15] published a series of 2053 open carpal tunnel release procedures; 1.6% required reexploration for recurrence. Concannon et al. [16] reported a 1% recurrence rate after endoscopic carpal tunnel release, whereas Chow [17] published one (0.96%) recurrence in 104 wrists treated endoscopically.

Vasiliadis et al. [18] published a systematic review and meta-analysis to evaluate recurrence and reoperation rates, comparing endoscopic carpal tunnel release with the traditional open approach. The meta-analysis revealed no statistical difference in recurrence between open and endoscopic release, and the cumulative meta-analysis illustrates a decreased odds ratio for endoscopic release versus open since 1992, which suggests a learning effect over the years. In terms of reoperation, endoscopic release had to be converted to open release in 15 cases, in five studies of the 16 included, due to intraoperative difficulties, but there were no differences in the incidence of reoperation between endoscopic and open release.

Schmelzer et al. [19] suggested that recurrence may be due to multiple factors besides incomplete release of the transverse carpal ligament, such as fibrous proliferation, scarring within the tunnel, entrapped palmar cutaneous nerve, reflex sympathetic dystrophy, painful scars, and psychological or legal motivation. Baranowski et al. [20] found that of 50 revision procedures following open carpal tunnel release, 31 had a wall of scar tissue around the median nerve and 28 had incomplete transection of the retinaculum (a combination of results was possible). Büchler et al. [21] described 35 cases of incomplete carpal tunnel release in 56 revisions following open procedure. They found, in 8 patients, an "early epineural fibrosis" which was the result of excess scar tissue. In the other 8 cases, they found "late fibrosis," as a result of the formation of a wall of scar tissue around the epineurium.

Consequently, multiple recent reports have shown a similar incidence of recurrence, incomplete release, and reoperation around 1% in patients that underwent an open or endoscopic carpal tunnel release, without statistical difference between these techniques.

17.4 Major Complications

Since the rise of endoscopic carpal tunnel release in literature, attention has focused on the increased risk of neurologic complications of the endoscopic technique reported in the available studies. Therefore, this technique is not exempt of potential complications, and special attention must be drawn to the higher risk of nerve injury compared to the traditional open approach. Sayegh et al. [5] amongst others described in their meta-analysis, comparing open versus endoscopic carpal tunnel release, a relative risk of nerve injury in the endoscopic approach compared to the open approach of 2.84 (1.08–7.46), though the majority were transient nerve neurapraxia, not showing a significant difference when comparing the two-portal technique versus the one-portal technique.

In order to avoid nerve injury, we must bear in mind the anatomic landscape of the median nerve and its anatomical variations. The thenar motor branch, sometimes described as the million-dollar nerve, as it is a source of litigation, was studied in depth by Poisel and further on by Lanz.

Lanz et al.'s [22] studies resulted on a classification system of median nerve motor branch anatomical variations. They included a scheme of the different nerve curses. Group 0 belongs to the extra-ligamentous thenar branch pattern; group 1 describes a series of variations that range from a sub-ligamentous branch, a trans-ligamentous branch, an ulnar-wards branch and a supra-ligamentous branch. Group 2 belongs to the distal accessory thenar branch and group 3 to the high median division which can be avascular, with artery or with lumbrical muscle. Finally, group 4 is the proximal accessory thenar branch, intramuscular or conjoint.

Table 17.2 Prevalence of the anatomical variations of the thenar branch of the median nerve classified by Lanz [22]

0: extra-ligamentous	1: thenar branch variations	2: distal accessory	3: high median division	4: proximal accessory
75.2%	24.8%	4.6%	2.6%	2.3%

Henry et al. [23] published in 2015 a systematic review and meta-analysis to determine the prevalence of the anatomical variations of the median nerve described before. His results showed that the rates of extra-ligamentous, sub-ligamentous, and trans-ligamentous courses were 75.2%, 13.5%, and 11.3%, respectively. The prevalence of Lanz groups 2, 3, and 4 were 4.6%, 2.6%, and 2.3%, respectively. Ulnar-side branching of the thenar motor branch was found in 2.1%. They also reported that the trans-ligamentous course of the thenar motor branch was more commonly found in the hands with hypertrophic thenar muscles compared to those without hypertrophic musculature and an identical bilateral course of thenar motor branch in 72.3% of patients. Therefore, Gould et al. [24] recommend an open ulnar approach with a layer-to-layer skin dissection, because unless clearly visualized, the rates of motor thenar branch injury can be as high as 25%. Table 17.2 shows the prevalence of the anatomical variations of the thenar branch of the median nerve classified by Lanz [22].

In Benson et al.'s [25] review of 80 articles describing complications of open and endoscopic carpal tunnel release, they divided major complications in four distinct categories: transient neurapraxias, major nerve injuries, tendon injuries, and arterial arch injuries.

17.4.1 Transient Neurapraxias

Benson et al. found that transient neurapraxias were reported in 1.45% of cases of endoscopic release and in 0.25% cases of open releases with a statistically higher proportion on the endoscopic release side [25].

It is clear from the literature that transient neurapraxias are present in a significantly higher proportion of endoscopic releases, relative to open releases. Despite this, if we further analyze the endoscopic release technique, we find that the transbursal approach to the carpal tunnel—which was popular when the endoscopic technique was first developed—is associated with higher complication rates of neurapraxia. As the transversal approach has fallen out of favor since the mid-1990s and the extrabursal approach has since then evolved as a more standard technique (whether a single-portal or two-portal system was used), there has been a reduction of this complication. It is clear that a high percentage of neurapraxias is related to the transbursal approach due to pressure applied to the median or ulnar nerves while the endoscope is manipulated through a transbursal path. For this reason, we believe that it is important to subdivide endoscopic cases according to the surgical approach to the flexor tendon bursa. When only extrabursal endoscopic release procedures are considered in the comparison, a significantly larger proportion of open release procedures are associated with complications as compared with the endoscopic release procedure [25].

Benson et al. [25] analyzed a number of conditions which could be a source of neurapraxia in the endoscopic carpal tunnel release technique. Conditions that may be the cause of ulnar neurapraxia are excessive pulling of a retractor on the ulnar side in the insertion site with compression of the superficial branch of the ulnar nerve, compression of the ulnar nerve when advancing the dilator, accidental entry in Guyon's canal, and friction on the ulnar nerve when the blade attachment is pulled back. They suspect that the actual cause is most probably the result of the insertion of the instruments in the flexion groove of the wrist where the entry point is on the ulnar side and results in the compression of the proximal ulnar nerve. To ensure that the instrument is not inserted into Guyon's canal, after the incision is made, the median nerve should be revealed and followed from distal to proximal, to the border of the retinaculum. This guarantees the correct entry into the carpal tunnel. In the literature, a greater number of complications are reported with Chow's method than with Agee's one. The question remains unanswered whether this is due to technical aspects of the procedure, or whether it is because Chow's method is more commonly used. Finally, the experience of the surgeon certainly is a decisive factor.

When transient neurapraxias were eliminated from the analysis and complications were redefined as structural injury to the nerves, arteries, or tendons, results from the comparison of the two techniques showed that a statistically significant larger proportion of open release procedures was associated with complications, as compared with endoscopic release procedures [25].

17.4.2 Major Nerve Injuries

Major nerve injuries, defined as damage to the median or ulnar nerve, were reported in 0.13% of endoscopic release cases and in 0.10% of open release cases; digital nerve injuries were reported in only 0.03% of endoscopic release cases and in 0.39% of open release cases [25]. Other studies show a rate of major nerve injuries of 0.11% in the open approach versus a 0.13% in endoscopic release. This difference does not achieve statistical significance. Boeckstyns et al. [26], who directly compared 9516 endoscopic and 1203 open releases regarding permanent structural injury, reported a 0.3% rate of complications for the endoscopic approach and a 0.2% complication incidence for the open technique. Structural complications from endoscopic and open techniques were numerically close with no statistical difference.

In Vasiliadis et al.'s [18] review, major nerve complications where scarcely found; of the 25 studies included, there were no differences between the open and endoscopic approach. The major complications recorded in these studies included one injury to the deep motor branch of the ulnar nerve in an open treated patient [27] and a case treated with endoscopic approach who developed symptoms compatible with common digital nerve injury [28]. Müller et al. [29] reported 14 lesions of nerve structures of the 31 complications that were found in his study. Albers et al. [30] (Chow technique) reported an instance in which the median nerve was completely severed. De Smet et al. [31] (Agee technique) also described one instance of the motor branch of the ulnar nerve being injured.

Several authors have reported injuries to the nerve arcade between the median and ulnar nerves causing neuromas [32]. According to Ferrari et al. [32], this superficial nerve arcade, formed by sensitive fibers from the ulnar to the median nerve (or the common middle hand nerve of the third and fourth fingers) is found in 90% of cases (45 of 50 cases in their cadaver study). They innervate part of the radial side of the ring finger and in 24% of cases run less than 4 mm parallel to the distal border of the retinaculum. They conclude this nerve arcade is a possible source of postoperative pain and neuroma formation.

17.4.3 Tendon and Artery Injuries

Benson et al. [25] found that tendon injuries were noted in 0.008% of endoscopic release cases as compared with none in open release cases. Similarly, arterial arch injuries occurred in 0.02% of endoscopic release cases and none in open release cases. Boeckstyns et al. [26] found similar results when comparing the two groups for other complications including tendon and arterial injuries. Atroshi et al. [33], in another comparative study, reported no nerve, vascular, or tendon injuries and no wound complications at 1-year follow-up.

The overall proportion of complications was 0.74% for the open release technique and 1.63% for the endoscopic release technique. This difference was statistically significant [25]. Nevertheless, Schmelzer et al. [19], in their large analysis of 54 publications, demonstrated that open carpal tunnel release and endoscopic carpal tunnel release have similar rates of complications. Therefore, it is clear that endoscopic release carries a similar rate of major complications compared with the open approach, but it is also clear that the endoscopic release carries a statistically higher rate of transient neurapraxia of the median or ulnar nerve compared with the open approach.

17.5 Minor Complications

Minor complications were analyzed by Benson et al. [25] in a meta-analysis, revealing that endoscopic release resulted, on average, in a lower rate of minor complications compared with the open release. The summary effect indicated that endoscopic release is associated with an average relative decrease in odds of minor complication of 50% compared to the open approach. However, in-depth analysis of minor complications revealed that endoscopic release was associated with a higher rate of transient nerve problems, such as neurapraxia, numbness, or paresthesia, when compared to the open release. Nonetheless, all the cases reported in this meta-analysis were transient and subsided within 2–3 weeks. Also, open release was associated with a higher rate of wound complications compared to the endoscopic release. The incision in the endoscopic approach does not harm the overlying subcutaneous nerves of the palm which could explain the fewer painful scars following endoscopic techniques. By contrast, the palmar incision used in open release results in an incision through the skin and subcutaneous tissue, increasing the risk of painful neuromas. Schmelzer et al. [19] reported that 12% of the patients complained of occasional scar tenderness and 4% complained of hypersensitivity over the scar to touch, cold, or heat. On postoperative day 84, 61% of open carpal tunnel release patients had painful scars, whereas only 36% of endoscopic carpal tunnel release patients had similar complaints.

Therefore, endoscopic release seems to be significantly superior to the open release in terms of minor complications, especially the ones related to wound problems. The endoscopic approach has been associated with reduced postoperative pain and an early return to work. Table 17.3 shows the complications after endoscopic versus open carpal tunnel release [34].

Table 17.3 Complications after endoscopic vs open carpal tunnel release. ECTR: endoscopic carpal tunnel release. OCTR: open carpal tunnel release. Modified from Palmer and Toitoven [34]

Complication	ECTR (n: 708)	OCTR (n: 616)
Median nerve injury	100	147
Palmar cut branch injury	17	117
Ulnar nerve injury	88	29
Digital nerve injury	77	54
Tendon injury	69	19
Superficial palmar arch injury	86	21
Ulnar artery injury	34	11
Total complications	708	616

17.6 Return to Work

The endoscopic surgical technique, with minimal incisions and minimal soft tissue damage, would theoretically provide improved results in terms of scar tenderness, less discomfort for patients, less postoperative pain, and subsequently earlier return to work and higher patient satisfaction.

Vasiliadis et al.'s [18] systematic review and meta-analysis revealed a statistically significant reduction of time out of work or daily activities with endoscopic release; hence, patients treated with endoscopic release returned to work or to daily activities on an average of 10 days earlier than those with an open release. The greater surgical trauma of open release is associated with increased pain, and therefore, it increases time out of work. However, inconsistency is likely to arise from the different definitions used, social and economic factors (the generosity of the public system in terms of sick leave), and the occupation of the participants enrolled in the studies. Concordantly, in Benson et al.'s [25] study, 3 months after the operation they observed a very high rate of patient satisfaction (average score 1.7) and a short absence from work (average 16.2 days). In the available literature the average reported recovery time until the patient returns to work is 40–50 days. As the length of time that a patient was absent from work depends on many sociomedical variables (e.g., type of insurance and individual motivation), it cannot be considered a reliable parameter. It does, however, play an important role in hand surgery, where absence from the workplace accounts for approximately two-thirds of the costs.

Therefore, although the recovery time until the patient is able to work is a variable difficult to be objectively measured, as many subjective factors have merged (individual motivation, insurance, psychological issues, etc.), the reported literature tends to agree that the endoscopic carpal tunnel release provides a clear advantage in terms of reducing the recovery period, allowing a faster return to working duties when compared to the open release technique.

17.7 Reporting Bias/Learning Curve

It is interesting to note that in the published studies since 1966, there are twice as many cases of endoscopic carpal tunnel release than open carpal tunnel surgery cases, even though the endoscopic approach has been used only since the past decade. In addition, we can find higher numbers of studies on. Moreover, the debate about their safety and complications as a novel technique could have possibly led to overreporting of its complications. All these facts suggest that a reporting bias exists regarding this issue.

Another explanation could be the lack of experience in performing a technically demanding novel technique that led to an increase in the rate of complications. It has been suggested that endoscopic carpal tunnel release has a relatively long learning curve. Meticulous training is mandatory before starting clinical practice in order to complete a safe procedure. Institutional courses and practice in cadavers are highly recommended and have shown to reduce the incidence of complications. Similarly, Schmelzer et al. [19] dictate that the risk of complications seems to be somewhat dependent on the experience of the surgeon. Several clinical studies such as Serra et al. [35] have shown that decreased complication rates correlate with increased surgical experience.

17.8 Costs

When analyzing the controversies of choosing between two treatments that have demonstrated to be safe and clinically and methodologically well accepted in the literature, it is of special importance to spend some time talking about costs and efficiency.

Koehler et al. [36] scrutinized costs related to the endoscopic and open carpal tunnel release techniques. He emphasized in his study that the total intraoperative time was found to be significantly longer in the endoscopic procedure (44.8 min) than in the open procedure (40.5 min) ($P < 0.05$). The main difference in resource consumption between the endoscopic and the open surgery was recognized for the orthopedic surgeon (32.7 min vs 21.3 min) and the central sterilization employees. The total procedural cost for the endoscopic carpal tunnel release was 43.9% greater ($841.64) than the open technique ($2,759.70 vs $1,918.06). This cost difference was primarily driven by the disposable endoscopic blade assembly ($217.14), direct operating room costs related to procedural duration ($582.12 vs $457.32), and orthopedic surgeon fees ($213.53 vs $139.09). Endoscopic equipment costs and the additional labor required for sterilization were not significant cost drivers.

Endoscopic carpal tunnel release was found to be more expensive than open carpal tunnel release, compared with the time-driven activity-based costing methodology at an academic medical center employing resident trainees. The cost of the disposable endoscopic blade assembly, direct operating room costs related to the procedural duration, and the attending surgeon labor costs were the greatest drivers of the identified cost discrepancy. The authors believed that the statistically significant difference recognized in procedural duration is also meaningful because it results in a substantive difference in the collective intraoperative labor costs ($118.52) and direct operating room costs ($120.71). The realization of cost savings from reduced labor requirements depends upon each institution's ability to reallocate and redistribute those labor resources. They demonstrated that open carpal tunnel release is less expensive than endoscopic release, but their analysis did not include downstream complications because the study was not designed, nor powered, to detect differences in complications between these two surgical techniques.

In order to achieve cost neutrality between the two techniques for carpal tunnel release, Koehler et al. stated that the duration of the endoscopic procedure would have to be decreased by 20.2 min. An alternative cost reduction strategy could be for the institution to seek a reduction in the purchase price of the disposable endoscopic blade assembly. If the institution was able to negotiate a 50% decrease in the price of the blade assembly, the endoscopic procedure would have to be decreased by 14.8 min to reach cost neutrality. Finally, cost containment could be achieved by strategically optimizing the time the attending orthopedic surgeon spends in the operating room. This can potentially be achieved by delegating noncritical portions of the care cycle to residents or advanced practice personnel. Differences in training level not captured by the study design may have an impact on the duration of attending supervision, as it pertains to the endoscopic procedure; however, the variation observed in the present study was relatively limited.

Another recent study [24] highlighted the cost of open versus endoscopic carpal tunnel release performed in the clinic versus in the operating room. They found operating time to be 60 min in the operating room and 30 min in the clinic and that the opportunity cost of using the operating room was approximately $2700. The cost per patient in the clinic was $985 for endoscopic versus $670 for open carpal tunnel release. In the operating room, endoscopic surgery was cheaper, $2273 versus $3469 for open surgery.

Chung et al. [37] examined cost, long-term quality of life, and costs of complications. They noted a cost of $2202 for open versus $2944 for endoscopic carpal tunnel release. The adjusted cost differential was $46 for endoscopic versus open release, which included the cost from Medicare relative value units, adjusted for outcomes. The same authors acknowledged differences in quality of life by decade for patients, meaning that benefits for endoscopic surgery are higher for younger patients. Here was a marginal benefit (for all age groups) of cost for endoscopic versus open release, which was feasible in the hypothetical case in which the rate of median nerve injury was 1% lower for endoscopic versus open surgery (this has not been reported in the literature). The authors concluded that if 70% of carpal tunnel release were performed in the clinic instead of the operating room, it could translate to a cost saving of $400 to $500 million per year.

As we have seen, cost estimates vary widely in the available literature, but there are certain statements in which most authors agree. Those statements that seem to be well accepted in literature are that overall costs of open carpal tunnel release are less than endoscopic tunnel release, performing a carpal tunnel release in the clinic is cheaper than in the hospital, and costs should include potential complications of the procedure selected.

17.9 Conclusions

Controversy continues when deciding the "gold standard" surgical technique for surgical carpal tunnel syndrome. Traditionally, open surgical release has proven excellent clinical results with a very low incidence of complications and acceptable postoperative recovery time. Nonetheless, the endoscopic technique has proven to achieve equal excellent clinical results with the advantage of an accelerated postoperative recovery and patient satisfaction. It is still in debate whether the observed higher incidence of transient neurapraxia experienced in the endoscopic surgical release is a decisive factor to restrain the use of this procedure or if it is an acceptable risk.

References

1. Padua L, Coraci D, Erra C, Pazzaglia C, Paolasso I, Loreti C, et al. Carpal tunnel syndrome: clinical features, diagnosis, and management. Lancet Neurol. 2016;15:1273–84.
2. Okutsu I, Ninomiya S, Takatori Y, Ugawa Y. Endoscopic management of carpal tunnel syndrome. Arthroscopy. 1989;5:11–8.
3. Chow J. The chow technique of endoscopic release of the carpal ligament for carpal tunnel syndrome: four years of clinical results. Arthroscopy. 1993;9:301–14.
4. Shi Q, MacDermid J. Is surgical intervention more effective than non-surgical treatment for carpal tunnel syndrome? A systematic review. J Orthop Surg Res. 2011;6(1):17.
5. Sayegh E, Strauch R. Open versus endoscopic carpal tunnel release: a meta-analysis of randomized controlled trials. Clin Orthop Relat Res. 2015:4731120–32.
6. Pajardi G, Pegoli L, Pivato G, Zerbinati P. Endoscopic carpal tunnel release: our experience with 12,702 cases. Hand Surg. 2008;13(1):21–6.
7. Tsuruta T, Syed S, Tsai T. Comparison of proximal and distal one portal entry techniques for endoscopic carpal tunnel release. J Hand Surg. 1994;19:618–21.
8. Levy H, Soifer T, Kleinbart F, Lemak L, Bryk E. Endoscopic carpal tunnel release: an atomic study. Arthroscopy. 1993;9:1–4.
9. Seiler J, Barnes K, Gelberman R, Chalidapong P. Endoscopic carpal tunnel release: an anatomic study of the two-incision method in human cadavers. J Hand Surg. 1992;17:996–1002.
10. Chow J. Endoscopic release of the carpal ligament: a new technique for carpal tunnel syndrome. Arthroscopy. 1989;5:19–24.
11. Lee D, Masear V, Meyer R, Stevens D, Colgin S. Endoscopic carpal tunnel release: a cadaveric study. J Hand Surg. 1992;17(6):1003–8.
12. Van Heest A, Waters P, Simmons B, Schwartz JT, Ramon S. A cadaveric study of the single portal endoscopic carpal tunnel release. J Hand Surg. 1995;20:363–6.
13. Shinya K, Lanzetta M, Conolly WB. Risk and complications in endoscopic carpal tunnel release. J Hand Surg Br. 1995;20:222–7.
14. Cobb TK, Cooney WP. Significance of incomplete release of the distal portion of the flexor retinaculum. Implications for endoscopic carpal tunnel surgery. J Hand Surg Br. 1994;19:283–5.
15. Langloh N, Linscheid R. Recurrent and unrelieved carpal-tunnel syndrome. Clin Orthop Relat Res. 1972;83:41–7.
16. Concannon MJ, Brownfield ML, Puckett CL. The incidence of recurrence after endoscopic carpal tunnel release. Plast Reconstr Surg. 2000;105:1662–5.
17. Chow JC. Endoscopic carpal tunnel release. Clin Sports Med. 1996;15:769.
18. Vasiliadis H, Nikolakopoulou A, Shrier I, Lunn M, Brassington R, Scholten R, et al. Endoscopic and open release similarly safe for the treatment of carpal tunnel syndrome. A systematic review and meta-analysis. PLoS One. 2015;10(12):e0143683.
19. Schmelzer R, Rocca G, Caplin D. Endoscopic carpal tunnel release: a review of 753 cases in 486 patients. Plastic Reconstruct Surg. 2006;117:177–85.
20. Baranowski D, Klein W, Grünert J. Revisions-Operationen beim Karpaltunnelsyndrom. Handchir Mikrochir Plast Chir. 1993;25:127–32.
21. Büchler UD, Goth D, Haußmann P, Lanz U, Martini AK, Wulle C. Karpaltunnelsyndrom: Bericht über 56 Nachoperationen. Handchirurgie. 1983;15(Suppl):3–12.
22. Lanz U. Anatomical variations of the median nerve in the carpal tunnel. J Hand Surg Am. 1977;2(1):44–53.
23. Henry B, Zwinczewska H, Roy J, Vikse J, Ramakrishnan P, Walocha J, et al. The prevalence of anatomical variations of the median nerve in the carpal tunnel: a systematic review and meta-analysis. PLoS One. 2015;10(8):e0136477.
24. Gould D, Kulber D, Kuschner S, Dellamaggiorra R, Cohen M. Our surgical experience: open versus endoscopic carpal tunnel surgery. J Hand Surg. 2018;43:853–61.
25. Benson L, Bare A, Nagle D, Harder V, Williams C, Visotsky J. Complications of endoscopic and open carpal tunnel release. Arthroscopy. 2006;22:919–924. e2.
26. Boeckstyns ME, Sorensen AI. Does endoscopic carpal tunnel release have a higher rate of complications than open carpal tunnel release? J Hand Surg. 1999;24:9–15.
27. Agee JM, McCarroll HR Jr, Tortosa RD, Berry DA, Szabo RM, Peimer CA. Endoscopic release of the carpal tunnel: a randomized prospective multicenter study. J Hand Surg. 1992;17:987–95.
28. Ejiri S, Kikuchi S, Maruya M, Sekiguchi Y, Kawakami R, Konno S. Short-term results of endoscopic (Okutsu method) versus palmar incision open carpal tunnel release: a prospective randomized controlled trial. Fukushima J Med Sci. 2012;58:49–59.
29. Müller L, Rudig L, Degreif J, Rommens P. Endoscopic carpal tunnel release: results with special consideration to possible complications. Knee Surg Sports Traumatol Arthroscopy. 2000;8:166–72.
30. Albers M. Die endoskopische Spaltung des Lig. carpi transversum. Arthroskopie. 1995;8:299–301.

31. De Smet L, Fabry G. Transection of the motor branch of the ulnar nerve as a complication of two-portal endoscopic carpal tunnel release: a case re-port. J Hand Surg. 1995:2018–9.
32. Ferrari GP, Gilbert A. The superficial anastomosis on the palm of the hand between the ulnar and median nerves. J Hand Surg. 1991;16:511–4.
33. Atroshi I, Hofer M, Larsson GU, Ornstein E, Johnsson R, Ranstam J. Open compared with 2-portal endoscopic carpal tunnel release: a 5-year follow-up of a randomized controlled trial. J Hand Surg. 2009;34:266–72.
34. Palmer A, Toivonen D. Complications of endoscopic and open carpal tunnel release. J Hand Surg. 1999;24:561–5.
35. Serra L, Panagiotopoulos K, Bucciero A, Mehrabi F, Pescatore G, Santangelo M, et al. Endoscopic release in carpal tunnel syndrome: analysis of clinical results in 200 cases. Minim Invasive Neurosurg. 2003;46:11–5.
36. Koehler D, Balakrishnan R, Lawler E, Shah A. Endoscopic versus open carpal tunnel release: a detailed analysis using time-driven activity-based costing at an academic medical center. The J Hand Surg. 2019;44:62.e1–9.
37. Chung KC, Walters MR, Greenfield ML, Chernew ME. Endoscopic versus open carpal tunnel release: a cost-effectiveness analysis. Plast Reconstr Surg. 1998;102:e1089–99.

Distal Radioulnar Joint: Resection Arthroplasty or Prosthetic Arthroplasty

18

Ciara Fox and Patrick Groarke

18.1 Introduction

Arthritis of the distal radioulnar joint (DRUJ), whether it be primary osteoarthritis, post-traumatic or inflammatory, is a difficult condition to adequately manage. This is due to the complexity of the anatomy and biomechanics of the joint and our inability as surgeons to truly replicate those factors in any operation. It is also not a very common pathology to encounter in the clinical setting, and therefore, studies comparing surgical options are relatively few with small numbers.

Resection of the DRUJ was performed as early as 1855 [1]. It provided good pain relief and was the mainstay of management for many years. Over time, it was acknowledged that the rate of longer-term pain, limitation of movement and potential for distal radioulnar convergence was relatively high. This sparked the development of prostheses for the DRUJ in order to enhance stability and function while reducing pain. Prostheses have also evolved from interposition implants to replacement of the ulnar head to total DRUJ replacement. Early results of arthroplasty are somewhat encouraging but studies are lacking in sample size and longevity. Therefore, the management of DRUJ pathology remains controversial.

C. Fox · P. Groarke (✉)
Department of Orthopaedic Surgery, Connolly Hospital, Blanchardstown, Dublin, Ireland

18.2 Distal Radioulnar Joint (DRUJ) Anatomy

The DRUJ is composed of the bony articulation between the styloid notch of the distal radius and the ulnar head. There is a significant mismatch in the radius of curvature of these two bony components with the styloid notch having a much greater radius of curvature than that of the ulnar head [2]. There can also be variability in both the sagittal and coronal plane alignment of the joint. In the axial plane, a "flat face" sigmoid notch is present in about 42% of patients and predisposes to instability [3]. With regard to the sagittal plane, differences in the slope of the articular surface of the sigmoid notch in comparison to the long axis of the ulna do not have a direct impact on DRUJ function but are one of the challenges that need to be addressed when considering the use of a prosthesis [3, 4]. Regardless of the morphology of the sigmoid notch or distal ulnar/radial articulation, the bony structures provide little mechanical stability.

Most of the stability of the DRUJ is attributable to the surrounding soft tissue structures, including the triangular fibrocartilage complex (TFCC) [5]. The TFCC is comprised of the dorsal and volar radioulnar ligaments, ulnocarpal ligaments, meniscus homologue, articular disc and tendon sheath of the extensor carpi ulnaris (ECU). The TFCC originates on the distal radius at the styloid notch and inserts at the base of the

E. C. Rodríguez-Merchán, A. Moreno-Garcìa (eds.), *Controversies in Orthopedic Surgery of The Upper Limb*, https://doi.org/10.1007/978-3-031-04907-1_18

ulnar styloid both dorsally and volarly [6]. Anatomical studies have shown a role not only of the TFCC, but also of the interosseous membrane and pronator quadratus muscle in providing stability to the joint [7, 8]. Interestingly, sectioning of any one of these components in isolation does not result in DRUJ instability, suggesting that there is very much a shared role of all of the soft tissue elements in maintaining stability [7–9]. Therefore, it is important in performing any surgical intervention to the DRUJ; that respect is given to, not only addressing the articular surfaces, but also preserving the soft tissue structures if possible.

18.3 DRUJ Biomechanics

The DRUJ is important in both weight-bearing and forearm rotation. Forearm rotation occurs through an axis of rotation from the centre of the radial head proximally to the centre of the distal ulnar fovea distally. The ulna is constrained proximally in the ulnohumeral joint; therefore, the forearm rotation occurs by rotation of the mobile radius around the fixed ulna [10]. Mismatch between the larger axis of rotation of the shallow sigmoid notch of the radius and the smaller ulnar head results in movement at the DRUJ occurring due to a combination of rotation and sliding. The ulna moves from the dorsal position in pronation to the volar position in supination as well as moving longitudinally relative to the radius.

The distal radius usually takes 80% of the load on axial weight-bearing with the distal ulna taking 20% when the forearm is in neutral position [11, 12]. The percentage of weight-bearing through the ulna varies depending on the position of the forearm (20% axial load through the ulna in neutral position but up to 50% in pronation and ulnar supination) [11, 12]. Load transmission through the ulna also varies depending on the ulnar length [13]. Shortening the ulna by 2.5 mm reduces its axial load to 4%, while lengthening by 2.5 mm increases it to 42% [12]. While ulnar shortening can increase peak pressure within the DRUJ, it may also aid in stability of the DRUJ by increasing TFCC tension [14, 15].

18.4 Management of Distal Radioulnar Joint Arthritis

The DRUJ can be affected by post-traumatic osteoarthritis (OA), primary OA or inflammatory arthropathies. Abnormalities of the joint surfaces can result in painful forearm rotation, limitation in range of movement, tenderness over DRUJ and instability. Given the complexity of the anatomy required to maintain the normal biomechanics of the DRUJ, surgical management is challenging.

As with any other pathology of any other joint in the body, the first step in management should be non-operative. In the case of DRUJ arthritis, conservative management includes activity modification, gentle physiotherapy, splinting, steroid injections and analgesia. When these measures fail, operative intervention is broadly divided into resection arthroplasty or prostheses. There are benefits and complications of each surgical option. The definitive treatment approach should be determined on a patient-to-patient basis by a highly skilled upper limb surgeon.

18.4.1 Resection Arthroplasty

Resection arthroplasty for the DRUJ was first performed in 1855 [1]. Overall, proponents would argue that patient satisfaction rates are relatively high. There are multiple long-term studies [16–18].

Pitfalls of resection procedures are persistent pain, instability of ulnar stump and radioulnar impingement. Opponents to the resection arthroplasty would suggest that these procedures do not reconstruct the complex anatomy of DRUJ.

These complications are relatively high but conversion to ulnar implant is an option.

18.4.1.1 Darrach Procedure

Description and History

Excision of the distal end of the ulna was first described as a technique for open DRUJ dislocation in the 1800s [1, 19]. It was later utilised as a method for addressing distal radial malunions [20–22]. Finally, it was popularised by Darrach

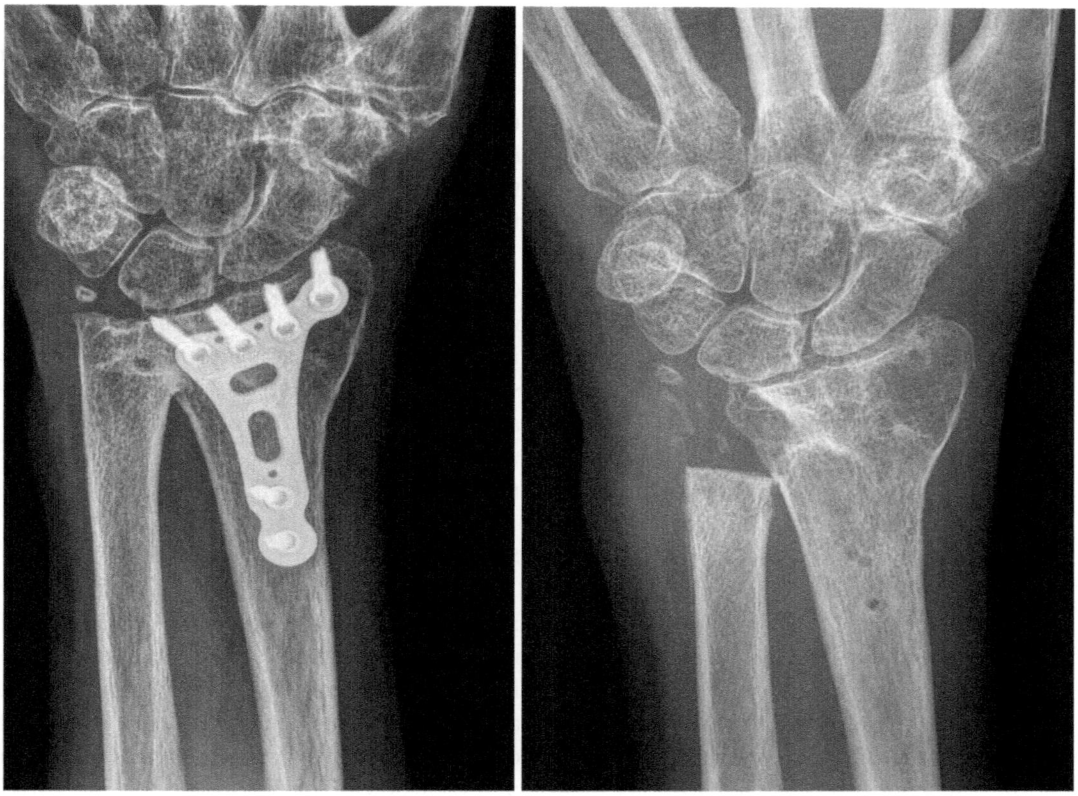

Fig. 18.1 Preoperative (left) and postoperative (right) imaging of Darrach resection arthroplasty

in 1912 as a management for rheumatoid arthritis and post-traumatic DRUJ OA [23].

Darrach's procedure is an excision arthroplasty of the ulnar head through the neck but with attempt at preservation of the ulnar styloid and TFCC attachments (Fig. 18.1).

Intended Benefits

Good longer-term studies exist for resection arthroplasty. Patient satisfaction is high. Range of movement is satisfactory in the longer term. Though radiological follow-up can show a significant percentage of radioulnar impingement, this does not directly correlate with clinical outcomes [16]. Darrach has a role to play particularly in older patients as outcomes in younger more active patients are less favourable.

Potential Complications

There are multiple potential downsides to performing a DRUJ resection arthroplasty. These include instability of the distal ulnar stump, impingement of the stump on the distal radius (radioulnar convergence) and ulnar carpal translation.

Outcomes

Good results are observed in post-traumatic and chronic DRUJ OA [18] as well as after distal radius fracture. Retrospective case series report satisfactory patient outcomes in more than 75% of patients undergoing the Darrach procedure for post-traumatic OA of the DRUJ after distal radius fracture [24].

Multiple studies have shown satisfactory or good long-term outcomes both from objective measures and patient-related subjective outcomes [16, 18].

High levels of postoperative dynamic ulnar convergence are present but do not seem to influence clinical outcomes [16].

Boretto et al. reviewed elderly patients with acute DRUJ instability secondary to concomitant distal ulna and distal radius fractures [25]. They compared open reduction and internal fixation (ORIF) of the distal ulnar fracture to resection of the distal ulna in patients greater than 70 years of age. Overall, there was no significant difference in either objective (active range of movement and grip strength) or subjective measures (pain and Mayo wrist score) between the two groups but complication rates were significantly higher in the ORIF group.

Several methods have been suggested to address the issue of stump instability and radioulnar impingement including the use of a slip of ECU or flexor carpi ulnaris (FCU) to stabilise the stump and interposition soft tissue to reduce impingement pain [17, 26, 27]. There are also reports of the use of Achilles tendon allograft used in the interosseous space to aid stability [28]. None of these alterations to the original described procedure have been shown to be clinically effective.

Studies have shown that the use of an ECU tendon slip to stabilise the remaining stump do not show superiority when compared to cases in which no tendon is used.

Barret et al. describe a technique of performing matched distal ulnar resection in combination with reconstruction of the sixth dorsal compartment and dorsalisation of the ECU tendon in order to improve stability [29]. They looked at 50 wrists in three groups—isolated matched distal ulnar resection (12), distal ulnar resection in combination with total wrist arthrodesis (21) and distal ulnar resection in combination with radius to proximal row arthrodesis (17). The majority of their patients had rheumatoid arthritis. With a mean follow-up of 8.2 ± 5.4 years, 72% of patients were pain-free and 90% would have the procedure performed again. Only two patients (4%) had both clinical and radiological instability with ulnar convergence. This was attributed to an excessively proximal resection of the distal ulna. Two other patients (4%) suffered from ulnocarpal impingement post-op due to a too-distal resection. Range of motion and grip strength were similar across all three groups postoperatively.

Tips

It is important to avoid the dorsal sensory branch of the ulnar nerve on approach. While one can use a strip of ECU or FCU to stabilise the stump, however, these do not bear out in the literature as truly aiding stability and therefore are not performed in our unit.

Rather than a completely horizontal cut, the cut of the distal ulna can be shaped in order to match the opposing surface of the radius. It is important to try to maintain static and dynamic stabilisers of the DRUJ as much as possible—anchor the TFCC to the cut surface of the distal ulna and preserve the interosseous membrane by not cutting too proximally.

Summary

There is very much a role still for distal ulnar resection in treating DRUJ pathology. Rates of radioulnar convergence and persistent stump instability remain high; however, this does not appear to correlate directly with poorer patient outcomes. Several soft tissue methods have been utilised in order to improve stability of the DRUJ post-resection [29] with varying success. Perhaps the most important factor is to be mindful both of the length (not too long—impingement or too short—instability) and shape of the distal ulnar cut as well as an attempt to preserve as much native soft tissue structure as possible.

Similar Procedures

Similar resection arthroplasty procedures include the hemiresection with interposition of the tendon (HIT) first described by Bowers in 1985 [30] and the "matched ulna" resection arthroplasty described by Watson in 1986 [31]. The hemiresection with interposition of the tendon theoretically reduces distal ulna instability as it maintains the ulnar border of the distal ulna and the soft tissue attachments (TFCC). It can be useful for younger patients with intact TFCC. These procedures have comparable outcomes to the Darrach procedure. Additional soft tissue-stabilising procedures do not result in better clinical outcome [32].

18.4.1.2 Sauvé-Kapandji Procedure

Description and History

The Sauvé-Kapandji procedure involves the fusion of the sigmoid notch of the distal radius with the distal ulna along with a more proximal ulnar osteotomy to allow pseudoarthrosis at the ulnar neck. This radioulnar fusion with metaphyseal resection was first described by Kapandji in 1936 [33].

Intended Benefits

There are multiple theoretical benefits of the Sauvé-Kapandji procedure over the Darrach resection. It maintains normal force transmission through the wrist and preserves the ulnar support of the carpus. It allows for the ulna to be shortened if needed and, as long as fusion does occur, results in a stable distal joint. As the distal ulnar attachments are left in situ, the TFCC and distal radioulnar ligaments are preserved.

The Sauvé-Kapandji procedure has been highlighted as an option for inflammatory arthropathy patients as it, theoretically, avoids the distal ulnar instability of a Darrach procedure. It has also been used in younger patients with post-traumatic OA of the DRUJ as it claims to provide better weight-bearing in the joint.

Potential Complications

The potential complications in performing a Sauvé-Kapandji procedure are similar to the Darrach procedure in that ulnar stump instability and radioulnar convergence can still be an issue. Many authors argue that impingement/convergence, present in almost all cases of any kind of resection arthroplasty, is not clinically significant.

As the procedure depends on a successful distal fusion, issues with non-union or delayed union can arise. In addition, the development of a fibrous or osseous union at the ulnar neck pseudoarthrosis site is a concern.

Outcomes

Studies looking at the Sauvé-Kapandji procedure are primarily small in number and retrospective. Overall, the trend suggests that the majority of patients have good pain relief which improves up to 1 year postoperatively, improved grip strength and preservation of movement at the wrist. There is a high rate of successful union at the DRUJ. However, complication rates remain very high.

A group from Switzerland have reported high levels of ulnar instability following the Sauvé-Kapandji procedure [34]. They reported that 6 out of 15 patients, at a mean follow-up of 13 years, required revision surgery for persistent instability of the ulnar stump. They also found that increased ulnar instability (when measured sonographically) was strongly correlated with worse DASH (Disabilities of the Arm, Shoulder and Hand) and PRWE (Patient-Rated Wrist Evaluation) scores as well as lower grip strength and supination torque. There was no significant difference in outcomes between those patients who had soft tissue stabilisation (FCU or retinacular flap) or no soft tissue stabilisation at the time of index surgery. Despite these issues, the pro-supination range in all patients was good. As a result of these findings, this group restricts the use of the Sauvé-Kapandji procedure to only very selected cases.

To minimise ulnar instability, minimal resection of the distal ulna with a very distally based pseudoarthrosis has been proposed. Lluch et al. performed the pseudoarthrosis at the level of the ulnar head and only removed 5 mm of the bone in 70 patients [35]. Despite these adjustments, all patients had ulnar stump instability. However, the instability was painless.

Complication rates following the Sauvé-Kapandji procedure have been reported to be as high as 58% [36] and 63% [37].

Munaretto et al. reviewed 35 patients with a mean follow-up of 49.5 months following the Sauvé-Kapandji procedure [38]. Pain scores were significantly improved postoperatively. Ninety-one percent of the patients had improvement in pain with 64% having complete resolution of pain. However, 9% had either no change or worsening of their pain following the procedure.

The mean grip strength improved in patients. They noted reduced wrist flexion in their patients postoperatively and attributed this to dorsal capsular plication which is performed routinely in their group to aid stability. Otherwise, there was some improvement in pronation, supination and wrist extension which did not reach statistical significance. Again, complication rates were high at 34%. Two cases had persistent ulnar stump instability, one case had persistent DRUJ pain and there was one case of painful heterotrophic ossification which all required re-operation. The other complications were described as "minor", including pin tract infection and prominent hardware. All patients had successful arthrodesis of the DRUJ.

Giberson-Chen et al. retrospectively reviewed 57 patients showing that patient-related outcome measures (QuickDASH score) improved up to 12 months postoperatively for both OA and inflammatory arthritis patients [39]. Interestingly, at 6 weeks postoperatively, QuickDASH scores were worse than those preoperatively for both groups but declined below the preoperative mean by 3 months and continued to improve until 12 months. While QuickDASH scores improved over time from pre- to post-op for OA patients, they remained lower than those for inflammatory arthritis patients at all time points. Supination improved significantly postoperatively, while range of movement in other planes of the wrist was unchanged.

Overall, there was a high revision rate of 21% including removal of hardware and revision osteotomy. Only one patient had ulnar stump instability requiring a revision stabilisation procedure. The group suggests that the low rate of instability of the ulnar stump post-op can be attributed to their surgical technique of a distal site of pseudoarthrosis only just proximal to the DRUJ articulation, thereby preserving soft tissue-stabilising structures such as the periosteum, pronator quadratus and interosseous membrane.

This paper is particularly helpful in counselling patients preoperatively regarding expected outcomes and recovery following the Sauvé-Kapandji procedure. Patients can expect that pain will worsen in the initial postoperative period but improve by 3 months. Functional improvements will continue for up to 12 months. The Sauvé-Kapandji procedure can also improve supination, for those patients with limited preoperative prosuppination, without compromising other wrist movements.

Tips

It can decrease the risk of non-union/delayed union at arthrodesis by ensuring good clearance of soft tissue/periosteum between the styloid notch and distal ulna, debridement down to the bleeding subchondral bone and good alignment + compression at arthrodesis site with the use of a compression screw.

It decreases the risk of fibrous or osseous union at the pseudoarthrosis site by carrying out minimal soft tissue retraction at that site and remove bone debris and periosteum.

By making pseudoarthrosis as close as possible to the head of the ulna, it can minimise ulnar stump painful instability by leaving the smallest bone defect as possible.

Summary

Different types of resection/Sauvé-Kapandji procedure all have similar benefits/perform the same function (no one procedure superior to others), but the rate of post-op pain is high and the range of movement is decreased.

Distal radioulnar convergence and impingement are ongoing issues. Most papers argue that radioulnar convergence does not correlate with clinical symptoms. However, measurement of ulnar stump instability as measured by ultrasound (as opposed to weight-bearing plain films) suggests that stump instability is significantly correlated with poorer outcomes on both objective and subjective measures [34]. Perhaps we are measuring the impingement/convergence inaccurately and should be using ultrasound studies more routinely.

The only statistically significant predictor of poor outcome is a high body mass index (BMI). Patients with raised BMI are found to have higher rates of persistent post-op pain. Other postoperative complications such as limited range of movement and need for revision surgery are not easily predictable. As such, it suggests that resection procedures for the DRUJ are poor options in themselves rather than the technique utilised or the comorbidities of the patients that result in poorer outcome [32].

There is still a role for both the Darrach and Sauvé-Kapandji procedures as surgical options for patients with DRUJ arthritis with careful patient selection, adequate preoperative education as to expected outcomes and correct surgical technique.

18.4.1.3 Comparison of the Darrach Versus Sauvé-Kapandji Procedure

There is paucity of literature directly comparing the outcomes of the Darrach versus Sauvé-Kapandji procedure. Those studies that seek to compare the two procedures are retrospective with small sample sizes. However, those that are out there show comparable long-term outcomes between the two procedures. Both the Sauvé-Kapandji and Darrach procedures have similar outcomes. No significant difference has been shown between the Sauvé-Kapandji and Darrach procedure [32, 36]. However, the Sauvé-Kapandji procedure is more complex and technically more demanding.

When patients less than 50 years of age underwent either the Darrach or Sauvé-Kapandji procedure to address post-traumatic DRUJ arthritis following distal radius fractures, no significant difference in grip strength or ulnar carpal shift was found [36]. Verhiel et al. showed similar outcomes for pain and function between the Darrach and Sauvé-Kapandji groups in post-traumatic DRUJ OA from both distal radius fractures and other causes [40]. Complication rates were higher in the Sauvé-Kapandji group (50% in patients who underwent the Sauvé-Kapandji procedure versus 30% in Darrach cases), but this was not statistically significant.

Yayac et al. reviewed 117 patients with DRUJ OA (post-traumatic, primary and inflammatory arthritis) at a mean follow-up of 70.6 months who underwent either the Darrach, Bowers (distal ulna hemiresection) or Sauvé-Kapandji procedures [32]. Overall, 25.6% of the patients experienced persistent pain postoperatively and 19.7% were limited in their range of movement postoperatively. The patients who underwent the Sauvé-Kapandji procedure were significantly younger than the Bower's hemiresection and Darrach groups (42.4 years versus 60 years). This age difference likely represents surgeon choice. DRUJ arthrodesis provides greater stability which is theoretically beneficial for the younger higher-demand patient. However, there was no significant difference between the groups with regard to pain or function. The study did highlight that patients with a raised body mass index (BMI) were at a significantly increased risk of persistent postoperative pain.

Traditionally, the Darrach procedure is highly utilised in the elderly population, while the Sauvé-Kapandji procedure is used in younger patients or manual labourers. The Sauvé-Kapandji procedure is more technically demanding. Multiple studies have shown that when patients are age-matched, pain, strength, range of movement, patient satisfaction and stump instability do not differ between the two procedures [41]. However, surgical revision rates were significantly higher in the Sauvé-Kapandji group.

Given the lack of superiority of the resection procedures discussed, it is difficult to advise on one rather than another. The traditional thinking that a Sauvé-Kapandji procedure was a better option for younger higher-demand patients as it resulted in greater stability has not been borne out in the current literature. Studies are limited by small numbers and retrospective design. Given that the Sauvé-Kapandji procedure is associated with a higher rate of revision surgery and is a more technically demanding procedure, should we be doing it at all?

Nikkhah et al. have called for a multicentre prospective study to be performed in the UK to determine the role of each operation given that there is no clear superiority of either [42]. Until a properly powered and well-designed study is carried out, the authors cannot advocate for one type of resection procedure over another. However, overall, pain seems to improve in majority of patients regardless of the procedure carried out.

18.4.2 Prosthetic Arthroplasty

The pitfalls of resection arthroplasty of the DRUJ, including persistent pain and radioulnar convergence, stimulated the introduction of prosthetic implant arthroplasty. Theoretically, prosthetic implants maintain more normal joint kinematics. They allow for restoration of the normal axis and rotation of the forearm as well as act to resist tensile and compressive forces across the wrist. The goal of any DRUJ implant arthroplasty is to reestablish the distal pivot joint necessary for the sufficient or adequate tensioning of the IOM allowing optimal transfer of load between the radius and ulna.

DRUJ implants are of three main types: Silastic, ulnar replacement alone and total DRUJ replacement with components on both the radius and ulna. Silastic implants are historical in perspective. Their use was related to significant bone resorption and silicon synovitis. They are no longer used due to high failure rates [43, 44]. The distal ulnar head prosthesis can be a partial or complete ulnar head replacement. In total DRUJ arthroplasty, the device is semi-constrained with components on both the distal radius and distal ulna.

Despite the advances in technology, it remains difficult for any prosthesis to fully address all aspects of the complex DRUJ anatomy and truly restore normal biomechanics. Surgeons should also be aware of the learning curve associated with the use of the newer prosthetic implants.

18.4.2.1 Partial or Complete Ulnar Head Replacement

Description and History

Ulnar head prostheses were introduced to address the limitations of resection arthroplasty at the DRUJ. Their aim was to improve patient's pain and maintain the normal DRUJ biomechanics while addressing the issues of radioulnar convergence and instability seen with resection procedures. They can be utilised when the distal radius sigmoid notch is well maintained and the joint is stable in cases of primary pathology. They are also indicated for use in salvage operations following resection arthroplasty with ongoing distal ulnar stump pain and radioulnar convergence.

In partial ulnar head replacement, the ulnar styloid, and its soft tissue attachments, is left intact. In a complete ulnar head replacement, the entirety of the distal ulna is excised (Fig. 18.2). However, the excision is performed sub-TFCC in order to protect the soft tissues. The complete ulnar head prosthesis is designed with a hole distally to allow the passage of sutures from the ulnar capsule and TFCC to the implant in order to maintain stability from the soft tissues.

Intended Benefits

An ulnar head replacement (UHR) allows for normal weight-bearing through the DRUJ. It aims to restore a normal axis and forearm rotation while resisting the tensile and compressive forces across the wrist joint. By maintaining the soft tissue-stabilising structures around the DRUJ, it also addresses the issue of instability. The benefit of an ulnar head replacement over a resection arthroplasty is to prevent stump pain, radioulnar convergence and instability. Multiples studies have shown that ulnar head replacement is a successful operation, and superior to distal ulnar resection, in restoring normal kinematics of the forearm [45–47].

Potential Complications

Despite adherence to careful surgical technique and repair of soft tissues, instability of the implant can be an issue particularly if the morphology of the native sigmoid notch is quite flat. This can be addressed by a gentle and careful "shaping" of the sigmoid notch at the time of ulnar head implant using a burr.

Sigmoid notch erosion and stress shielding are other concerns with UHR. The metallic ulnar head may erode into the sigmoid notch of the distal radius over time. While the distal ulnar replacement enables normal weight-bearing through the DRUJ, the force transmission on loading passes down the implant stem to the more proximal ulnar diaphysis, thus bypassing the remaining more distal ulnar diaphysis. This can result in stress shielding and osteolysis around the implant.

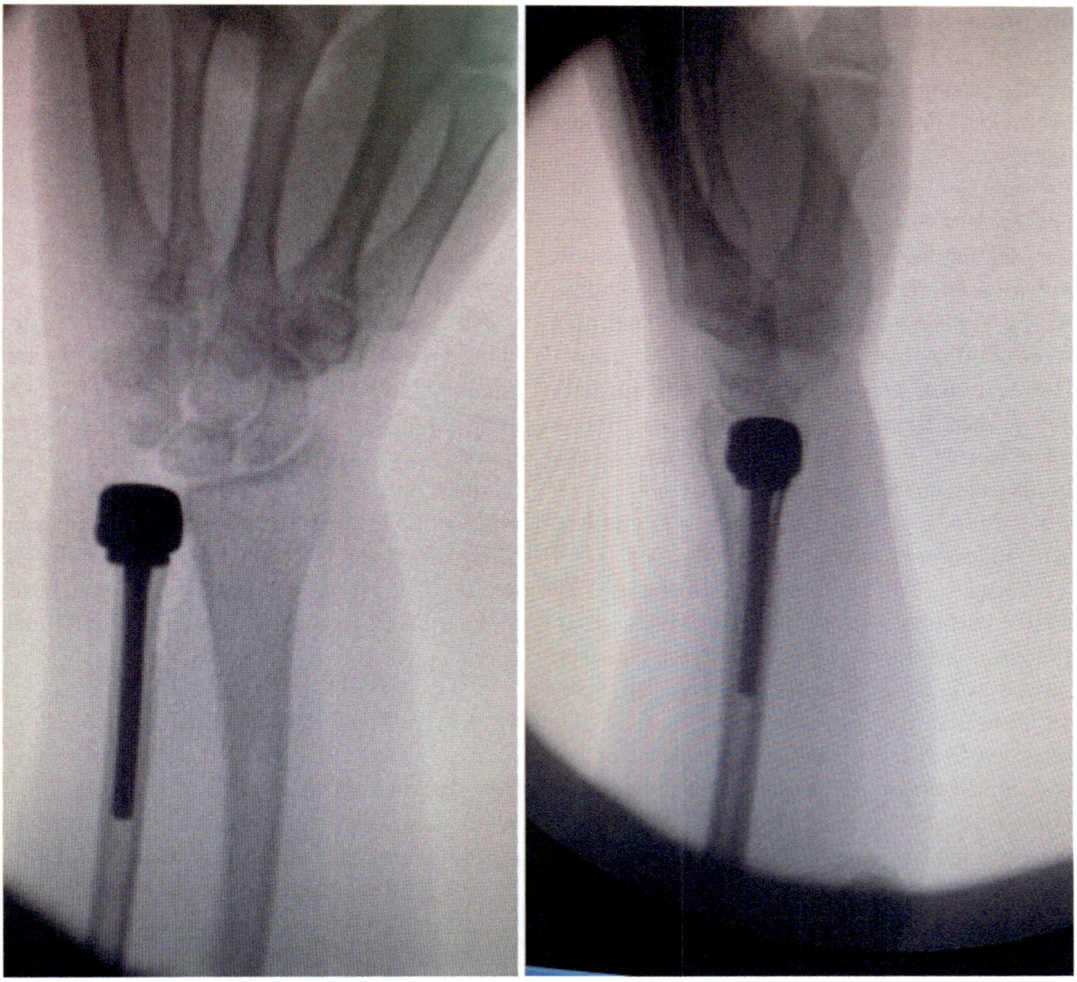

Fig. 18.2 Anteroposterior (left) and lateral (right) images of total ulnar head replacement (UHR)

Stress shielding of the distal ulna can produce significant osteolysis around the implant at short-term follow-up. This has been reported to occur in 90%–100% of patients [48, 49]. Although it is argued that the radiological presence of stress shielding and osteolysis does not directly correlate with clinical outcome [50]. However, one paper does suggest that the presence of a "pedestal" at the tip of the ulnar stem correlates with a worse functional result [51].

Outcomes

In reviewing the outcomes of UHR implants, there are only relatively small studies that are retrospective in nature. However, patient satisfaction and outcomes are generally good.

Baring et al. looked at 10 patients who underwent distal ulnar replacement with mixed aetiologies (primary OA, post-traumatic OA, rheumatoid and failed Darrach procedure) [50]. Nine out of ten patients had developed osteolysis of the distal ulna at a mean follow-up of 48 months. Despite this, the patient-related outcome measures were good. The mean visual analogue scale (VAS) for pain was 2.7 and the mean DASH score was 37. Of the nine patients with osteolysis, eight felt their condition was either "better" or "much better". Though this was a small single-surgeon study with some limitations (no clearly defined preoperative functional or pain measurements and no postoperative measurement of grip strength), it is important in discussing the relevance of stress shielding of these implants. The majority of patients seem to develop distal ulnar osteolysis but the radiological findings do not directly correlate with patient outcomes.

Sauerbier et al. reviewed 25 patients who underwent UHR either as a primary procedure for DRUJ arthritis or as a salvage procedure post resection arthroplasty [48]. There was a statistically significant improvement in pain and pain scores during stress of the DRUJ in both groups. However, patient outcomes were significantly better when the procedure was done as a primary operation rather than as salvage. This may be due to the meticulous maintenance of soft tissue structures when the ulnar head implant in utilised as an index procedure.

Warwick et al. presented their results of 56 UHRs performed in 52 patients with a mean follow-up of 60 months [52]. The mean pain score was 2.2, while the mean DASH score was 18. While there were no preoperative scores recorded to allow a direct evaluation of objective improvement, patient satisfaction was high. Forty-seven of the patients would have undergone the same procedure again. There were five complications reported, of which three required surgical interventions (two-stage revision for infected loosening, impaction grafting for aseptic loosening, tendon transfers for delayed extensor tendon rupture). There were five radiologically confirmed patients with styloid notch erosion, but all of these patients were asymptomatic. Overall, this study reports low pain scores, good function and high patient satisfaction with UHR.

Tips

Regardless of which specific implant is utilised, careful dissection and protection of the TFCC and surrounding soft tissue structures should be a priority. If the corresponding styloid notch of the distal radius is particularly flattened, it can be contoured by gently and carefully using a burr to develop a more "C-shaped" notch to improve stability of the implant.

Summary

There is a lack of robust studies regarding UHRs. However, the small retrospective studies that are available all report high levels of patient satisfaction and improvement in pain postoperatively. The best outcomes are when a UHR is carried out as an index procedure rather than as a salvage procedure after a failed resection. This is likely due to the integrity of the soft tissues.

No significant difference has been documented between partial or total UHR. Partial UHRs show some decrease in range of movement but higher grip strength and rotational force postoperatively when compared to total UHRs, but these differences do not reach statistical significance [53]. As no firm evidence has shown a benefit for total UHR over a partial UHR, we advise that surgeons would use whichever implant they are most familiar and comfortable with.

18.4.2.2 Total DRUJ Arthroplasty

Description and History

While ulnar head replacements were a benefit in restoring normal forearm kinematics in DRUJ pathology, complications such as instability and styloid erosion due to the implant drove the development of a total distal ulnar replacement. The main implant that we refer to in our discussion here is the Scheker or Aptis implant. Schuurman also developed a total DRUJ replacement. While the Schuurman implant has been adapted over time and later designs show superiority over earlier devices, studies have shown better longevity with the Aptis prosthesis when compared to the Schuurman [54, 55]. Most of the current literature available relates to the Aptis implant and it is the prosthesis we use in our unit. The Aptis implant is a semi-constrained, modular implant. It is designed to replace the function of the ulnar head, sigmoid notch of the radius and TFCC. It can be used in inflammatory arthritis, primary OA, post-traumatic OA and congenital DRUJ pathology and has also been shown to be of benefit in failed resection arthroplasty cases (Figs. 18.3 and 18.4).

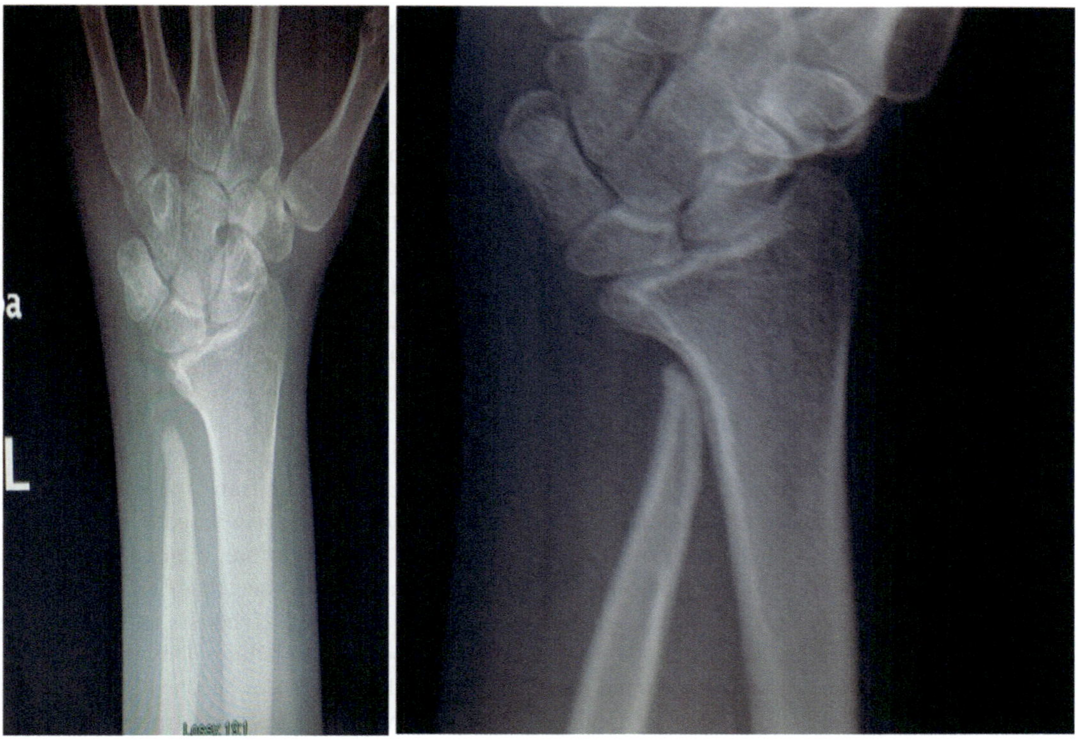

Fig. 18.3 Anteroposterior (left) and lateral (right) preoperative images of patient post-failed Darrach procedure for post-traumatic distal radioulnar joint (DRUJ) osteoarthritis with ongoing significant pain

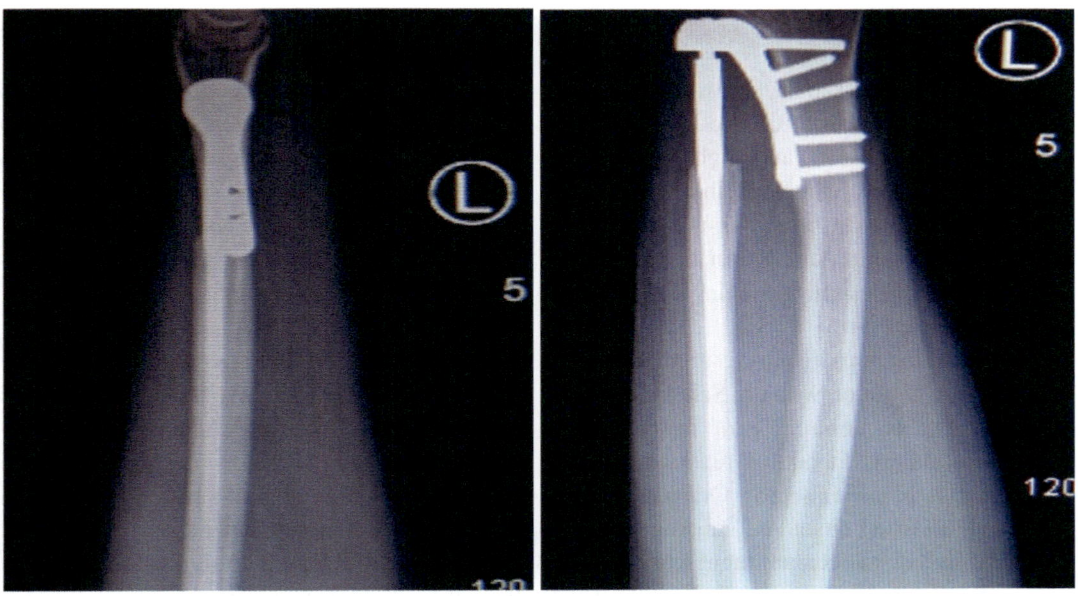

Fig. 18.4 Postoperative images of the same patient following conversion to total distal radioulnar joint (DRUJ)—Scheker prosthesis—with improvement in pain and function

Intended Benefits

The aim of performing a total distal radioulnar joint replacement is to reproduce a stable painless joint and restore normal biomechanics allowing full pronation and supination, radial migration and variable angle of rotation. It has a particularly significant role as a salvage implant for previous failed operations on the DRUJ.

Potential Complications

The total DRUJ arthroplasty theoretically addresses both instability and restores normal biomechanics of the DRUJ but it is not a panacea for all of DRUJ arthritis. It involves significant soft tissue dissection which could lead to injuries of the DRUJ stabilisers. As a semi-constrained device, the Aptis implant attempts to overcome these issues and maintain stability. However, the semi-constrained design may predispose young active patients to loosening over time.

Stress shielding and osteolysis around the ulnar component, similar to UHRs, is another concern. While it has a role as a salvage implant in patients who have failed previous DRUJ operations, concern exists over what options are available if the Aptis itself fails. This is a particular worry in younger patients.

Outcomes

Overall high patient satisfaction rates and good survival are reported with the Aptis implant but high complication rates and high rates of re-intervention are also recorded. There is concern that using this implant in young active patients may predispose to loosening over time given its semi-constrained design. Loosening was reported with early studies [54].

Late complications requiring secondary surgery are very common with the Scheker implant and shown to occur in 21% of patients [55]. Synovitis of the ECU tendon is reported to occur in up to 44% of patients [56]. Other complications include irritation of the superficial radial nerve and first dorsal compartment tenosynovitis which may occur secondary to the length of the radial screws.

The Aptis implant has a wide range of indications for use with good outcomes reported across the board. Galvis et al. report on its benefit in rheumatoid patients [57]. Pain scores and range of movement were both improved postoperatively. Axelsson et al. have reported positive outcomes when the Aptis is used for failed previous DRUJ surgery [58]. DASH scores are significantly improved. Other objective parameters, such as grip strength, are improved but do not reach significance. Significant bone resorption was noted at the distal ulna in most patients but there was no evidence of implant loosening. However, the mean follow-up was only 3.7 years [58].

Frost in 1994 described stress shielding as relating to Wolff's law and bone's structural adaptations or remodelling based on the stresses applied to it [59]. Therefore, if an implant results in force bypassing the bone, the bone will become weaker and less dense as there is no stimulus for continued bone remodelling. This is seen commonly with hip prostheses but can also be present in upper limb prostheses such as humeral stems and even in the distal radius following wrist arthroplasty. While we have noted evidence of stress shielding with the UHRs and total DRUJ replacements, it is not clear whether there is any clinical significance to this finding and whether it can act as a predictor of aseptic loosening in longer-term follow-up.

Rampazzo et al. reviewed the use of the Aptis prosthesis in younger patients [60]. This group looked at 46 arthroplasties performed at a mean age of 32 years with a mean follow-up of 61 months. Both objective and subjective parameters were significantly improved postoperatively, including grip strength, pain scores, DASH scores, PRWE scores and range of movement. The overall survival rate was 96% at 5 years.

Calcagni et al. in Europe reviewed his results of the Aptis implant at both midterm and longer-term follow-up [55, 61]. This group again reported good pain relief and patient satisfaction with significant improvement in strength and weightlifting. There was no significant change in the range of movement. Their overall survival was 80% at 5 years. Calcagni et al. report that, despite it being a "delicate" procedure with careful dissection of soft tissues and the need for a meticulous surgical technique, the learning curve with this implant is quite flat.

Multiple studies have shown very good results with regard to patient satisfaction and functional scores with a mean implant survival of 96%–100% at 5 years [60, 62–64]. However, longer follow-up and assessment are needed to truly assess the outcomes of this implant.

Tips
While the Aptis total DRUJ replacement has very good early results, the surgical technique is somewhat challenging and requires a good deal of soft tissue dissection. We feel that its primary role at present is as a salvage implant as a last option for patients. Therefore, we would suggest attempting other surgical options first. Preoperative planning is important for this implant. It is essential to have high-quality radiological imaging, anteroposterior (AP) and lateral views of the full length of the forearm, in order to plan for the most appropriate implant insertion. Care should be taken to protect soft tissues intraoperatively. It is essential to ensure adequate soft tissue flap to cover the prosthesis and protect the ECU in order to reduce the complications of ECU irritation.

Summary
Overall, 5-year survival rates are good with DRUJ arthroplasty. However, the difficulty then becomes options for revision when the implants do fail. This is particularly relevant in the setting of DRUJ arthritis in a young person.

The National Institute for Health and Care Excellence (NICE) guidelines published in November 2017 suggest that this is a useful prosthesis but that it should be used in very limited setting and by a very small number of surgeons in order to accrue the specialist technique [65].

Even with comprehensive review, very few papers with proper pre-/post-op data are available and very few reached statistical significance. Therefore, it is difficult to comment.

By not addressing the ulnocarpal joint with total DRUJ replacement, we are increasing the axial load to the radiocarpal joint similar to what would occur with an excision arthroplasty.

These need to be added to the National Joint Registry in order to truly calculate accurate preoperative and postoperative outcomes and to compare different prostheses. Without standardised follow-up, early identification of complications and major issues with these implants is very difficult particularly given that they are performed in such small numbers.

Calcagni et al. performed a systematic review of the literature surrounding DRUJ arthroplasty with implants in 2017 [55]. This review highlighted the paucity of data available for review. Very few papers have complete preoperative and postoperative data collection. There are no large studies to reference, and therefore, very few reach statistical significance given the small patient numbers. However, this review did show a patient satisfaction rate of 95% with UHRs and 98% with the Aptis total DRUJ replacement. The UHRs were found to have a 95% survival at or beyond 5 years and the total DRUJ had a survival rate of 98% at or beyond 5 years.

A further systematic review by Moulton et al. in 2017 reviewed both distal ulnar replacements and total DRUJ replacements [66]. Fourteen studies had shown an implant survivor rate of 93% at a mean of 45 months for the ulnar head replacements and 97% survivorship for the total DRUJ prosthesis (primarily Aptis implant) at 56 months.

Certainly the shorter-term results with DRUJ implant arthroplasty are very encouraging but we are somewhat cautious with the use of these implants in younger patients given the lack of long-term outcome data. We feel that a prospective multicentre trial is needed in order to most accurately assess the outcomes in these implants.

18.4.3 Authors' Preferred Treatment Methods

In general, we prefer a Darrach procedure in older less-demanding patients. It is a relatively straightforward procedure with overall high satisfaction rates. As a local group, we do not tend to do Sauvé-Kapandji procedure as we feel that, in our hands, the high complication rates and rates of revision surgery outweigh the benefits. In the younger patient, we would tend to favour an ulnar head replacement. We have found that some of these implants are becoming increasingly difficult to obtain and to have adequate surgical rep support as larger companies take over smaller ones and drop these from their portfolio as they are utilised in a much smaller volume than other upper limb implants. In cases of prior failed surgery as a salvage operation or for that subset of patients with concomitant DRUJ arthritis and instability, we favour a Scheker total DRUJ prosthesis.

While the newer implants for either ulnar head or total DRUJ replacements show good outcomes in the short term and hold great potential, there is certainly an added cost issue with their use. In the current age of careful resource utilisation, each surgeon needs to decide what is best for their patient based on the resources available in their unit as well as their own surgical expertise while still maintaining a focused individualised optimal patient care.

18.4.4 Conclusions

It is difficult to propose an algorithm to aid with treatment options in DRUJ arthritis. It remains an area of great controversy. We would recommend that surgeons decide management options on a case-by-case basis dependent on both patient factors (i.e. BMI, function, age) and joint factors (stability, congruency, morphology).

We need robust, prospective long-term studies to assess the true outcome of these procedures. These are all done in such a small number; it is difficult to reach statistical significance. Our understanding may always be somewhat limited as a result.

The authors hesitate to suggest a rigid algorithm of management for these cases. There is definite potential for the prostheses; however, their complication rate is high and the number of studies, long-term follow-up and rigid pre- and post-op data are limited. Prosthetic replacement of the DRUJ is not something for the "casual" hand surgeon to undertake. If done, they should be carried out in very specialist centres by a very small number of surgeons in order to improve the learning curve of any newer technology.

It is perhaps one of those conditions where arthritis in a young patient does not have an easy management option and conservative measures should be employed first at all costs.

We think it is important when considering any of the surgical options for DRUJ arthritis that we counsel patients appropriately. Most of these options (resection and prosthesis) will provide pain relief and functional improvement. However, when we discuss supposedly "good" outcomes, we must emphasise to our patients that no surgical procedure offers 100% pain relief in all patients. Functional range of movement is still considered flexion/extension of 40°/40°, radial-ulnar deviation combined of 40° [67] and pronation/supination of 50°/50° [68]. These may be very disappointing figures for some young and active patient's, particularly in this contemporary age where the use of computer keyboards or smart phones requires a greater degree of pronation [69].

In this age, particularly with younger patients, expectations are high. It is important to explain what we interpret as "good" results.

References

1. Malgaigne J. Traites des fractures et des luxations. Paris; 1855.
2. af Ekenstam F. Anatomy of the distal radioulnar joint. Clin Orthop Relat Res. 1992;275:14–8.
3. Tolat AR, Stanley JK, Trail IA. A cadaveric study of the anatomy and stability of the distal radioulnar joint in the coronal and transverse planes. J Hand Surg. 1996;21:587–94.
4. Sagerman SD, Zogby RG, Palmer AK, Werner FW, Fortino MD. Relative articular inclination of the distal radioulnar joint: a radiographic study. J Hand Surg. 1995;20:597–601.
5. Stuart PR, Berger RA, Linscheid RL, An KN. The dorsopalmar stability of the distal radioulnar joint. J Hand Surg. 2000;25:689–99.
6. Palmer AK, Werner FW. The triangular fibrocartilage complex of the wrist—anatomy and function. J Hand Surg 1981;6:153–162.
7. Cole DW, Elsaidi GA, Kuzma KR, Kuzma GR, Smith BP, Ruch DS. Distal radioulnar joint instability in

distal radius fractures: the role of sigmoid notch and triangular fibrocartilage complex revisited. Injury. 2006;37:252–8.
8. Watanabe H, Berger RA, Berglund LJ, Zobitz ME, An KN. Contribution of the interosseous membrane to distal radioulnar joint constraint. J Hand Surg. 2005;30:1164–71.
9. Gofton WT, Gordon KD, Dunning CE, Johnson JA, King GJ. Soft-tissue stabilizers of the distal radioulnar joint: an in vitro kinematic study. J Hand Surg. 2004;29:423–31.
10. af Ekenstam F, Hagert CG. Anatomical studies on the geometry and stability of the distal radio ulnar joint. Scand J Plastic Reconstruc Surg. 1985;19:17–25.
11. Palmer AK, Werner FW. Biomechanics of the distal radioulnar joint. Clin Orthop Relat Res. 1984;187:26–35.
12. Palmer AK, Werner FW, Glisson RR, Murphy DJ. Partial excision of the triangular fibrocartilage complex. J Hand Surg. 1988;13:391–4.
13. Nygaard M, Nielsen NS, Bojsen-Moller F. A biomechanical evaluation of the relative load change in the joints of the wrist with ulnar shortening: a 'handbag' model. J Hand Surg Eur. 2009;34:724–9.
14. Nishiwaki M, Nakamura T, Nagura T, Toyama Y, Ikegami H. Ulnar-shortening effect on distal radioulnar joint pressure: a biomechanical study. J Hand Surg. 2008;33:198–205.
15. Nishiwaki M, Nakamura T, Nakao Y, Nagura T, Toyama Y. Ulnar shortening effect on distal radioulnar joint stability: a biomechanical study. J Hand Surg. 2005;30:719–26.
16. Grawe B, Heincelman C, Stern P. Functional results of the Darrach procedure: a long-term outcome study. J Hand Surg. 2012;37(2475–80):e1–2.
17. Tulipan DJ, Eaton RG, Eberhart RE. The Darrach procedure defended: technique redefined and long-term follow-up. J Hand Surg. 1991;16:438–44.
18. Jochen-Frederick H, Pouyan Y, Khosrow BA, Christoph H, Berthold B, Ulrich K, et al. Long-term functional outcome and patient satisfaction after ulnar head resection. J Plastic Reconstruct Aesthetic Surg. 2016;69:1417–23.
19. EM M. Three cases illustrating luxation of the ulna in connection with Colles' fracture. Medical Records 1880;17:305–308.
20. L VL. Zur behandlung fehrerhaft gehlilter bruche der karpalen radiusepiphuse. Centralblatt fur Chirurgie 1887;14:265–269.
21. C L. Zur Fraser der derangement interne des kniegelenks. Deutsche Medizinische Wolhenschrift 1840;16:169–170.
22. Buck-Gramcko D. On the priorities of publication of some operative procedures on the distal end of the ulna. J Hand Surg. 1990;15:416–20.
23. Darrach W. Anterior dislocation of the head of the ulna. Ann Surg. 1912;56
24. Coulet B, Onzaga D, Perrotto C, Boretto JG. Distal radioulnar joint reconstruction after fracture of the distal radius. J Hand Surg. 2010;35:1681–4.
25. Boretto JG, Zaidenberg EE, Gallucci GL, Sarme A, De Carli P. Comparative study of internal fixation of the ulna and distal ulna resection in patients older than 70 years with distal radius and distal metaphyseal ulna fractures. Hand. 2019;14:540–6.
26. Breen TF, Jupiter JB. Extensor carpi ulnaris and flexor carpi ulnaris tenodesis of the unstable distal ulna. J Hand Surg. 1989;14:612–7.
27. Sotereanos DG, Gobel F, Vardakas DG, Sarris I. An allograft salvage technique for failure of the Darrach procedure: a report of four cases. J Hand Surg. 2002;27:317–21.
28. Allende C. Allograft tendon interposition and brachioradialis tendon stability augmentation in revision surgery for failed Darrach distal ulna resections. Tech Hand Upper Extremity Surg. 2010;14:237–40.
29. Barret H, Lazerges C, Chammas PE, Degeorge B, Coulet B, Chammas M. Modification of matched distal ulnar resection for distal radio-ulnar joint arthropathy: analysis of distal instability and radioulnar convergence. Orthop Traumatol Surg Res. 2020;106:1597–603.
30. Bowers WH. Distal radioulnar joint arthroplasty: the hemiresection-interposition technique. J Hand Surg. 1985;10:169–78.
31. Watson HK, Ryu JY, Burgess RC. Matched distal ulnar resection. J Hand Surg. 1986;11:812–7.
32. Yayac M, Padua FG, Banner L, Seigerman DA, Beredjiklian PK, Aita DJ, et al. Treatment outcomes in patients undergoing surgical treatment for arthritis of the distal radioulnar joint. J Wrist Surg. 2020;9:230–4.
33. M SLaK. Nouvelle technique de traitement chirurgical des luxations recidivantes isolees de l'extremite inferieure du cubitus. J Chirurgie (Paris). 1936;47:589–94.
34. Reissner L, Schweizer A, Unterfrauner I, Estermann L, Nagy L. Long-term results of Sauve-Kapandji procedure. J Hand Surg Eur. 2021;46:626–31.
35. Lluch A. The sauve-kapandji procedure. J Wrist Surg. 2013;2:33–40.
36. George MS, Kiefhaber TR, Stern PJ. The Sauve-Kapandji procedure and the Darrach procedure for distal radio-ulnar joint dysfunction after Colles' fracture. J Hand Surg. 2004;29:608–13.
37. Carter PB, Stuart PR. The Sauve-Kapandji procedure for post-traumatic disorders of the distal radio-ulnar joint. J Bone Joint Surg Br. 2000;82:1013–8.
38. Munaretto N, Aibinder W, Moran S, Rizzo M. Sauve-Kapandji remains a viable option for distal radioulnar joint dysfunction. Hand. 2020 Nov;22:1558944720966725.
39. Giberson-Chen CC, Leland HA, Benavent KA, Harper CM, Earp BE, Rozental TD. Functional outcomes after Sauve-Kapandji arthrodesis. J Hand Surg. 2020;45:408–16.
40. Verhiel S, Ozkan S, Ritt M, Chen NC, Eberlin KR. A comparative study between Darrach and Sauve-Kapandji procedures for post-traumatic distal radioulnar joint dysfunction. Hand. 2021;16:375–84.

41. Roulet S, Williot A, Sos C, Mazaleyrat M, Marteau E, Laulan J, et al. Comparison of subjective outcomes of Darrach and Sauve-Kapandji procedures at a minimum 2 years' follow-up. Orthop Traumatol Surg Res. 2021;107(5):102974.
42. Nikkhah D, Rodrigues J, Dejager L. Do patients really do better after the Sauve-Kapandji procedure when compared to the Darrach procedure? A systematic review. J Hand Surg Eur. 2011;36(7):615.
43. Sagerman SD, Seiler JG, Fleming LL, Lockerman E. Silicone rubber distal ulnar replacement arthroplasty. J Hand Surg. 1992;17:689–93.
44. McMurtry RY, Paley D, Marks P, Axelrod T. A critical analysis of Swanson ulnar head replacement arthroplasty: rheumatoid versus nonrheumatoid. J Hand Surg. 1990;15:224–31.
45. Gordon KD, Dunning CE, Johnson JA, King GJ. Kinematics of ulnar head arthroplasty. J Hand Surg. 2003;28:551–8.
46. Berger RA, Cooney WP 3rd. Use of an ulnar head endoprosthesis for treatment of an unstable distal ulnar resection: review of mechanics, indications, and surgical technique. Hand Clin. 2005;21:603–20.
47. Masaoka S, Longsworth SH, Werner FW, Short WH, Green JK. Biomechanical analysis of two ulnar head prostheses. J Hand Surg. 2002;27:845–53.
48. Sauerbier M, Arsalan-Werner A, Enderle E, Vetter M, Vonier D. Ulnar head replacement and related biomechanics. J Wrist Surg. 2013;2:27–32.
49. Herzberg G. Periprosthetic bone resorption and sigmoid notch erosion around ulnar head implants: a concern? Hand Clin. 2010;26:573–7.
50. Baring TK, Popat R, Abdelwahab A, Ferris B. Short- to mid-term results of ulna head replacement as both a primary and revision implant. J Clin Orthop Trauma. 2016;7:292–5.
51. Kakar S, Swann RP, Perry KI, Wood-Wentz CM, Shin AY, Moran SL. Functional and radiographic outcomes following distal ulna implant arthroplasty. J Hand Surg. 2012;37:1364–71.
52. Warwick D, Shyamalan G, Balabanidou E. Indications and early to mid-term results of ulnar head replacement. Ann R Coll Surg Engl. 2013;95:427–32.
53. Estermann L, Reissner L, Rosskopf AB, Schweizer A, Nagy L. Clinical, radiological and patient-rated outcome comparison between total and partial ulnar head implants. J Hand Surg Eur. 2021:17531934211048406.
54. Schuurman AH, Teunis T. A new total distal radioulnar joint prosthesis: functional outcome. J Hand Surg. 2010;35:1614–9.
55. Calcagni M, Giesen T. Distal radioulnar joint arthroplasty with implants: a systematic review. EFORT Open Rev. 2016;1:191–6.
56. Savvidou C, Murphy E, Mailhot E, Jacob S, Scheker LR. Semiconstrained distal radioulnar joint prosthesis. J Wrist Surg. 2013;2:41–8.
57. Galvis EJ, Pessa J, Scheker LR. Total joint arthroplasty of the distal radioulnar joint for rheumatoid arthritis. J Hand Surg. 2014;39:1699–704.
58. Axelsson P, Sollerman C. Constrained implant arthroplasty as a secondary procedure at the distal radioulnar joint: early outcomes. J Hand Surg. 2013;38:1111–8.
59. Frost HM. Wolff's law and bone's structural adaptations to mechanical usage: an overview for clinicians. Angle Orthod. 1994;64:175–88.
60. Rampazzo A, Gharb BB, Brock G, Scheker LR. Functional outcomes of the Aptis-Scheker distal radioulnar joint replacement in patients under 40 years old. J Hand Surg. 2015;40(1397–403):e3.
61. Fuchs N, Meier LA, Giesen T, Calcagni M, Reissner L. Long-term results after semiconstrained distal radioulnar joint arthroplasty: a focus on complications. Hand Surg Rehab. 2020;39:186–92.
62. Sander AL, Ebert F, Marzi I, Frank J. Outcome after implantation of the Aptis total distal radioulnar joint replacement prosthesis. Handchirurgie, Mikrochirurgie, plastische Chirurgie : Organ der Deutschsprachigen Arbeitsgemeinschaft fur Handchirurgie: Organ der Deutschsprachigen Arbeitsgemeinschaft fur Mikrochirurgie der Peripheren Nerven und Gefasse. 2015;47:306–11.
63. Bizimungu RS, Dodds SD. Objective outcomes following semi-constrained total distal radioulnar joint arthroplasty. J Wrist Surg. 2013;2:319–23.
64. Kachooei AR, Chase SM, Jupiter JB. Outcome assessment after Aptis distal radioulnar joint (DRUJ) implant arthroplasty. Arch Bone Joint Surg. 2014;2:180–4.
65. Excellence NIfHaC. Total distal radioulnar joint replacement for symptomatic joint instability or arthritis 2017. Available from: https://www.nice.org.uk/guidance/ipg595.
66. Moulton LS, Giddins GEB. Distal radio-ulnar implant arthroplasty: a systematic review. J Hand Surg Eur. 2017;42:827–38.
67. Ryu JY, Cooney WP 3rd, Askew LJ, An KN, Chao EY. Functional ranges of motion of the wrist joint. J Hand Surg. 1991;16:409–19.
68. Valone LC, Waites C, Tartarilla AB, Whited A, Sugimoto D, Bae DS, et al. Functional elbow range of motion in children and adolescents. J Pediatr Orthop. 2020;40:304–9.
69. Sardelli M, Tashjian RZ, MacWilliams BA. Functional elbow range of motion for contemporary tasks. J Bone Joint Surg Am. 2011;93:471–7.

Controversies in the Treatment of Fingertip Amputations in Adults: Conservative Versus Surgical Reconstruction

19

Elena Bravo and E. Carlos Rodríguez-Merchán

19.1 Introduction

It is the most common amputation injury treated by hand surgeons. It is estimated that approximately 45,000 fingers amputations are performed in the USA per year with an incidence rate of 7.5/100,000 people [1]. This results in some 4.8 million visits to emergency departments each year. The highest rates of fingertip injuries are usually seen in children under 5 years of age and in working-class adults, due to occupational activities.

Multiple treatments are available, but none is the gold standard. However, the goals of treatment of these injuries are clear: minimize pain, optimize healing time, preserve sensation and digit length, prevent painful neuromas, avoid or limit nail deformity, minimize lost time at work, and achieve an acceptable cosmetic appearance. The face and hand are the most looked at part of our body [2].

Fingertip is defined as the part of the digit distal to the insertion of the extensor and flexor tendons at the distal phalanx. Injuries to this area can present in various forms including lacerations, avulsions, and crush injuries and result in post-traumatic fingertip amputation. The severity of soft tissue, bone, artery, and nerve damage will depend on the mechanism and will guide therapeutic decision-making [1].

The fingertip is vital for sensation, as it has a high concentration of sensory receptors, and therefore, the restoration of sensation is the most important goal of treatment. The three main goals of treatment are restoration of sensation, durability of the tip, and ensuring adequate bone support to allow nail growth. Many complications can arise after fingertip amputation, such as delayed wound healing, nail deformities with poor aesthetic results, hypersensitivity, residual pain, cold intolerance, scar retraction, flexion contractures, chronic ulceration, infection, and flap loss.

The treatment algorithm can often be complex, as a wide variety of physicians, including orthopedic surgeons, general surgeons, plastic surgeons, and emergency physicians, may care for these injuries, depending on the location and local culture. Sindhu et al. stated that in the United States, up to 90% of fingertip amputations were treated with techniques without replantation. However, most amputations are replanted in Asian countries due to moral values and the importance of bodily integrity [3]. Tip amputation injuries can be managed with local debridement, complex reconstruction, or simply with irrigation and application of a sterile dressing. The precise management of a fingertip injury in

E. Bravo
Department of Plastic and Reconstructive Surgery, "La Paz" University Hospital-IdiPaz, Madrid, Spain

E. C. Rodríguez-Merchán (✉)
Department of Orthopaedic Surgery, "La Paz" University Hospital-IdiPaz, Madrid, Spain

E. C. Rodríguez-Merchán, A. Moreno-Garcìa (eds.), *Controversies in Orthopedic Surgery of The Upper Limb*, https://doi.org/10.1007/978-3-031-04907-1_19

adults will depend on the extent of the injury itself, and various surgical and nonsurgical techniques can be successfully employed. Psychosocial factors and clinician experience are determinant in selecting the most appropriate option. Psychosocial factors to be considered are occupation, hobbies, cultural norms, socioeconomic status, secondary motive, and clinician bias.

In this chapter we will present the various therapeutic options available for the management of injuries to the fingertips and the data available to support them.

The first step should be a physical examination to assess the sensitivity, mobility, and capillary refill of the injured finger. In addition, anteroposterior, lateral, and oblique radiograph views should be requested to detect dislocations, fractures, or foreign bodies.

19.2 Nonoperative Management

This treatment promotes secondary healing by granulation with occlusive dressing. Nonoperative management achieves a fast recovery and do not normally experience functioning issues with the fingers. Its results may be aesthetically superior to graft or flap reconstruction, without incurring donor site morbidity [4]. For fingertip amputations that have less than 1 square centimeter skin loss and no exposed bone and tendon, nonoperative treatment is recommended because healing by secondary intention is an effective and simple procedure. It remains a preferred treatment and multiple publications support this management.

19.2.1 Occlusive Dressing

In 1977, Fox et al. published a study on the nonsurgical treatment of 18 fingertip pulp amputations in adult patients. After wound cleansing and debridement, the wound was covered with an occlusive dressing. Healing of the amputated fingertip occurred within 4 weeks. The healed fingertips showed excellent sensory perception, a normal range of motion, and an acceptable cosmetic appearance. These satisfactory results were achieved with less than 10 days lost from work [5].

Even exposed bone and tendon promote granulation, which supports healing through secondary intention [6]. Farrell et al. in 1977 published a study of 17 patients (21 amputations), evaluating a nonoperative management for fingertip amputations which allowed spontaneous healing of the defects. Six patients had exposed bone in the lesion. These lesions healed with excellent results in terms of maintenance of maximum finger length, minimal aesthetic, and functional deformity. Rapid return to work was possible in most cases. In addition, morbidity associated with surgery was avoided [7].

In 2014, Krauss and Lalonde stated that conservative wound treatment with dressings and protective splints allowed patients to avoid immobilization and donor site morbidity; furthermore, good results were usually achieved with near-normal sensibility, minimal cold intolerance, and tip durability; early return to work was possible, which reduced overall healthcare costs and burden to society [8].

Champagne et al. support that fingertip amputation with exposed bone take the longest time to heal. Nonetheless, gradual formation of a granulation pad covers the exposed bone and healing is achieved. The wound begins to contract with time and the surrounding skin expands, resulting in a scar that covers the amputated finger. To perform this secondary healing treatment, a digital block is sometimes necessary to relieve acute pain and clean the wound. The bone should not be shortened to minimize the deformity of the nail even if it protrudes slightly above the amputation level. It is not necessary to cover the exposed end of the distal phalanx with soft tissue. Any nonadherent dressing material is adequate, and wound care is simple, with soap-and-water cleansing and dressing changes once or twice a week. Initial tenderness usually diminishes greatly by 7–10 days, and comfort, rather than healing, will indicate when patients will be ready to return to work. Complete healing usually occurs in 4–6 weeks. These authors stated that conservative healing was more likely to result in a sensate, nontender, and cosmetically acceptable fingertip than surgical treatment in many clinical scenarios. They also presented a classification that allowed prognosis and prediction of the need for secondary corrective surgery, Champagne classification [9].

There are multiple classifications to describe fingertip lesions and to guide us in choosing the appropriate therapeutic option. The most commonly used are the Allen [10] and Urbaniak [11] classifications. Other classifications are those of Merle and Dautel [12].

Boudard et al. in 2019 analyzed a series of patients who underwent a distal finger amputation and who were treated with occlusive dressing. They performed a retrospective study of 19 patients. At evaluation, an independent examiner assessed the time required for wound healing, the number of occlusive dressings used, fingertip trophic skin changes, epicritic sensibility using the Weber two-point discrimination (2PD) test, sensitivity based on the monofilament test, complications, the presence of dysesthesia or cold intolerance, and the QuickDASH score. The mean follow-up was 12.6 months. A mean of 3.2 occlusive dressings were used per patient, and the mean healing time was 4.3 weeks. The skin texture, fingertips, and nail bed were good to excellent in 18 cases. The 2PD test was good or normal in 16 cases. Eighteen patients were satisfied or very satisfied with the outcome. The mean QuickDASH score was 5.53. In the literature, the recovery of tactile sensation was good after the use of occlusive dressings (2PD from 2.5 to 4 mm). The mean sensitivity reported in various studies is better than that observed after the use of a skin flap. Although the sample size of this study was small, the functional outcome and appearance were good. Therefore, Boudard et al. preferred to use occlusive dressings in zone 1 and 2 fingertip amputations, and flaps in zones 3 and 4 according to the Merle and Dautel classification to ensure better fingertip viability and sensation [13].

In 2021, Masaki et al. presented the case of a 36-year-old woman suffering from Allen type III fingertip amputation injury with her right middle finger crushed in a thick iron door. The amputated fingertip was not recovered. The attending plastic surgeon initially recommended reconstructive surgery to the patient. However, the patient opted for conservative treatment. Conservative management with moist wound dressings (Plus moist™) was performed, and the wound healed after 12 weeks, with outstanding aesthetic and functional results. Therefore, conservative management with moist wound dressings can be a successful treatment modality for Allen type III fingertip amputation injury [14].

19.2.2 Semiocclusive Dressing and Splint Caps

In 2020, Ng et al. described a method for treating fingertip amputation injuries consisting of a semiocclusive dressing and splint cap and presented their short-term results. They performed a retrospective study of patients with isolated fingertip amputation injuries who were treated with the aforementioned method. The semiocclusive dressing used was UrgoTul. The splint cap was a three-dimensional thermoplastic splint to cover the semiocclusive dressing of the injured finger. Twenty-eight patients (31 fingers) were analyzed. The mean age was 39.9 years. Further, 89.3% were men, 75% were foreign workers, 96.4% were blue-collared workers, 40% had injuries in the dominant hand, and 25.8% had nail bed involvement. The mean duration of follow-up was 66 days and the mean duration of hospital leave was 6.5 weeks. The splint cap was applied for a mean of 18.1 days. Total tissue regrowth time was 27.5 days. Residual nail deformities were 14.8% and return of sensation took 31.5 days. Grip strength was 82.5% of the unaffected hand. The mean ROM at the distal interphalangeal, proximal interphalangeal, and metacarpophalangeal joints was 58.8°, 86.9°, and 81.4°, respectively, and 63.9° and 66.3° at the interphalangeal and metacarpophalangeal joint of the thumb, respectively. In short, fingertip amputation injuries had a potential for regeneration through healing by secondary intention under semiocclusive dressing conditions. The splint cap provided an easy to fashion, cost-efficient, and comfortable addition to semiocclusive dressings for fingertip injuries [15].

In spite of simplicity and good results of nonoperative management, it requires a few basic principles: not to remove bone length to avoid hook nail and to have adherence to dressings to avoid infection. Finally, there will be cases that will be managed surgically because of the type of lesion and patient choice (fear of having an open wound or thinking that surgery achieves better results).

19.3 Surgical Treatment

19.3.1 Primary Closure

This procedure usually entails shortening the protruding bone to close the wound. This management achieves fast return to work (Fig. 19.1). However, the process involves losing part of the skin, digital length, and fingernail deformities. This treatment occasionally causes function

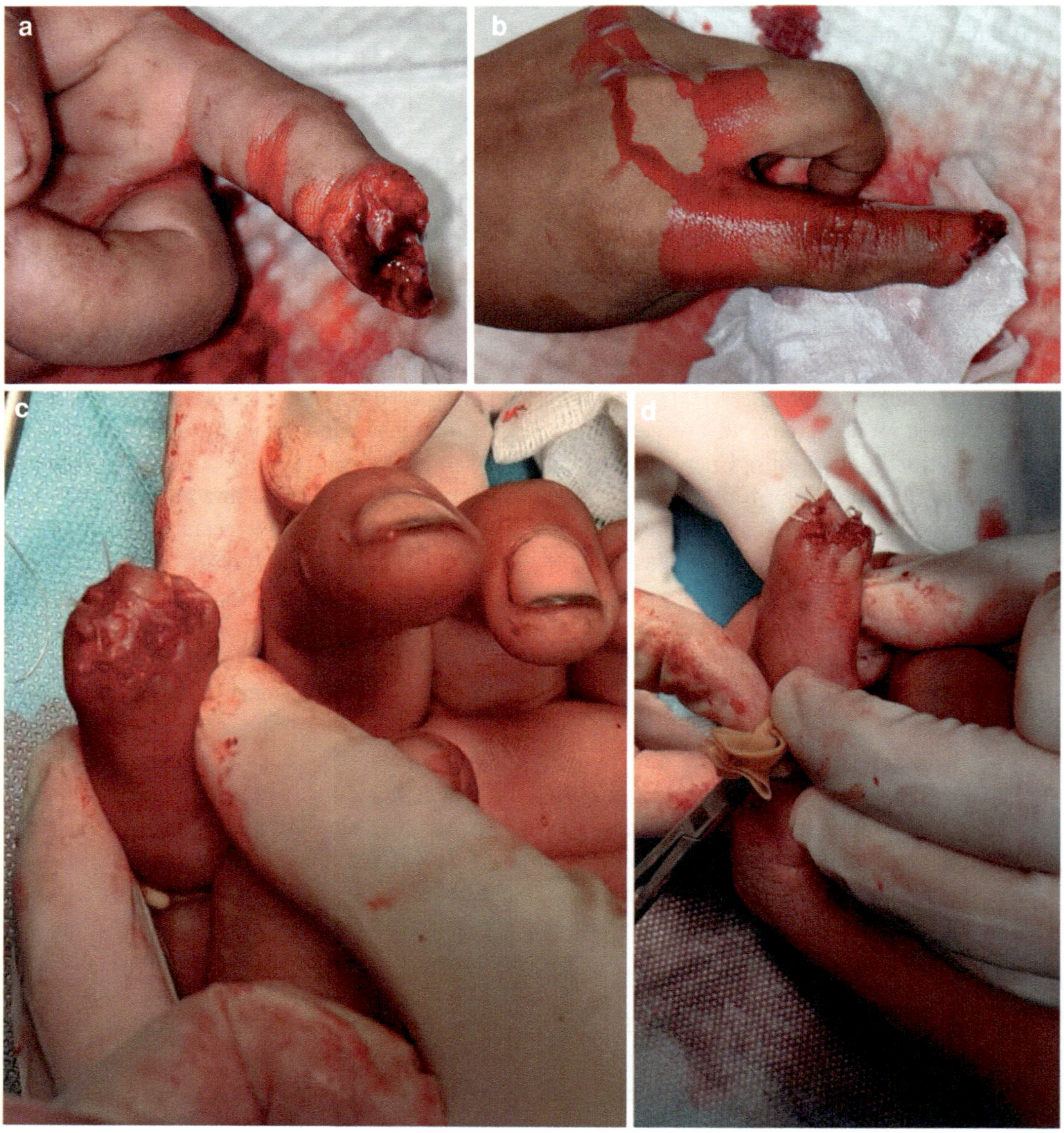

Fig. 19.1 (**a**–**d**) Amputation of the second finger without bony exposure. (**a**) Palmar view after trauma. (**b**) Dorsomedial view after trauma. (**c**) and (**d**) Direct closure

issues related to cold intolerance. Cold intolerance may be caused by the damaged nerves at the time of the injury rather than the treatment procedure [1].

19.3.2 Grafts

19.3.2.1 Composite Grafting

The outcome of composite graft is generally predictable in young children [16] but outcomes were less predictable in adults [17]. In adults, the appearance of contour distortion and nail deformity is common, but if the patient accepts these limitations of the technique, it is a good surgical option without donor site morbidity.

In 2003, Adani et al. stated that the treatment of very distal finger amputations when the amputated portion is saved remains controversial. Both reattachment of the amputated portion as a composite graft and microvascular anastomosis may fail in this distal location. In fact, replantation is often associated with technical difficulties, risk of failure due to poor venous drainage, and high costs. Except for children, amputations at the level of the lunula tend to survive poorly direct replantation. To solve this problem Adani used the replantation model without vascular anastomosis described by Hirase or cooling composite graft. It consists of using ice water and aluminum foil to enhance survival of the composite graft. Cooling the entire recipient site retarded cellular degeneration in the graft until neovascularization occurred [18].

Adani et al. used the Hirase method in seven cases in which a finger amputation had occurred between the tip and the lunula. In four cases, the method was completely satisfactory; however, in two cases, an area of tip necrosis was observed. The Hirase method proved to be a simple and reliable surgical technique for fingertip reattachments [19].

In 2016, Idone et al. published their experience with the Hirase technique considering it a reliable alternative to microsurgery implantation. They analyzed eight patients and reported their clinical results after a 10-month follow-up. The amputated part survived almost completely in six patients; in these cases, the finger amputations were classified according to Allen's classification as level I in two cases, level II in three cases, and level III in one case [10]. Ultimately, Idone et al. considered that reattachment of an amputated finger with the Hirase technique was possible and could provide good distal soft tissue coverage and recovery of sensory and motor functions. Therefore, they stated that reattachment of the amputated portion as a composite graft represented an important alternative to microsurgery [20].

In 2011, Chen et al. stated that composite grafting was often used to treat nonreplantable fingertip amputations and that this technique had a high success rate and good results in the treatment of finger amputations in children, although in adults the success rate was lower. The authors analyzed 27 patients with 31 fingers with traumatic fingertip amputation. All 31 injured fingers had a nonreplantable distal amputated fingertip and underwent composite grafting. The surgical technique was refined by excising the bony segment, defatting, deepithelialization, tie-over suturing, and finger splinting to increase graft survival. The mean age of the patients was 40.5 years. The mean lesion size was 2.4 cm. Twenty-one fingers (67.7%) had been injured by crushing injury and the other 10 fingers (32.3%) by cutting injury. The overall graft survival rate was 93.5% (29 of 31). The average two-point discrimination was 6.3 mm at 6 months postoperatively. The aesthetic outcome assessed by a self-report questionnaire was 93.1% satisfaction, and 86.2% of patients were able to use their injured finger normally in daily work. In short, for Chen et al. a one-stage surgical procedure of easy performance was a reliable method for treating microsurgically nonreplantable fingertip amputations caused by hand trauma. The high success rate, satisfactory aesthetic outcome, and good functional preservation allowed patients to quickly return to their daily lives [17].

In 2016, Lai et al. published their experience using composite grafting with pulp adipofascial advancement flaps for treating nonreplantable fingertip amputations and thus improving fingertip contour. They analyzed 14 patients (16 digits).

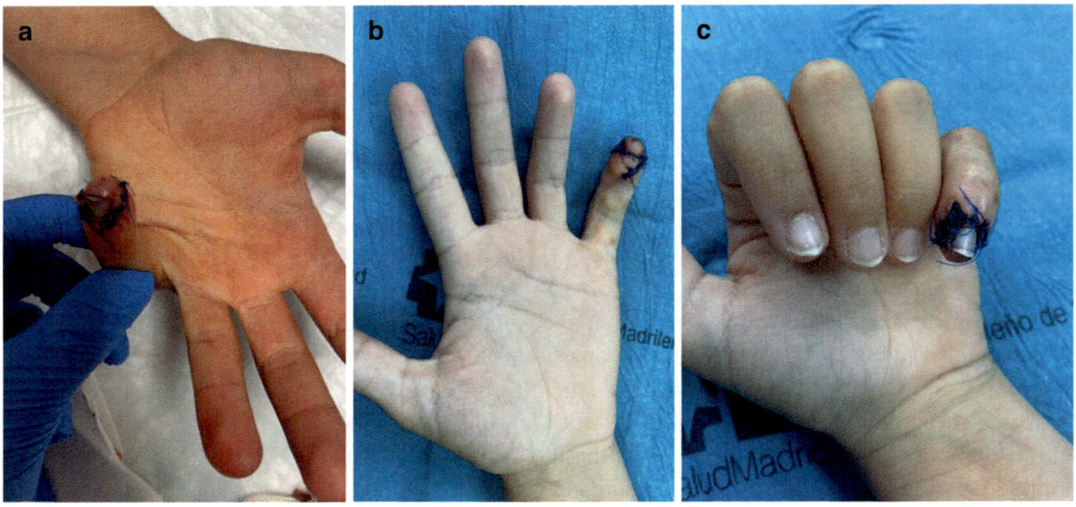

Fig. 19.2 (a–c) Composite pulpal graft: (**a**) Palmar view after surgery; doubtful viability of grafted tissue. (**b**) Palmar view 3 weeks after surgery. Viability of grafted tissue is visualized. (**c**) Dorsal view 3 weeks after surgery

The mean age of the patients was 43.9 years. All patients underwent the procedure under digital block anesthesia. First, a pulp adipofascial advancement flap for better soft tissue coverage of bone exposure stump was performed. The amputated parts were defatted, trimmed, and reattached as composite graft. The age and sex of the patients, injured finger, Hirase classification, mechanism of trauma, overall graft survival area, two-point discrimination (2PD) (mm) at 6 months, finger shortening length, average Disabilities of the Arm, Shoulder, and Hand (DASH) score, and subjective self-evaluation questionnaire score at 6 months were recorded. The mean graft survival was 89%. The mean shortening length was 2.2 mm. The 2PD at 6 months postoperatively was 6.3 mm on average (5–8 mm). The mean DASH (Disabilities of the Arm, Shoulder, and Hand) score at 6 months was 1.45. The self-assessed cosmetic results showed that 12 patients (85.7%) were very satisfied, and no patient was completely dissatisfied. Ultimately, in Hirase's [18] traumatic amputation of finger zone IIA, in which replantation is difficult, the modified technique of composite grafting with pulp adipofascial advancement flap provided an alternative option with a high success rate and acceptable functional and aesthetic results [21].

In 2021, Elzinga et al. stated that after a fingertip amputation, if vessels are present and in adequate condition, microsurgical replantation is the preferred therapeutic technique. Also, composite grafting has a limited role in the treatment of fingertip amputations due to its unreliable nature, but may be an option when the amputated fingertip is not replantable and the patient wishes to restore the length and aesthetics of the fingertip (Fig. 19.2). When composite grafting is selected as the treatment of choice for a particular patient, there are methods to optimize the chances of revascularization and graft survival, such as early grafting, graft cooling, and a moist wound healing environment [22].

19.3.2.2 Skin Grafts

Fingertip skin grafts are rarely used and must be full-thickness skin graft (FTSG). It is well known that a thin graft over bony prominence is the cause of tenderness and sensitivity [23, 24]. FTSG can be reliably and useful for pulp reconstruction [25], but sometimes loss of pulp contour and hypo- or hyperesthesia may appear [26]. The ulnar aspect of the hand has been used as a donor site, but we would avoid it because it is often a surface on which the hand rests during activity [27]. Skin grafts are associated with more tenderness, diminished sensitivity, and cold intolerance than what is seen after secondary healing [9].

19.3.3 Flap Reconstruction

There are a large number of flaps that can be used for fingertip reconstruction. Most fingertip amputations are adequately treated with V-Y advancement flaps and cross-finger flaps. The choice of flap is based on the type and location of injury, surgeon experience, and patient characteristics. Heterodigital flaps are usually avoided to limit the lesion to a single finger, and cross-finger flaps are avoided in older patients because of the risk of joint stiffness. Dissection and mobilization of the neurovascular bundle up to the common digital artery bifurcation with or without adjacent arterial division is routinely performed to facilitate flap advancement of 15–20 mm. Flexion of the IFP joint should be avoided and early mobility facilitated to minimize joint stiffness. Retrograde or reverse-flow flaps offer good coverage and thumb flexion and always check that the palmar arch is well preserved. Local flaps are tedious to perform and are associated with risk of flap failure and iatrogenic sensory loss is common even when experienced hand surgeons perform the surgery [9].

19.3.3.1 Volar V-Y Plasty

V-Y plasty can be used from the volar (Fig. 19.3), unilateral (Fig. 19.4), or bilateral side of the finger. Limited length is the major disadvantage of this technique [28, 29]. In 1985, Tupper et al. stated that V-Y plasty was a well-accepted method for the treatment of transverse fingertip amputations. Some authors had suggested that fingertip sensation was almost normal after the procedure. Tupper et al. analyzed 16 patients with 20 fingertip injuries, who reported a mean sensitivity estimate of 73% of normal. There was decreased sensitivity in two-point discrimination and/or von Frey monofilament testing in all fingertips compared with the digitocontralateral. Eight patients (12 digits) reported hypersensitivity, especially cryalgia. In almost all fingertips treated by V-Y plasty for transverse amputations, the sensitivity was not normal [30].

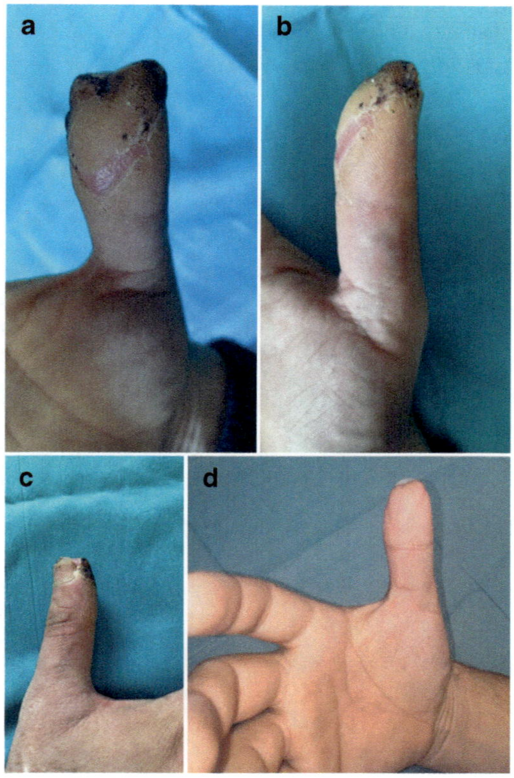

Fig. 19.3 (**a**–**d**) Palmar V-Y flap for first finger: (**a**) Palmar view 3 weeks after trauma. (**b**) Lateral view 3 weeks after trauma. (**c**) Dorso-medial view 3 weeks after trauma (**d**) Result 2 months after surgery

19.3.3.2 Advancement Flap

These are flaps such as V-Y plasty that use tissue close to the amputated area to cover the loss of substance. Their design and shape are variable. Dissection consists of releasing the structures that attach the cutaneous and subcutaneous tissue to the deep structures without injuring the neurovascular bundles of the digit (Fig. 19.5).

19.3.3.3 Cross-Finger Flap and Thenar Flap

These flaps require a two-stage surgery. Between two operations, patients must use a short-arm splint for approximately 3 weeks. The major dis-

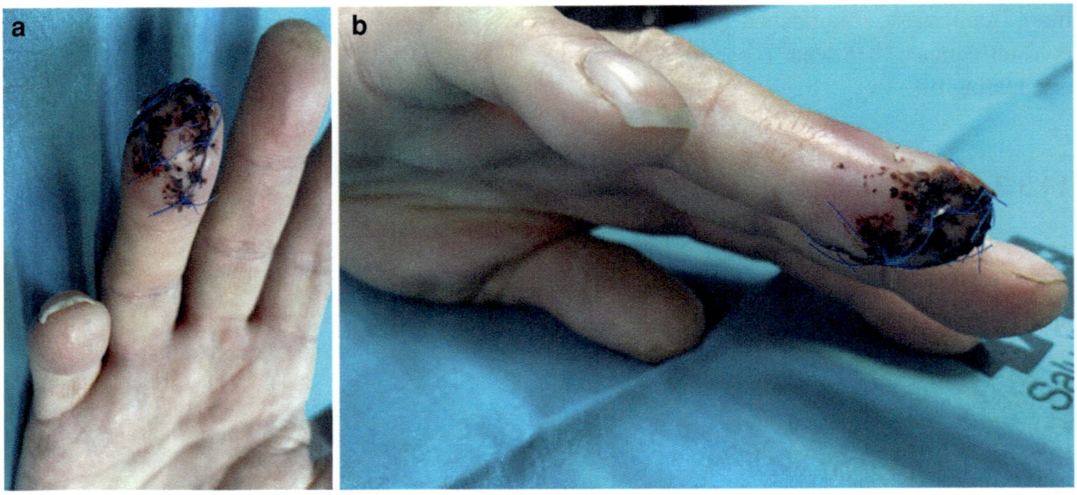

Fig. 19.4 (**a**, **b**) Palmar V-Y flap: (**a**) Palmar view 1 week after trauma. (**b**) Medial view 1 week after trauma

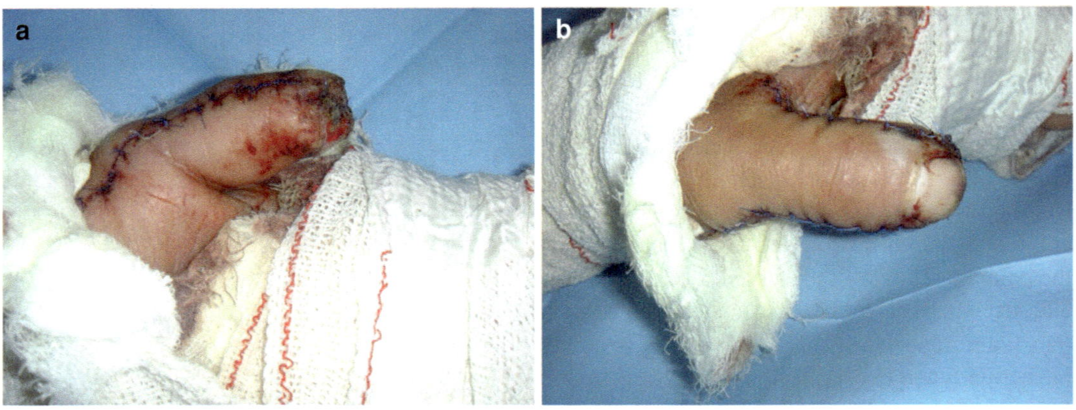

Fig. 19.5 (**a**, **b**) Moberg advancement flap for first finger: (**a**) Palmar view 1 week after trauma. (**b**) Medial view 1 week after trauma

advantage of the splint is joint stiffness [29, 31–33].

In 2016, Rabarin et al. performed a level IV evidence study in which they evaluated the long-term clinical outcomes of the use of cross-finger flap (CFF). It was a retrospective analysis of 28 patients operated on for fingertip amputation: 16 type III, 8 type II, and 4 type IV. The CFF was obtained from an adjacent finger on the dorsal side of the middle phalanx down to the epitenon. A dorsopalmar hinge was retained to ensure vascularization. The CFF was divided a mean of 18.7 days later. The following parameters were assessed: pulp volume (injured compared to contralateral finger), presence of neuroma, occurrence of complications (necrosis, infection, and donor site morbidity), cold discomfort, static and tactile discrimination, and patient satisfaction (from 0 to 10 on the VAS). The mean follow-up was 19.7 years; 22 patients (78.6%) were reexamined in person or contacted by telephone. The mean ratio of healthy to reconstructed pulp was 1.03. No postoperative complications, such as neuromas, were found. Cold sensitivity was present in seven patients. The flap was resensitized in all patients. There was no morbidity at the donor site. The mean patient satisfaction score was 9 (range 8–10). Ultimately, in the long term, the use of CFF resulted in near-normal fingertip metabolism, no complications, and good distal sensitization without pain or neuromas. CFF was found to be a simple, reliable, and durable reconstruction technique [34].

In 2017, Kwon et al. stated that although the thenar flap for single-finger amputation was a common and popular surgical technique, the double thenar flap technique for patients with two-finger amputations had rarely been published in the literature. In their case-control study, they presented the double thenar flap technique and compared the clinical outcomes between single thenar flap and double thenar flap surgical treatments. Over a 10-year period, 92 patients with single-finger amputations were treated with single thenar flap (group I) and 28 patients with two-finger amputations were treated with double thenar flap (group II). All 120 patients were followed up for a minimum of 12 months after surgery. At the last assessment, pain, cold intolerance in the reconstructed finger, functional outcomes according to Chen's criteria [35], and subjective patient satisfaction were evaluated in the two groups. At the last evaluation, all flaps in both groups had survived. No flap failure occurred. There were no significant differences in cold intolerance, donor site pain, fingertip pain, or paresthesia between the two groups. A total of 100 (83.3%) patients were completely or fairly satisfied. There was no significant difference in satisfaction between the two groups. According to Chen's criteria, 102 (85%) patients had excellent or good results. Ultimately, this study demonstrated that the double thenar flap technique used in patients with two-finger amputations produced complete survival with functional outcomes comparable to those of the single thenar flap technique [36].

19.3.3.4 Vascular and Neurovascular Island Flap

Vascular island flaps offer good skin coverage and are usually distant from the amputated area. They require experience in hand surgery for their dissection (Fig. 19.6). Direct-flow neurovascular island flap have better results in terms of sensitivity, providing direct blood flow without sacrificing a major artery. This technique is more favorable than reverse-flow flaps [37, 38] and it is elevated from the area close to the defect.

In 1986, Tsai and Juen analyzed 16 patients who had been treated with a neurovascular island flap for volar-oblique fingertip amputations with at least 2 years of follow-up. The mean active/passive ROM was 54/55 degrees at the DIP joint, 96/98 degrees at the PIP joint, and 83/83 degrees at the MP joint. Twelve of the 16 flaps (75%) had a two-point discrimination less than 10 mm. Moderate and severe problems included cold intolerance (6 patients), hypersensitivity (3 patients), stiffness (3 patients), and numbness (2 patients). Of the 16 patients treated with this technique, 14 were satisfied with the surgical outcome. This technique was safe and reliable for reconstructing volar-oblique fingertip amputations [39].

19.3.3.5 Reverse Homodigital Artery Flap Coverage

In reverse-flow flaps, the blood supply comes from the contralateral digital artery and has higher flow insufficiency rates. It requires dissection and transection of the major digital artery, has higher rate of insufficiency, and is elevated distantly from the defect area [37]. This flap is not indicated when direct-flow flap is possible [38].

In 2006, Alagoz et al. performed homodigital artery flaps to cover the bone and nail bed grafts taken from the amputation to restore fingertip function with acceptable results. They chose this flap because it provides vascularization of the grafts. Alagoz et al. mentioned how important it was to take into account venous insufficiency, as it could increase the likelihood of flap failure. They proposed to preserve a certain amount of soft tissue around the vascular pedicle to overcome venous insufficiency; they further opined that to preserve the length of the finger and the aesthetic appearance of the nail would mean sacrificing the digital artery [40].

In 2018, Sir et al. used reverse homodigital artery flap to cover the naked bone-nail complex and called it reposition flap [41], with good results as with homodigital artery flap.

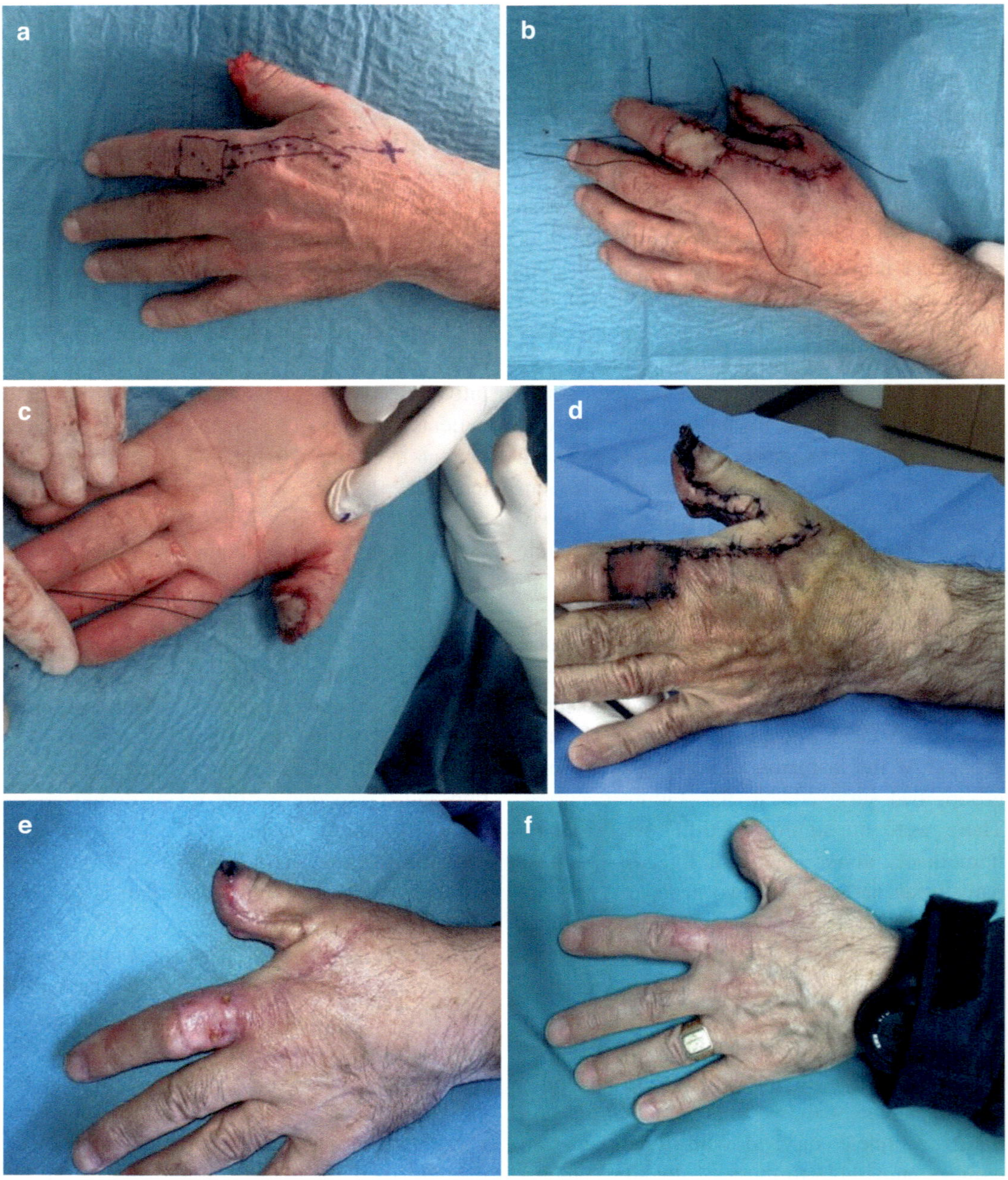

Fig. 19.6 (**a**–**g**) Comet distal pedicled flap for first finger: (**a**) Injury and flap design. (**b**) Immediate postoperative period. Graft in donor site. (**c**) Immediate postoperative period. Flap in the thumb. (**d**) Result 1 week after surgery. (**e**) Result 1 month after surgery. (**f**) and (**g**) Result 4 months after surgery

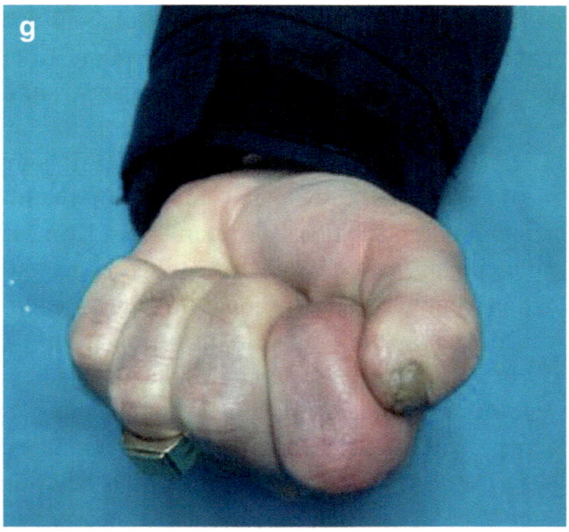

Fig. 19.6 (continued)

19.3.4 Purse-String Suture as a Complementary Technique with Conventional Flaps in Repairing Fingertip Amputation

In 2011, Hassanpour et al. analyzed the use of purse-string suture as a complementary technique accompanying conventional flap repair in fingertip amputation. They studied 54 patients with fingertip amputations on the nail bed who had been referred to their hospital for fingertip reconstruction. Of these, 41 patients with at least one-third of the nail remaining (to preserve the nail) were chosen to undergo the aforementioned technique. Patient satisfaction with the functional results (pain and motion) was as follows: 32 excellent, 8 good, and 1 fair. Likewise, patient satisfaction with regard to the esthetic results obtained was excellent in 7 and good in 2 women ($n = 9$) and excellent in 19, good in 7, and fair in 6 men ($n = 32$). Ninety-three percent of patients (38 patients) had a two-point discrimination of less than 3 mm. No flap necrosis was observed in this study. The flap donor site was covered by primary closure (in 24 cases), secondary intention (in 11 cases), and skin graft (in 6 cases). The nail and finger contours were important to achieve a satisfactory esthetic and functional result. Hassanpour et al. considered that this complementary technique could be an easy way to achieve such a result. It was recommended that this technique was applied to all fingertip injuries to preserve the nail [42].

19.3.5 The Palmar Pocket Method

This technique consists of making a palmar subcutaneous pocket to cover the exposed areas of the fingertip amputation. This flap requires a two-stage surgery as cross-finger or thenar flap.

Brent in 1979 described a reimplantation technique, without vascular anastomosis, using a subcutaneous pocket. Brent chose the contralateral chest wall as a pocket site [43]. However, other clinical reports had used the abdominal wall. Complications, such as stiffness in the wrist, elbow, and shoulder joints and anxiety about pulling out the pocketed finger, were published in both locations.

Arata et al. in 2001 published their results using the Brent technique. To overcome these problems, they chose the ipsilateral palm and named this method the palmar pocket method. They used this technique in 16 cases in which amputation of a finger other than the thumb had occurred between the tip and lunula. In 13 cases, the method was completely successful, and in 3, there was a small area of tip necrosis. According to Arata et al., the palmar pocket method was a simple and reliable operation for fingertip reattachment and more comfortable for patients than pocketing in the chest wall or abdominal wall [44].

In 2012, Jung et al. used the pocket principle to treat 10 patients. All patients were adults and underwent complete fingertip amputation from the tip to the lunula in a digit. In all patients, the amputation was due to a crush or avulsion-type injury, and a microsurgical replantation was not feasible. In these patients we used the palmar pocketing method following a composite graft and prepared the pocket in the subcutaneous layer of the ipsilateral palm. Of the 10 cases, nine had complete replantation survival and one had 20% partial necrosis. In all cases, nail preservation was achieved, resulting in acceptable cosmetic results. In conclusion, a composite graft and palmar pocketing in adult cases of fingertip injury constituted a simple, reliable operation for digital amputation extending from the tip to the lunula. This method had satisfactory results [45].

19.3.6 Fingertip Replantation

Replantation is the primary option for amputation in terms of preserving function of the finger and getting good aesthetic result [46]. It uses the missing part by utilizing its original tissue and minimizes donor site morbidity (Fig. 19.7).

As published in 2021 by Van Handel et al., fingertip replantation is technically challenging, although in motivated patients, excellent aesthetic and functional results can be achieved [47].

This technique can provide excellent results and possibly reduce the risk of cold intolerance and painful neuroma when it is successful [9]. However, after fingertip replantation, cold intolerance was reported in 0%–35% [48, 49]. Hattori et al. compared 23 patients who had undergone fingertip replantation and 23 patients with fingertip revision amputation and found no statistically significant difference ($P > 0.05$) between the two groups in cold intolerance: 35% for replantation and 40% in revision amputation [48].

It is important to note that cold intolerance is assumed to be the result of vascular insufficiency and peripheral nerve injury rather than as a result of treatment [50, 51].

The publication's results can aid surgeons and patients to choose the best surgery option. After finger revision amputation, sensation can be similar or better than following fingertip replantation. Cold intolerance as well as DIP and PIP joint motion is similar to outcomes reported in the literature for replantation. The return to work time is shorter than what is reported after fingertip replantation. Future studies should evaluate health-related quality of life of both treatments [52].

In 2019, Yoon et al. concluded that with patient selection, replantation of all finger amputation patterns, whether single-finger or multifinger injuries, may be cost-effective compared with revision amputation. Multifinger replantations had a higher probability of being cost-effective than single-finger replantation. Cost-effectiveness may depend on injury pattern and patient factors [53].

Careful preoperative patient and lesion selection is essential to develop an appropriate treatment plan that takes into account the following factors [54]: (1) patient factors (medical comorbidity, age, physical and occupational demands, social factors, cultural and personal values, and psychiatric disease), (2) injury factors (level of injury, digits involved, mechanism, injury to adjacent fingers, and incomplete or complete amputation), and (3) Circumstantial factors (time to presentation and availability of post-replantation care).

Early indications for replantation are injuries threatening a catastrophic functional deficit (hands, thumbs, multiple digits, pediatric) [54–57]. Contraindications to fingertip replantation are consistent with those for amputation at any level and include severely crushed or mangled parts, multilevel injury to the same digit, comorbid or otherwise injured patients, severe atherosclerotic disease, and mental illness. A prolonged warm ischemia time is also a traditional contraindication to replantation, but the absence of ischemia-sensitive muscle at the fingertip level makes these amputations less time-sensitive. The traditional limit of warm ischemia for a digit replantation is 6–12 h [58], but even in excess of 12 h, success rates of more than 90% have been reported [59].

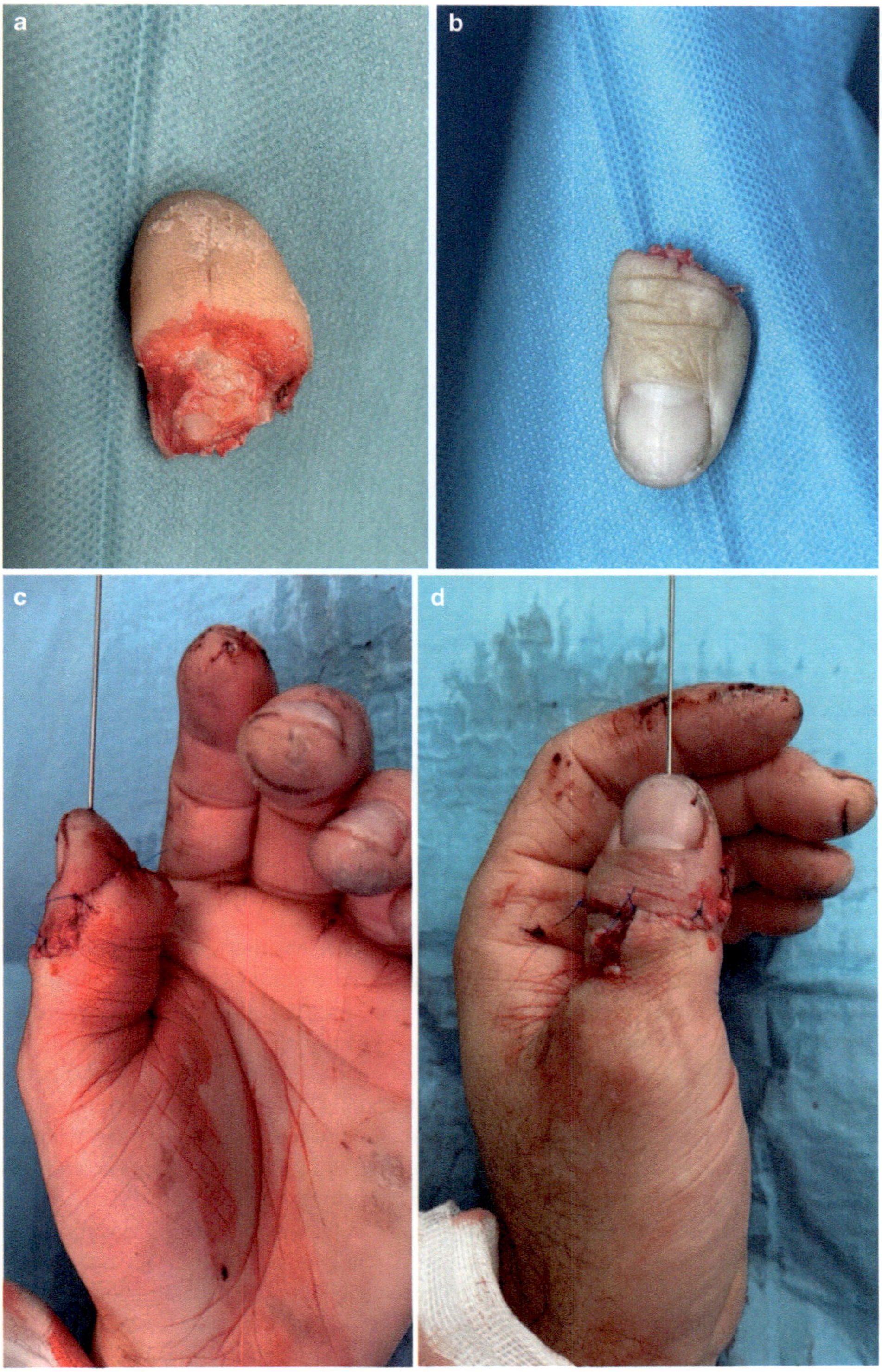

Fig. 19.7 (**a**, **f**) Reimplantation of the thumb: (**a**) Palmar view of the amputated fragment. (**b**) Dorsal view of the amputated fragment. (**c**) Radio-palmar view of the immediate postoperative result. (**d**) Dorsal view of the immediate postoperative result. (**e**) Palmar view 5 weeks after surgery. (**f**) Dorsal view 5 weeks after surgery

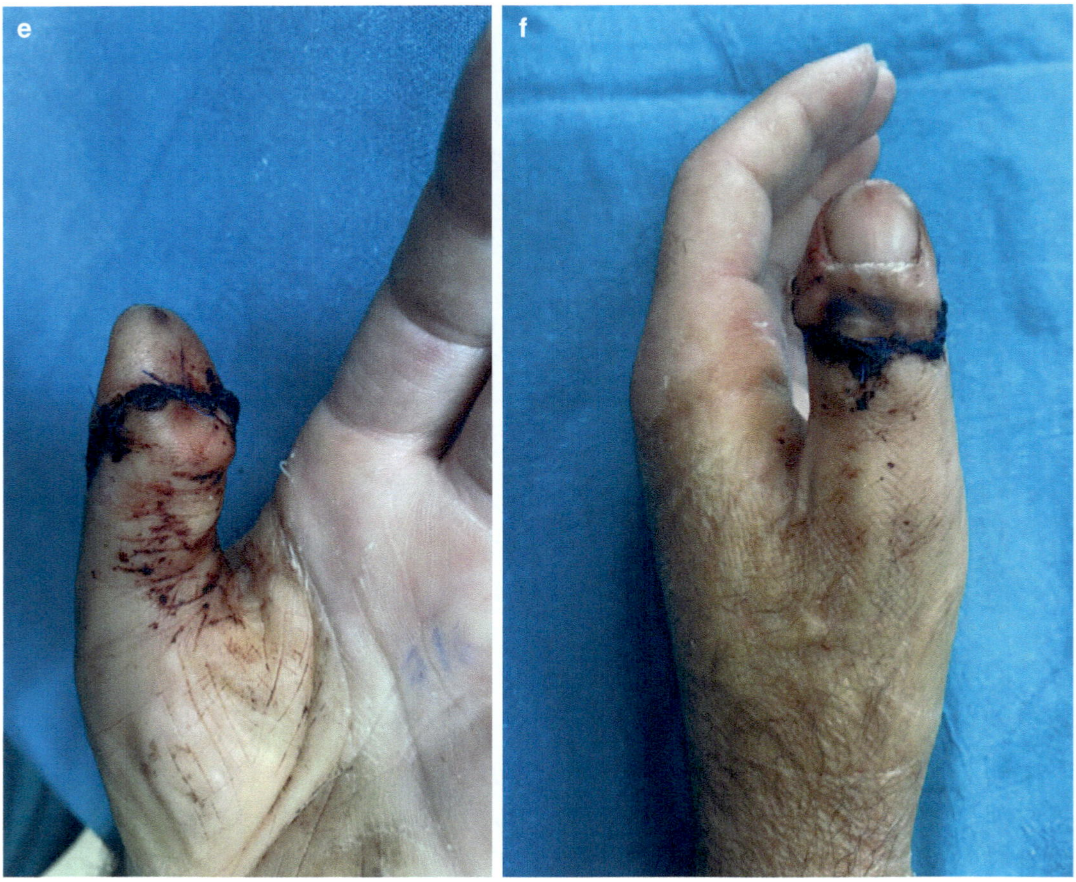

Fig. 19.7 (continued)

19.4 Do We Need to Repair the Nerves When Replanting Distal Finger Amputations?

In 2010, Wong et al. stated that distal replantation was an excellent model to study the results of nerve repair. In their study they attempted to demonstrate the differences in aesthetic, sensory, and functional outcomes in fingertip replantation, with and without nerve repair. They analyzed 28 fingers in 28 patients who underwent successful distal replantation over a 5-year period. Nerve repair was performed in half of the fingers. The mean follow-up was 39 months. Symptoms of pain, numbness, cold intolerance, scar hypersensitivity, pulp atrophy, and weakness were reported. Nail width, pulp length, two-point discrimination, Semmes-Weinstein test, and power were evaluated. No significant association was found between nerve repair and symptoms. No significant differences were found between groups, with and without nerve repair. All fingers showed a mean two-point discrimination of 5.6 mm, and Semmes-Weinstein test results were green in 3 fingers and blue in 17. There was no significant difference in the overall results when repairing or not repairing the nerve in distal finger replantation. Both groups had satisfactory results. Possibly spontaneous neurotization took place and nerve repair was not necessary [60].

19.5 Digit Tip Regeneration

This is a very promising field under study. The distal tip of the human is capable of endogenous regeneration after amputation and the identification of critical components of this response has led to treatments that expand the regenerative capabilities of nonregenerative amputation wounds. It is necessary to know the regeneration component cells and morphogenetic agents which are present at traumatic injury wound sites to stimulates a multi-tissue response that culminates in structural regeneration. Currently, regenerative failure is caused by a toxic wound environment that minimally lacks the signaling profile of a morphogenetic agent necessary to coordinate a multi-tissue regenerative response [61].

19.6 Conclusions

Injuries to the fingertips cause some 4.8 million visits to emergency departments in the USA each year. Multiple treatments are available (surgical and nonsurgical), but none is currently the gold standard. However, the goals of treating these injuries are clear: minimize pain, optimize healing time, preserve sensation and digit length, prevent painful neuromas, avoid or limit nail deformity, minimize lost time at work, and achieve an acceptable cosmetic appearance. Nonsurgical treatments include occlusive dressings and splint caps. Surgical techniques include the following: volar V-Y plasty, neurovascular island flap for volar oblique fingertip amputations, reconstruction of fingertip amputations with full-thickness perionychial grafts from the retained part and local flaps, cooling composite graft (Hirase technique), reverse homodigital artery flap coverage for bone and nail bed grafts, purse-string suture as a complementary technique with conventional flaps in repairing fingertip amputation, composite grafting, cross-finger flap, thenar flap, the palmar pocket method, reconstruction of incomplete distal thumb amputations, graft reposition on flap in Allen type IV amputation, and fingertip replantation.

Currently with the development of microsurgery, if the amputated part is in good condition, replantation is the favored intervention. If replantation is not performed, multiple chirurgical/non-surgical options are available depending on the type of injury, patient characteristics, and surgeon preferences. The development of regenerative medicine would offer an ideal solution that is still in its very early stages.

References

1. Kawaiah A, Thakur M, Garg S, Kawasmi SH, Hassan A. Fingertip injuries and amputations: a review of the literature. Cureus. 2020;12(5):e8291.
2. Peterson SL, Peterson EL, Wheatley MJ. Management of fingertip amputations. J Hand Surg Am. 2014;39:2093–101.
3. Sindhu K, DeFroda SF, Harris AP, Gil JA. Management of partial fingertip amputation in adults: operative and non operative treatment. Injury. 2017;48:2643–9.
4. Lee LP. A simple end efficient treatment for fingertip injuries. J Hand Surg Br. 1995;20:63–71.
5. Fox JW 4th, Golden GT, Rodeheaver G, Edgerton MT, Edlich RF. Nonoperative management of fingertip pulp amputation by occlusive dressings. Am J Surg. 1977;133:255–6.
6. Simman R, Hermans MHE. Managing wounds with exposed bone and tendon with an esterified hyaluronic acid matrix (eHAM): a literature review and personal experience. J Am Coll Clin Wound Spec. 2018;9:1–9.
7. Farrell RG, Disher WA, Nesland RS, Palmatier TH, Truhler TD. Conservative management of fingertip amputations. JACEP. 1977;6:243–6.
8. Krauss EM, Lalonde DH. Secondary healing of fingertip amputations: a review. Hand (N Y). 2014;9:282–8.
9. Champagne L, Hustedt JW, Walker R, Wiebelhaus J, Nystrom NA. Digital tip amputations from the perspective of the nail. Adv Orthop. 2016;2016:1967192.
10. Allen MJ. Conservative management of finger tip injuries in adults. Hand. 1980;12:257–65.
11. Lefèvre Y, Mallet C, Ilharreborde B, Jehanno P, Frajmann JM, Penneçot GF, et al. Digital avulsion with compromised vascularization: study of 23 cases in children. J Pediatr Orthop. 2011;31:259–65.
12. Merle M, Dautel G. Amputations d'attente et amputations definitives. In: La main traumatique. Tome 1. Paris: Masson; 1997. pp. 251–253.
13. Boudard J, Loisel F, El Rifaï S, Feuvrier D, Obert L, Pluvy I. Fingertip amputations treated with occlusive dressings. Hand Surg Rehabil. 2019;38:257–61.

14. Masaki S, Kawamoto T. Fingertip amputation injury of Allen type III managed conservatively with moist wound dressings. Am J Case Rep. 2021;22:e928950.
15. Ng HJH, Sim J, Tey VHT, Selvaganesh S, Rebosura CKP, Rajaratnam V. Experience with the use of splint caps for the management of fingertip amputation injuries. J Hand Surg Asian Pac. 2020;25:199–205.
16. Butler DP, Murugesan L, Ruston J, Woollard AC, Jemcc B. The outcomes of digital tip amputation replacement as a composite graft in a paediatric population. J Hand Surg Eur. 2016;41:164–70.
17. Chen SY, Wang CH, Fu JP, Chang SC, Chen SG. Composite grafting for traumatic fingertip amputation in adults: technique reinforcement and experience in 31 digits. J Trauma. 2011;70:148–53.
18. Hirasé Y. Postoperative cooling enhances composite graft survival in nasal-alar and fingertip reconstruction. Br J Plast Surg. 1993;46:707–11.
19. Adani R, Marcoccio I, Tarallo L. Treatment of fingertips amputation using the Hirase technique. Hand Surg. 2003;8:257–64.
20. Idone F, Sisti A, Tassinari J, Nisi G. Cooling composite graft for distal finger amputation: a reliable alternative to microsurgery implantation. In Vivo. 2016;30:501–5.
21. Lai HT, Wu SH, Lai YW, Hsieh TY, Lee SS, David Wang HM, et al. Composite grafting with pulp adipofascial advancement flaps for treating non-replantable fingertip amputations. Microsurgery. 2016;36:651–7.
22. Elzinga K, Chung KC. Non-microsurgical composite grafting for acute management of fingertip amputation. Hand Clin. 2021;37:43–51.
23. Shepard GH. Treatment of nail bed avulsions with split-thickness nail bed grafts. J Hand Surg Am. 1983;8:49–54.
24. Young FC, Teoch LC. Nail bed reconstruction with split-thickness nail bed grafts. J Hand Surg Br. 1992;1:193–7.
25. Lee JH, Burn JS, Kang SY, Yang WY. Full-thickness skin grafting with de-epithelization of the wound margin for finger defects with bone or tendon exposure. Arch Plast Surg. 2015;42:334–40.
26. Yeo C, Sebastin SJ, Chong AKS. Fingertip injuries. Singap Med J. 2010;51:78–86.
27. Martin-Playa P, Foo A. Approach to fingertip injuries. Clin Plastic Surg. 2019;46:275–83.
28. Atasoy E, Ioakimidis E, Kasdan ML, Kutz JE, Kleinert HE. Reconstruction of the amputated finger tip with atriangular volar flap. A new surgical procedure. J Bone Joint Surg Am. 1970;52:921–6.
29. Evans DM, Martin DL. Step- advancement island flap for finger-tip reconstruction. Br J Plast Surg. 1988;41:105–11.
30. Tupper J, Miller G. Sensitivity following volar V-Y plasty for fingertip amputations. J Hand Surg Br. 1985;10:183–4.
31. Tempest MN. Cross-finger flaps in the treatment of injuries to the finger tip. Plast Reconstr Surg. 1946;1952(9):205–22.
32. Miller AJ. Single finger tip injuries treated by thenar flap. Hand. 1974;6:311–4.
33. Melone CP, Beasley RW, Carstens JH Jr. The thenar flap. An analysis of its use in 150 cases. J Hand Surg Am. 1982;7(291):297.
34. Rabarin F, Saint Cast Y, Jeudy J, Fouque PA, Cesari B, Bigorre N, et al. Cross-finger flap for reconstruction of fingertip amputations: Long-term results. Orthop Traumatol Surg Res. 2016;102(4 Suppl):S225–8.
35. Chen YC, Chan FC, Hsu CC, Lin YT, Chen CT, Lin CH. Fingertip replantation without venous anastomosis. Ann Plast Surg. 2013;70:284–8.
36. Kwon YJ, Ahn BM, Lee JS, Park YG, Ryu HJ, Ha YC. Reconstruction of two fingertip amputations using a double thenar flap and comparison of outcomes of surgery using a single thenar flap. Injury. 2017;48:481–5.
37. Kayalar M, Bal E, Toros T, Sügün ST, Ozaksar K, Gürbüz Y. The outcome of direct-flow neurovascular island flaps in pulp defects. Acta Orthop Traumatol Turc. 2011;45:175–84.
38. Kayalar M, Bal E, Toros T, Ozaksar K, Sügün ST, Ademoglu Y. The results of reverse-flow island flap in pulp reconstruction. Acta Orthop Traumatol Turc. 2011;45:304–11.
39. Tsai TM, Yuen JC. A neurovascular island flap for volar oblique fingertip amputations. Analysis of long-term results. J Hand Surg Br. 1996;21:94–8.
40. Alagoz MS, Uysal CA, Kerem M, Sensoz O. Reverse homodigital artery flap coverage for bone and nail bed grafts in fingertip amputations. Ann Plast Surg. 2006;56:279–83.
41. Sir E, Aksoy A, Aksoy MK. Comparisons between long-term outcomes of the reposition flaps and replantations in finger amputations. Ulus Trauma Acil Cerrahi Derg. 2018;24:462–7.
42. Hassanpour SE, Hosseini SN, Abdolzadeh M. Purse-string suture as a complementary technique with conventional flaps in repairing fingertip amputation. Tech Hand Up Extrem Surg. 2011;15:94–8.
43. Brent B. Replantation of amputated distal phalangeal parts of fingers without vascular anastomoses, using subcutaneous pockets. Plast Reconstr Surg. 1979;63:1–8.
44. Arata J, Ishikawa K, Soeda H, Sawabe K, Kokoroishi R, Togo T. The palmar pocket method: an adjunct to the management of zone I and II fingertip amputations. J Hand Surg Am. 2001;26:945–50.
45. Jung MS, Lim YK, Hong YT, Kim HN. Treatment of fingertip amputation in adults by palmar pocketing of the amputated part. Arch Plast Surg. 2012;39:404–10.
46. Mitsunaga N, Mihara M, Koshima I, Gonda K, Takuya I, Kato H, et al. Digital artery perforator (DAP) flaps: modifications for fingertip and finger stump reconstruction. J Plast Reconstr Aesthet Surg. 2010;63:1312–7.
47. Van Handel AC, Pet MA. Fingertip replantation: technique details and review of the evidence. Hand Clin. 2021;37:53–65.

48. HattoriY DK, Ikeda K, Estrella EP. A retrospective study of functional outcomes after successful replantation versus amputation closure for single fingertip amputations. J Hand Surg Am. 2006;31:811–8.
49. Ozcelik IB, Purisa H, Mersa B, Sezer I, Erturer E, Ergun O. Late results of replantations in tip amputation of the thumb. Acta Orthop Traumatol Turc. 2008;42:252–7.
50. Gelberman RH, Urbaniak JR, Bright DS, Levin LS. Digital sensibility following replantation. J Hand Surg. 1978;3:313–9.
51. Irwin MS, Gilbert SE, Terenghi G, Smith RW, Green CJ. Cold intolerance following peripheral nerve injury. Natural history and factors predicting severity of symptoms. J Hand Surg Br. 1997;22:308–16.
52. Wang K, Sears ED, Shauver MJ, Chung KC. A systematic review of outcomes of revision amputation treatment for fingertip amputations. Hand. 2013;8:139–45.
53. Yoon AP, Mahajani T, Hutton DW, Chung KC. Cost-effectiveness of finger replantation compared with revision amputation. JAMA Netw Open. 2019;2(12):e1916509. 1/14.
54. Pet MA, Ko JH. Indications for replantation and revascularization in the hand. Hand Clin. 2019;35:119–30.
55. Frykman GK, Wood VE. Saving amputated digits. Current status of replantation of fingers and hands. West J Med. 1974;121:265–9.
56. Manktelow RT. What are the indications for digital replantation? Ann Plast Surg. 1978;1:336–7.
57. O'Brien BM, MacLeod AM, Miller GD, Newing RK, Hayhurst JW, Morrison WA. Clinical replantation of digits. Plast Reconstr Surg. 1973;52:490–502.
58. Lin CH, Aydyn N, Lin YT, Hsu CT, Lin CH, Yeh JT. Hand and finger replantation after protracted ischemia (more than 24 hours). Ann Plast Surg. 2010;64:286–90.
59. Waikakul S, Sakkarnkosol S, Vanadurongwan V, Un-nanuntana A. Results of 1018 digital replantations in 552 patients. Injury. 2000;31:33–40.
60. Wong C, Ho PC, Tse WL, Cheng S, Chan DK, Hung LK. Do we need to repair the nerves when replanting distal finger amputations? J Reconstr Microsurg. 2010;26:347–54.
61. Dolan CP, Dawson LA, Muneoka K. Digit tip regeneration biology with regenerative medicine. Stem Cells Translational Med. 2018;7:262–70.

Metacarpophalangeal (MCP) and Proximal Interphalangeal (PIP) Joint Arthroplasty

20

Elena Bravo and E. Carlos Rodríguez-Merchán

20.1 Introduction

Arthritis (degenerative or inflammatory) of the small joints of the hand is a common problem. Nonsurgical treatment includes splinting, oral analgesics, and in some situations local injections. Pain is the main indication for arthroplasty and arthrodesis of small joints of the hand. Other indications are joint deformity, stiffness, and incongruity seen in degenerative and inflammatory arthritis.

Surgical treatment of arthritis of the metacarpophalangeal (MCP) and finger proximal interphalangeal (PIP) joints should be well indicated. Existing surgical options are debridement of painful osteophytes, arthroplasty, and arthrodesis. For an implant to function well, bone and soft tissue stability is essential. Therefore, the treatment of each patient will depend on the soft tissue envelope and the amount of joint destruction. In most cases arthrodesis is a better alternative to arthroplasty [1].

Silicone implant arthroplasty has been the most widely accepted and widely performed technique for the treatment of small joint deformities of the hand in patients with rheumatoid arthritis (RA). The implant is placed as a joint spacer without bony fixation to provide adequate stability and alignment until scar tissue forms. Several studies have confirmed the benefits of silicone MCP arthroplasty, including pain relief and improved functional and cosmetic appearance of the hand [2–7]. However, fractures of silicone implants are very common. This is because the implant is subjected to high stress concentrations during active flexion [8–10]. The published survival of silicone implants, considering implant fracture as the end point, is 58% at 10 years and 34% at 17 years. Although at 17 years two-thirds of the implants are ruptured on radiographs, the published survival rate considering revision surgery as the end point is 63% at 17 years [11]. The aforementioned disparity indicates that high silicone implant fracture rates are not necessarily associated with clinical failure rates. There are several silicone implants on the market. One-piece silicone implants (Swanson finger joint implants, Wright Medical Group NV, Memphis, TN, USA) have been used since the 1960s [12]. The volar hinge silicone implant (Small Bone Innovations, Inc., Avanta Orthopaedics, LLC, Morrisville, PA, USA) was introduced in 1987 [13]. Its center of flexion is palmar with respect to the longitudinal axis, unlike the Swanson type, in which the center of flexion is slightly dorsal with respect to the longitudinal axis. It has been published that the range of motion (ROM) after surgery and implant fracture rates vary depending on the type of implant used [13–17]. Several

E. Bravo
Department of Plastic and Reconstructive Surgery, "La Paz" University Hospital-IdiPaz, Madrid, Spain

E. C. Rodríguez-Merchán (✉)
Department of Orthopaedic Surgery, "La Paz" University Hospital-IdiPaz, Madrid, Spain

E. C. Rodríguez-Merchán, A. Moreno-Garcìa (eds.), *Controversies in Orthopedic Surgery of The Upper Limb*, https://doi.org/10.1007/978-3-031-04907-1_20

authors have reported that the volar hinge silicone implant is associated with better ROM than the one-piece silicone implant; however, reported fracture rates have been higher with the volar hinge silicone implant [9, 18].

Implant fracture has not been directly related to reoperation. Furthermore, it has been observed that the rate of reoperation is much lower than the rate of radiographic implant fracture [11]. However, patients with active hand use may have increased pain and deformity shortly after surgery due to implant fracture, a complication that will require a revision procedure [19]. Although prevention of early implant fracture is important to attain a satisfactory outcome and to avoid an early revision procedure, few publications have analyzed the risk factors for implant fracture [11, 18].

This chapter discusses the current controversies concerning the previously mentioned arthroplasties. Finally, it should be remembered that in most cases arthrodesis is a better alternative than arthroplasty.

20.2 Metacarpophalangeal (MCP) Joint Arthroplasty

Degeneration of the MCP joint is more often the result of rheumatoid arthritis (RA) than of OA. For this reason, MCP arthrodesis is poorly tolerated, and implant arthroplasty is the preferred surgical option [20].

20.2.1 Primary MCP Joint Arthroplasty

The most common implants used are the pyrocarbon and silicone implants, with the metal-plastic SRA a distant third [20].

20.2.1.1 Unconstrained MCP Joint Arthroplasties

Pyrocarbon MCP Joint Arthroplasty in Noninflammatory Arthritis

Due to its unconstrained design, its use is a valid option in OA. However, concerns have been raised in RA patients. Pyrocarbon implants have been associated with excellent pain relief, improved hand appearance, increased postoperative motion, and high patient satisfaction [21, 22].

In 2015, Dickson et al. published the results, complications, and survival of pyrocarbon MCP joint arthroplasty in noninflammatory arthropathy with a minimum follow-up of 5 years (level IV evidence study). They retrospectively analyzed 51 implants in 36 patients. Patient demographics, complications, subsequent surgeries, and implant revision were recorded. Objective outcomes were assessed by grip strength, ROM, and radiological assessment of alignment, loosening, and subsidence. Subjective outcomes were assessed by Patient Evaluation Measure, Quick Disabilities of the Arm, Shoulder and Hand, and Visual Analog Scale scores (0, best; 10, worst) for appearance, satisfaction, and pain. There were 35 index fingers and 16 middle fingers. The mean follow-up was 103 months. The mean ROM was 54°. There was no difference in grip strength between the operated and unoperated side. Six implants were revised, of which three required additional surgery. The average Patient Evaluation Measure and Quick Disabilities of the Arm, Shoulder and Hand scores were 27 and 29, respectively. The mean Visual Analog Scale (VAS) score for pain, satisfaction, and appearance were all 1, with ranges of 0–7, 0–4, and 0–6, respectively. The majority of the implants were Herren grade 1 lucency, while the remaining 5 proximal and 12 distal implants were grade 2. The mean subsidence was 2 mm in the proximal component and 1 mm in the distal component. The degree of loosening or subsidence did not correlate with the outcome. Implant survival evaluated by Kaplan-Meier analysis was 88% at 10 years. Ultimately, good pain relief, functional ROM, and high satisfaction were observed in most patients. All implant revisions were performed within 18 months of the initial procedure [21].

In 2017, Aujla et al. performed a systematic literature review on the outcomes of unconstrained MCP joint arthroplasty. They observed that pyrocarbon implants reduced pain by 85%, increased pinch grip by 144%, and improved ROM by 13° in both osteoarthritis (OA) and inflammatory arthritis (IA). Patients implanted with metal on polyethylene (MoP) arthroplasties showed a decrease in pinch strength. Satisfaction rates were 91% and 92% for the OA and IA groups, respectively. There were 9 failures in 87 joints (10.3%) during a mean follow-up of 5.5 years in the pyro-OA group. There were 18 failures in 149 joints (12.1%) during a mean period of 6.6 years in the pyro-IA group. Due to the heterogeneity of the studies and the limited presentation of the data, a meta-analysis was not possible [23].

Pyrocarbon arthroplasty of the MCP joint leads to better improvements in total arc motion as compared to arthroplasty of the PIP joint [24, 25], although complication rates after pyrocarbon arthroplasty tend to be greater than those after silicone arthroplasty [26, 27]. Drake and Segalman proposed that there is a well-defined patient who may benefit from this arthroplasty: young people with posttraumatic arthritis, no angular deformities, and adequate soft tissue coverage [28]. Srnec et al. considered pyrocarbon arthroplasty as the treatment of choice for OA MCP joint [20]. Generally speaking, this procedure should be avoided in RA for progressive destruction of capsuloligamentous support.

20.2.1.2 Silicone MCP Arthroplasty

Alfred B. Swanson first introduced the concept of a silicone rubber spacer for joint replacement in 1962 [29]. To this day, the Swanson finger joint silicone arthroplasty implant is the most widely used small joint arthroplasty [30].

The hinged MCP joint silicone implant is designed to maintain a joint space and alignment while relying on the formation of a capsule around the arthroplasty and proper tendon and ligament balance to maintain stability. Although silicone is generally well tolerated in the body, microscopic debris may cause pain and destruction secondary to local inflammatory response (Figs. 20.1 and 20.2).

In 2012, Chung et al. analyzed patients with rheumatoid arthritis (RA) treated with silicone MCP joint arthroplasty (SMPA). In a prospective multicenter study, 162 patients with severe subluxation and/or ulnar deviation of MCP joints were analyzed [31]. The long-term results of a group operated with SMPA ($N = 67$) were compared with those of a group of nonoperated patients ($N = 95$). Patients could choose whether to undergo SMPA or not. Results were assessed using the Michigan Hand Outcomes Questionnaire (MHQ), Arthritis Impact Measurement Scales 2 (AIMS2), grip/pinch strength, Jebsen-Taylor test, ulnar deviation, extensor lag, and ROM measurements at the MCP joints. There were no significant differences in mean age, race, education, and income at baseline between the two groups. Surgical patients had worse MHQ function and functional measurements at baseline. At 3 years, the mean MHQ global score and MHQ function, activities of daily living, aesthetics, and satisfaction scores were significantly better in the surgical group than in the nonsurgical group. Ulnar deviation, extensor lag, and arc of motion in the MCP and proximal interphalangeal (PIP) joints also improved significantly in the surgical group. No improvement in mean AIMS2 scores or grip/pinch strength was observed. Complications were minimal, and there was a fracture rate of 9.5%. Ultimately, compared with nonsurgical controls, AR patients had long-term improvement in hand function and appearance after SMPA treatment [31].

In a randomized controlled trial on silicone MCP joint arthroplasty, Chung et al. in 2015 demonstrated excellent patient satisfaction and better outcomes for the surgically treated group of RA patients with severe hand deformities [6].

Patients suffering from nonrheumatic arthritis also experience pain relief, increased ROM, and satisfaction with silicone arthroplasty [32].

Compared to PIP arthroplasties, MCP joint silicone ones show greater improvement in total range of motion [5]. Neral et al. reported a statistically significant 15° improvement in total arc of motion after MCP joint arthroplasty [32]. However, Hansraj et al. found a decrease in ROM after surgery [33] and Olsen et al. observed variable pain relief and satisfaction [34].

In 2013, Chetta et al. stated that RA patients with swan neck deformities have greater MCP joint ROM because of their need to flex the joint to make a fist, whereas the boutonniere deformity places the fingers into the flexed position, creat-

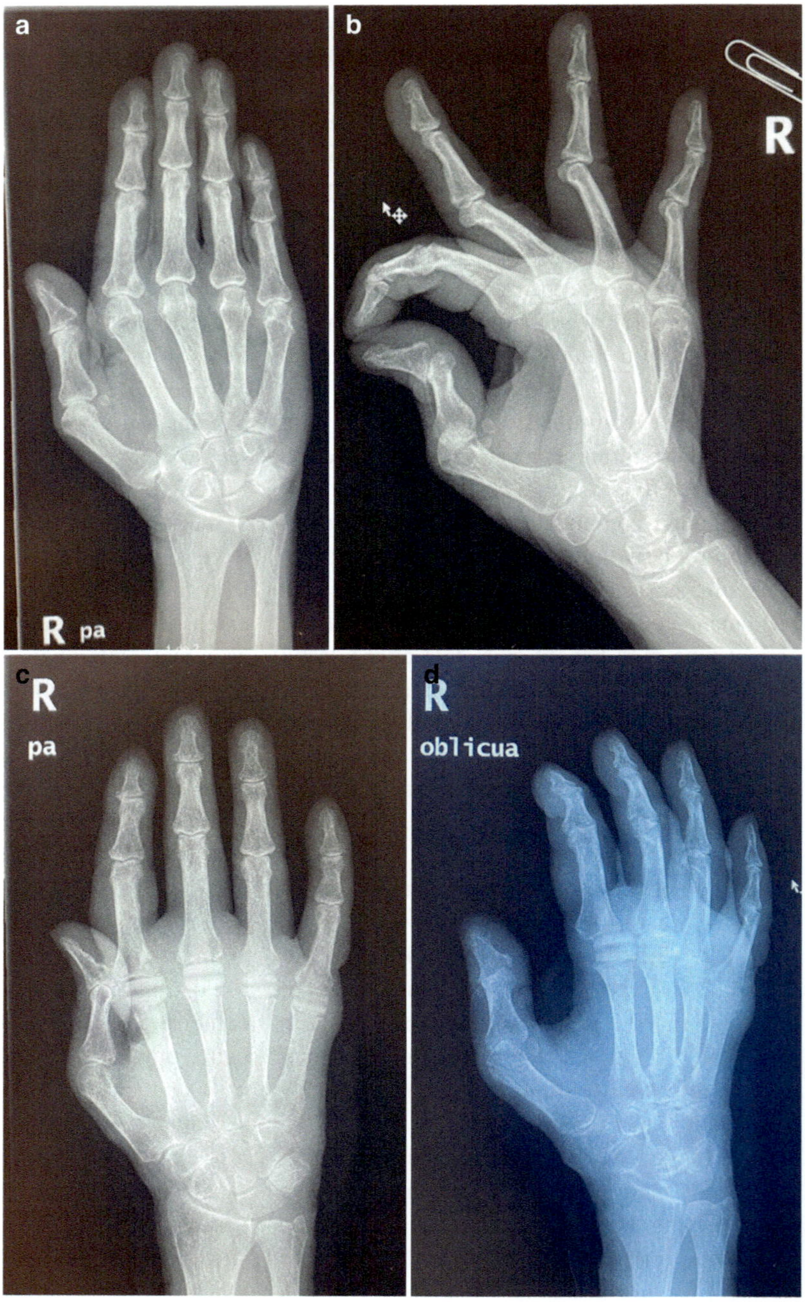

Fig. 20.1 (**a**–**d**) Rheumatic hand with metacarpophalangeal (MCP) joint subluxation operated with silicone prosthesis: (**a**) anteroposterior (AP) radiological view presurgery, (**b**) oblique radiological view presurgery, (**c**) AP radiological view 1 year postsurgery, and (**d**) oblique radiological view 1 year postsurgery

ing less demand on the joint for grip [35]. They conducted a study (level II evidence) in which they analyzed the effect of the aforementioned deformities on joint ROM and hand function. They measured the ROM of the MCP joint in 73 surgically treated patients. The data was distributed into groups according to finger and hand deformity. Functional outcomes were measured using the Michigan Hand Outcomes Questionnaire and the Jebsen-Taylor test. Nineteen fingers had boutonniere deformity, 95 had gooseneck deformity, and 178 had no deformity. The no deformity group had the lowest ROM at baseline (16 degrees) compared to the boutonniere (26 degrees) and swan neck (26 degrees) groups. The mean ROM in the no-

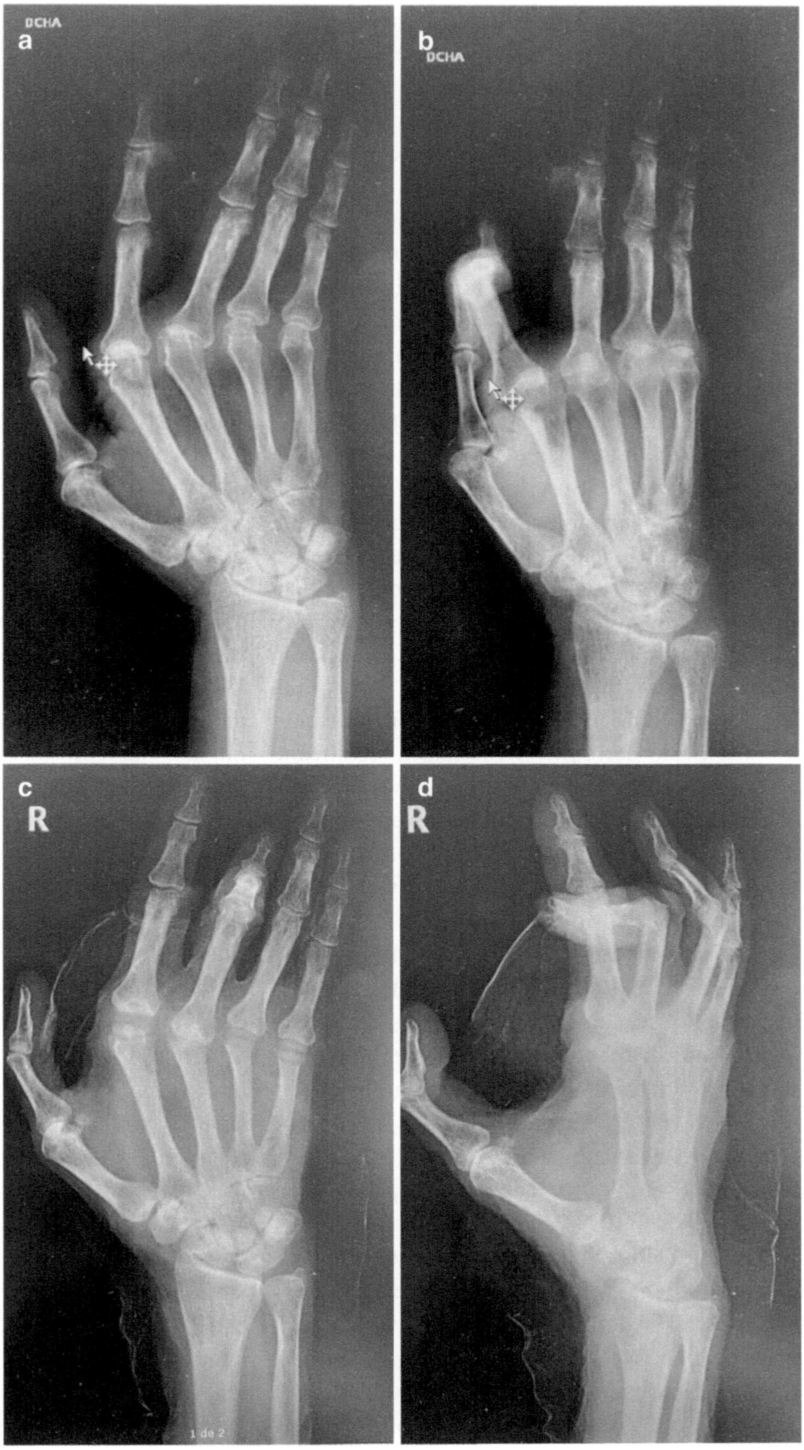

Fig. 20.2 (**a**–**d**) Rheumatic hand with joint metacarpophalangeal (MCP) dislocation and severe ulnar deviation operated with silicone prosthesis: (**a**) presurgical anteroposterior (AP) radiological view, (**b**) presurgical oblique radiological view, (**c**) AP radiological view 6 months postsurgery showing third-finger prosthesis dislocation, and (**d**) oblique radiological view 6 months postsurgery showing third-finger prosthesis dislocation

deformity group compared with the boutonniere group at baseline was statistically significant, but all groups had similar ROM at long-term follow-up. Only the mean Jebsen-Taylor test scores at baseline between the boutonniere and no-deformity groups were significantly different. Ultimately, the results did not support the hypothesis that swan neck deformity has a better ROM than boutonniere deformity. The boutonniere deformity had worse function at baseline, but in the long term there was no difference in function between groups [35].

Long-term results have been less satisfactory, often noting recurrence of deformity.

In 2018, Boe et al. published an analysis (level IV evidence) of 325 silicone MCP arthroplasties prospectively collected from a single institution's total joint registry over a 14-year period to assess long-term radiographic and functional outcomes [36]. Patients were followed for a mean of 7.2 years or until revision. Survival at 5, 10, and 15 years without revision was 98%, 95%, and 95%, respectively. Survival rates at 5, 10, and 15 years without radiographic implant fracture were 93%, 58%, and 35%, respectively. The 5-, 10-, and 15-year survival rates without coronal plane deformity greater than 10° were 81%, 37%, and 17%, respectively. Patients had significant improvements in postoperative pain levels and MCP joint ROM. Neither implant fracture nor coronal plane deformity >10° had a significant association with worse function. Overall, pain relief and functional improvement were reliable, although silicone implants did not protect against progression of coronal plane deformity and had a high fracture rate [36].

Implant fracture is a complication unique to silicone arthroplasty [37]. Fractures are typically caused by a tear in the implant from excessive wear from sharp bone edge. In the literature, implant fractures are reported to range from 0% to 63% [8, 11]. A fracture implant is not necessarily correlated with pain, decreased patient satisfaction, disability, or need for reoperation or revision [11].

In 2018, Morrell and Weiss set out a study to demonstrate that MCP silicone arthroplasty provides excellent long-term outcomes with a low complication rate in patients with osteoarthritis (OA) (therapeutic level IV evidence study) [38]. A group of 35 patients with OA of one or more MCP joints undergoing anatomically neutral MCP silicone arthroplasty was followed for a period of 15 years. Functional outcomes, including strength and ROM, as well as complications were recorded. All patients were available for long-term evaluation including radiographs and an outcome questionnaire. The mean follow-up of the 35 patients (40 implants) was 8.3 years. The mean age was 58 years, with 22 men and 13 women. Only one MCP joint was affected in 31 patients (middle finger, 20; index finger, 10; small finger). The dominant hand was affected in 23 patients. Seven (out of 14) patients underwent radial collateral ligament (RCL) reconstruction of the MCP joint of the index finger; no other fingers required collateral ligament reconstruction. The mean final VAS pain score was 0.3 over 10. The mean final active ROM was 4° to 73° of flexion. One patient underwent revision MCP arthroplasty with a clinical survival of 97%. Radiographs demonstrated implant fracture in 5 of 40 (12.5%) implants, but none showed instability, pain, or ROM impairment. The mean Michigan Hand Outcomes Questionnaire score was 82 (out of 100) at the end of follow-up. Ultimately, silicone arthroplasty was effective in the treatment of MCP joint OA. Long-term implant survival was 97% (clinical) and 88% (radiographic) [38].

In 2021, Iwamoto et al. attempted to identify risk factors associated with early fracture of the MCP silicone arthroplasty implant using the volar hinge silicone implant in patients with RA (therapeutic level IV evidence study) [39]. They retrospectively reviewed 113 fingers from 31 hands that underwent MCP arthroplasty, with a minimum follow-up of 3 years. An implant fracture within 3 years after surgery was considered an early implant fracture. Patient records were reviewed for possible risk factors of age, affected toes, ulnar drift angle, and ROM of the MCP joint before surgery and 1 year after surgery. Candidate risk factors were compared at the digit level and at the patient level. With implant fracture as the end point, the estimated Kaplan-Meier survival rate was 74.3% at 3 years and 67.9% at 5 years. Early implant fracture was detected in 29 fingers. Bivariate analyses showed significant associations between early implant fracture and MCP joint ROM before surgery, MCP joint flexion range 1 year after surgery, and MCP joint ROM 1 year after surgery. Multiple logistic regression analysis showed that increased MCP joint flexion range 1 year after surgery was an independent risk factor for early implant fracture. Ultimately, increased MCP joint flexion arc was associated with increased implant fractures. Iwamoto et al. proposed that the MCP joint flexion range should be restricted to less than 60° in postoperative rehabilitation. This required educating patients to avoid excessive MCP joint flexion [39].

In 2015, Squitieri et al. performed an economic evaluation of the long-term outcomes of silicone MCP arthroplasty in patients with RA [40]. In a 5-year prospective study, they analyzed 170 patients (73 surgical and 97 nonsurgical). They assessed objective functional measurements and patient-rated outcomes using the Michigan Hand Outcomes Questionnaire and the Arthritis Impact Measurement Scales 2 at 3 and 5 years. A cost-effectiveness analysis was performed using direct costs from Medicare outpatient claims data (2006–2010) to estimate incremental cost-effectiveness ratios for the Michigan Hand Outcomes Questionnaire and the Arthritis Impact Measurement Scales 2. At 5 years, a statistically significant difference in outcomes (Michigan Hand Outcomes Questionnaire) was observed between the two groups, with surgical patients having better outcomes. The costs associated with improved outcomes at 5 years after surgery ranged from $787 to $1150 when measured with the Michigan Hand Outcomes Questionnaire and from $49,843 to $149,530 when measured with the Arthritis Impact Measurement Scales 2. The incremental cost-effectiveness ratios did not increase substantially with the observed surgical revision rate of 5.5% (approximately 4% incremental cost-effectiveness ratio increase) or with previously published long-term revision rates of 6.2% (approximately 6% incremental cost-effectiveness ratio increase).

Ultimately, the short-term improvements in the outcomes of silicone MCP arthroplasty were maintained over the 5-year follow-up. Moreover, these results were achieved at a relatively low cost, even when the cost of potential surgical complications was added [40].

In 2020, Esterman et al. attempted to identify the causes of satisfaction of patients with inflammatory disease undergoing hand reconstruction with silicone MCP arthroplasty [41]. Their hypothesis was that patients taking biologic drugs would be more satisfied with the outcome. The minimum follow-up was 1 year. Patients rated their satisfaction with treatment outcome and hand appearance on a 5-point Likert scale, with a score of 5 indicating "very satisfied" and 1 indicating "very dissatisfied," and completed the brief Michigan Hand Outcomes Questionnaire (MHQ). MCP ROM, ulnar drift, and grip strength were measured. Forty-one patients with 118 operated fingers were available for follow-up after a mean of 5.6 years. Patients were satisfied with the overall treatment outcome (score 4.4), but only somewhat satisfied (score 3.3) with the appearance of their hand. The total ROM of the MCP was 61° with an ulnar deviation of 10°. Appearance and ulnar deviation were determinants of satisfaction. There was no difference in the results between patients who used biologic drugs and those who did not. The hypothesis that patients taking biologic drugs were more satisfied after surgery could not be proved. Hand appearance and ulnar deviation were the most important determinants of satisfaction after reconstruction of the MCP deformity [41]. Finally, with respect to MCP arthritis, silicone remains the gold standard for RA [20].

20.2.1.3 Surface Replacement Arthroplasty (SRA)

SRA was design to create a more anatomical joint. It tries to reproduce a physiologic articulation while preserving bone stock and collateral ligaments for stability. Preservation of collateral ligaments would decrease endosteal contact forces, minimizing osteolysis and subsidence [42]. The implant consists of a proximal cobalt chromium (CoCr) component and a distal metal-backed polyethylene-titanium component. The material properties of the implant allow better coronal plane deformity because of its modularity. However, it lacks the inherent stability of the hinged silicone implant that can be of interest in patients with poor soft tissue stabilizers.

In 2020, Claxton et al. investigated the results of surface replacement arthroplasty (SRA) in RA patients with MCP joint involvement. It was a retrospective study of 80 SRAs performed in 27 patients. The parameters analyzed were demographics, SRA revisions, reoperations, complications, pain, and ROM of the MCP joint. The mean follow-up was 9.5 years (minimum 2 years). Thirteen fingers (16%) required revision arthroplasty and 29 (36%) required reoperation. Survival rates at 5, 10, 15, and 20 years after implant revision were 95%, 85%, 80%, and 69%, respectively. Survival rates at 5, 10, 15, and 20 years from global reoperation were 80%, 65%, 55%, and 46%, respectively. MCP joint ROM, grip strength, and pain intensity were significantly improved after surgery. Ultimately, MCP joint SRA improved function and pain in patients with AR. However, the high overall reoperation rates were of concern, although most did not involve revision arthroplasty [43].

This procedure has limited use because of the high reoperation rate and its 5-year low survival rate of 67% compared to 85% for pyrocarbon and silicone implants [44].

20.2.1.4 Dorsal Capsule Interpositional Arthroplasty of the MCP Joint

In isolated MCP joint degenerative or traumatic arthritis, dorsal capsule interposition arthroplasty is a technique that provides short-term pain relief and has the advantage of preserving the bony anatomy, collateral ligaments, and volar plate, thus not excluding further implant arthroplasty.

In 2020, Walker et al. analyzed the results of a novel soft tissue arthroplasty technique that interposes the dorsal capsule, with a mean follow-up of 2 years [45]. They performed a retrospective review of 10 dorsal capsule interposition arthroplasties of the MCP joint in eight patients. Physical evaluation assessed MCP joint ROM, grip strength, and pain. The outcome tests used were the Michigan Hand Outcomes Questionnaire, Visual Analog Scale (VAS), and Quick Disabilities of the Arm, Shoulder, and Hand (QuickDASH) scores. The Kellgren and Lawrence classification assessed the severity of MCP joint osteoarthritis on preoperative radiographs. The mean follow-up was 29 months. The mean VAS score was 2/10 postoperatively and the mean postoperative ROM improved 7 degrees. The mean postoperative grip strength of the operated hand was 30 kg. The mean Michigan Hand Outcomes Questionnaire final score was 70. Patients with Kellgren's grade 2 or 3 osteoarthritis scored highest on the QuickDASH and Michigan Hand Outcomes Questionnaire. All patients who were working before surgery returned to work. No patient required a second surgery. Ultimately, this technique of dorsal capsule interposition arthroplasty was considered a viable technique for isolated degenerative or traumatic arthritis of the MCP joint after a mean follow-up of 2 years. Pain relief was more intense in patients with less severe radiographic findings. The advantage of this procedure is that it preserves the bony anatomy, collateral ligaments, and volar plate, thus not excluding further implant arthroplasty [45].

20.2.2 Revision MCP Arthroplasty

The main complications of MCP arthroplasty are subsidence, osteolysis, dislocation, and implant fracture. These complications are more frequent in patients with joint deformities and loss of joint stability and do not always require revision surgery. Different materials have been used and different techniques have been developed to achieve favorable results after revision MCP arthroplasty. It should not be forgotten that the main problem of this technically complex surgery is the loss of bone tissue and soft tissue support.

In 2007, Ikavalko et al. stated that MCP arthroplasty after silicone implant arthroplasty had frequent complications, such as severe bone loss, osteolysis, and diaphyseal perforations. Also, impacted, morselized allografts were frequently used to treat bone loss in revision surgery [46]. They described a new treatment method using a bioreconstructive poly-L/D-lactic acid (PLDLA) joint scaffold and allograft bone packing, after complete removal of the original silicone implants. This method restored bone deficiencies, corrected malalignment, and improved hand function. In a prospective, nonrandomized study, the authors presented the clinical and radiographic results of 21 patients with 52 MCP revision arthroplasties using PLDLA implants and allograft bone packing, with 1-year follow-up. Recurrent volar displacement of the proximal phalanges occurred in 33 of the 52 joints. No surgical wound healing problems were encountered. Some patients suffered transient loss of tactile sensation. Bone packing appeared to be successful in restoring host bone stock and PLDLA implantation provided a bioresconstructive scaffold for fibrous tissue ingrowth that promoted adequate stability and function. However, Ikavalko et al. also mentioned that the role of the described method should be assessed in the long term [46].

In 2012, Tiihonen et al. stated that revision arthroplasty of MCP joint in patients with chronic inflammatory arthritis after silicone implants was technically challenging due to severe bone loss and existing soft tissue deficiencies [47]. In their study they evaluated the results of the revision MCP arthroplasty using poly-L/D-lactic acid 96:4 (PLDLA) interposition implant and morcelized allograft or autograft bone packing in patients with failed MCP arthroplasties and severe osteolysis. They analyzed 15 patients (15 hands and 36 joints) with a mean follow-up of 7 years. They reviewed radiographs for osteolysis and incorporation of the grafted bone. The clinical parameters evaluated were active ROM, pain, subjective outcome, and grip power. The technique provided satisfactory pain relief, but function was limited. Radiographic analysis showed complete incorporation of the grafted bone into the diaphyseal portion of the metacarpal bones and into the host phalanges in 30 of 36 joints. All patients had very limited grip strength on both the operated and nonoperated sides. Ultimately, due to soft tissue deficiencies, long-term functional and alignment problems could not be resolved with the PLDLA interposition implant [47].

In 2019, Wagner et al., in a level IV evidence study, analyzed the results of 128 revision MCP arthroplasties performed in 64 patients [44]. The mean age of the patients was 62 years. Fifty nonconstrained (31 pyrocarbon and 19 surface-replacing arthroplasty) and 78 constrained silicone implants were used for revisions. With a mean follow-up of 6 years, 20 (16%) implants required secondary revision surgery. The 5- and 10-year survival rates were 81% and 79%, respectively. Postoperative dislocation occurred in 17 (13%) MCP joints. Subgroup analysis demonstrated a 5-year survival rate of 67% in surface-replacing arthroplasties, compared with 83% for both pyrocarbon and silicone implants. Postoperatively, improvements in pain and ROM of the MCP were observed in most patients. Ultimately, MCP revision arthroplasty was a difficult procedure, with one in five patients requiring a revision procedure at 5 years and a relatively high rate of postoperative dislocations. However, most patients who did not require secondary revision surgery improved in terms of pain and ROM. The worst results were obtained in patients with a history of MCP dislocations [44].

In 2020, Notermans et al. stated that MCP silicone arthroplasty had a high revision rate and that the preoperative degree of ulnar and radial wrist deviation had been suggested to influence the duration of revision [39]. They conducted a study to evaluate what factors were associated with reoperation after MCP silicone arthroplasty. They retrospectively evaluated 73 adult patients (252 arthroplasties). The treated fingers included 66 index, 67 long, 60 ring, and 59 small fingers. The overall reoperation rate was 9.1% ($N = 23$). Indications for reoperation were implant rupture ($N = 11$), instability ($N = 4$), soft tissue complications ($N = 4$), infections ($N = 3$), and stiffness ($N = 1$). Patients operated on a single finger showed a greater tendency to have higher revision rates (19% vs. 3.5%, $p = 0.067$). Radiographic follow-up demonstrated joint incongruity in 50% of cases, bone erosion in 58%, and implant breakage in 19%. There was a tendency to have a higher revision rate in patients without preoperative MCP joint subluxation (19% vs. 6.7%, $p = 0.065$). Implant survival rates at 1, 5, and 10 years were 96%, 92%, and 70%, respectively. Revision surgery occurred at the first 14 months in 15 patients (65%) and after 5 years in 8 (35%) patients. In short, revision surgery after MCP silicone arthroplasty appeared to be bimodal. Patients with greater preoperative hand function may be at greater risk of needing revision surgery [48]. This is consistent with Iwamoto's statement that increased arc of flexion of the MCP joint is associated with increased implant fractures [39].

20.3 PIP Joint Arthroplasty

The complexity of the PIP joint makes management particularly challenging.

Treatment of the PIP joint has evolved over time and requires an understanding of the biomechanics of the joint. Normal functional range of motion is between 23° and 87°. It is important to consider functional ROM when evaluating the results of arthroplasty. The PIP joint destruction is often related to OA or posttraumatic degeneration and to a lesser extent to RA. The most common implants used are silicone arthroplasty, metal-plastic SRA, and pyrocarbon arthroplasty.

20.3.1 Emergency Arthroplasty of the PIP Joint for Complex Fractures with Silicone Implant

Silicone arthroplasty usually provides good pain relief and patient satisfaction [49–52] (Figs. 20.3 and 20.4). However, ROM improvements are less predictable than in the MCP joint. Swanson reported a 35° increase in PIP joint arc of motion [12], but in a larger study he later noticed only a 10° increase in arc of motion [53]. Other studies reported little changes in total PIP range of motion [24, 49–51]. Conolly and Rath demonstrated that preoperative contracture was inversely related to the arc of motion that could be restored [54]. Long-term survivorship has been satisfactory, between 80% and 90% at 8–10 years [51, 52, 55]. This implant has been shown to be ineffective for the correction of boutonniere and swan neck deformities, subluxation, and ulnar and radial deviation [51].

In 2020, Laurent evaluated emergency finger silicone implants in complex and comminuted fractures of the PIP joint, as well as their clinical and radiological complications [56]. In comminuted fractures, arthroplasty with a silicone implant is a controversial therapeutic option in an emergency setting. Joint destruction is often accompanied by soft tissue injuries (skin, tendons, devascularization), which makes reconstruction even more complex. In their retrospective study they analyzed 13 patients undergoing emergency surgery with a PIP NeuFlex arthroplasty 1. PIP joint reconstruction was associated with soft tissue repair at the same time (skin cover, tendons, nerves) in all patients. The mean age of the patients was 57.7 years, and there was a predominance of male sex (92%). Injuries were caused by domestic accident in 61% of cases. The mean follow-up was 4.7 years. The mean total active ROM was 183°. The mean QuickDASH score was 24. There was one case of implant rupture without functional consequences. There were no cases of infection or instability. Arthroplasty with a silicone implant was a simple, reliable, fast, and durable solution for complex PIP joint fractures when conservative treatment was impossible. This solution is a good alternative to arthrodesis or even amputation of the finger and they stated that the PIP joint was particularly vulnerable to trauma [56].

The complications of this implant are instability, implant fracture, and synovitis.

As for instability or deviation of the postoperative axis, we will discuss it later with the SRA. Implant fracture varies between 0% and 55% according to the studies [49–52, 55].

A fractured implant is not necessarily associated with disability, pain, and revision surgery. Bales et al. reviewed 21 fractures of which only 3 required revision for pain and concluded that radiographic alterations did not correlate with prognosis [52].

Silicone synovitis and granuloma formation are another clinical problems that may require implant removal due to pain and bone loss. It has been reported but is rare (0%–24%) at the PIP and MCP joint in contrast to the higher incidence after silicone total wrist arthroplasty [50–52, 57].

Silicone arthroplasty has remained a good treatment option for PIP joint arthritis, and it has the longest follow-up studies of all available implant arthroplasties.

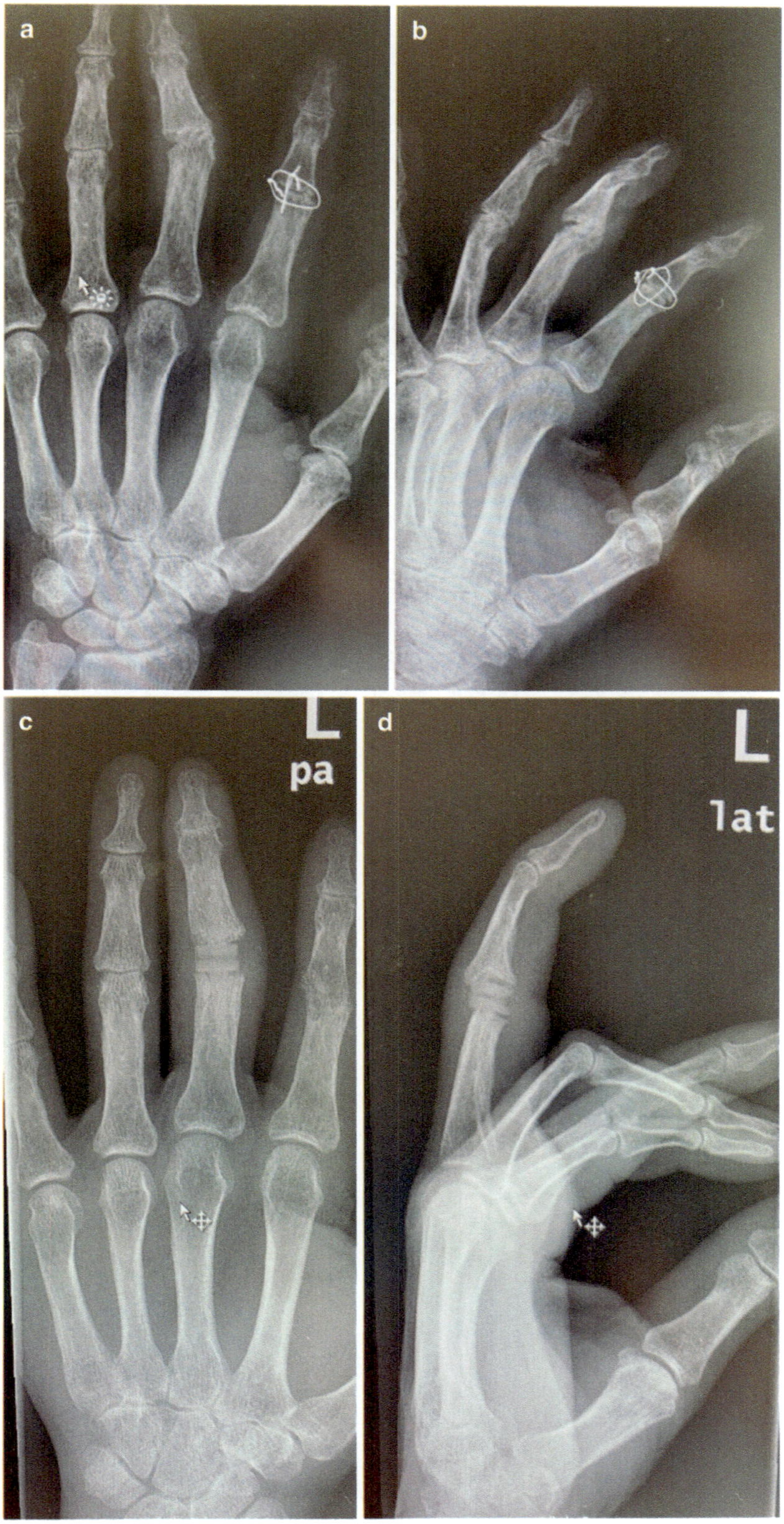

Fig. 20.3 (**a**–**d**) Posttraumatic lesion of the proximal interphalangeal (PIP) joint third finger operated with silicone prosthesis: (**a**) presurgical anteroposterior (AP) radiological view, (**b**) presurgical oblique radiological view, (**c**) AP radiological view 1 year postsurgery, and (**d**) lateral radiological view 1 year postsurgery

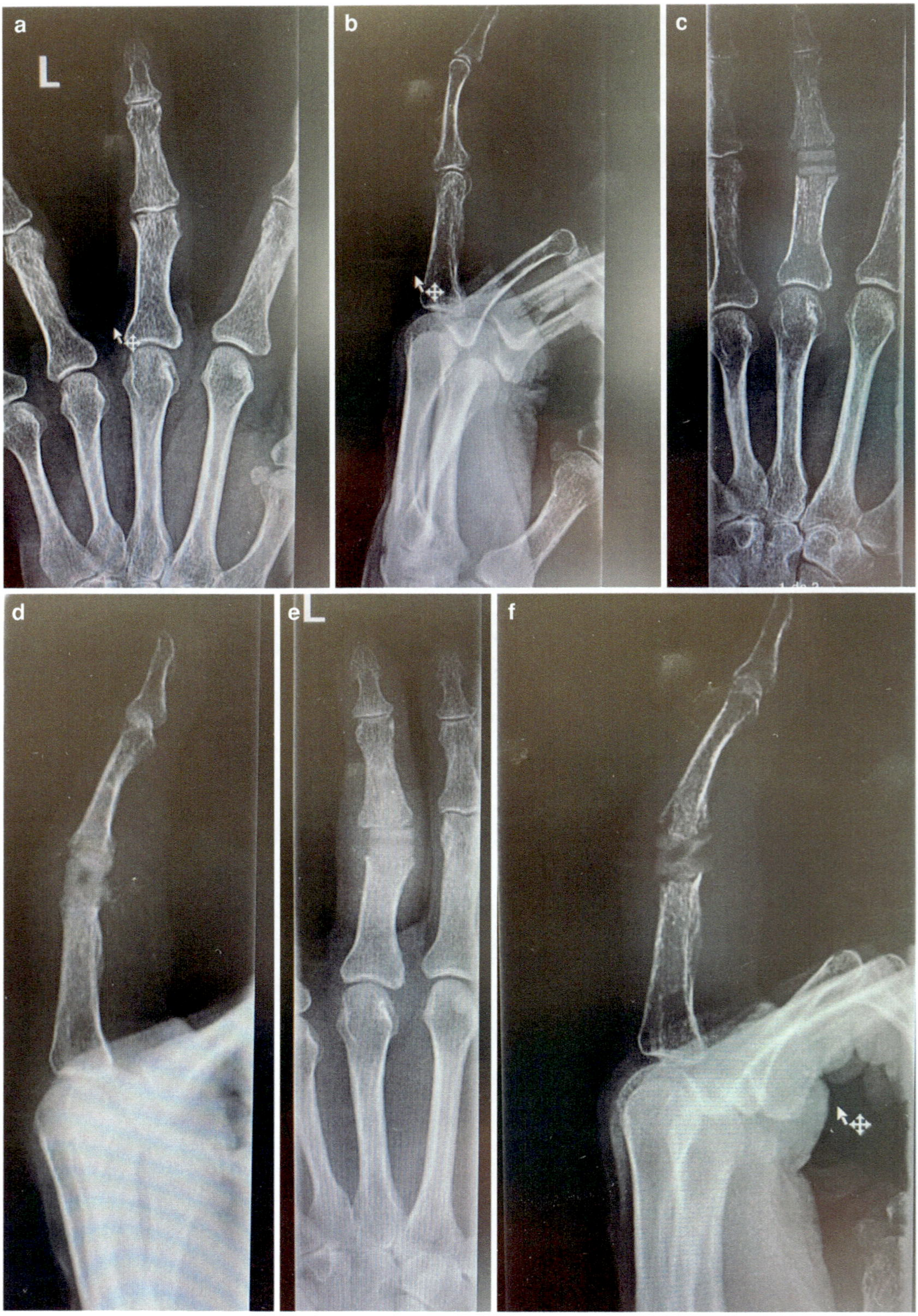

Fig. 20.4 (**a**–**f**) Posttraumatic arthritis of proximal interphalangeal (PIP) joint of the fourth finger treated with silicone prosthesis: (**a**) anteroposterior (AP) radiological view before surgery, (**b**) lateral radiological view before surgery, (**c**) AP radiological view 1 year postsurgery, (**d**) lateral radiological view 1 year postsurgery, (**e**) AP radiological view 2 years postsurgery, and (**f**) lateral radiological view 2 years postsurgery

20.3.2 Surface-Replacing Implant Arthroplasty

The aim of this procedure was to create an implant with more physiological articulation and stability, particularly with laterally directed tension [42]. Linscheid et al. reported their data using the SRA PIP implant, and total pain relief was achieved in 86.1% of patients and a 12° increase in mean total ROM [42]. Jennings et al. observed good pain relief but no improvement in PIP joint ROM [58]. Daecke et al. found a 2° loss of PIP joint motion at 3-year follow-up [26]. Stoecklein et al. reported a 27° increase in total ROM using a volar approach that maintains the integrity of the extensor mechanism allowing early postoperative motion [59].

In 2020, Bodmer et al. compared the results of volar, Chamay, and tendon-splitting approaches for PIP arthroplasty using a superficial replacement implant (CapFlex-PIP) (level IV evidence study) [60]. One thousand patients were studied prospectively, with a 2-year follow-up. PIP ROM, brief Michigan Hand Outcomes Questionnaire scores, and complications were analyzed. The mean PIP joint ROM increased in the volar (53° to 54°), Chamay (38° to 53°), and tendon-splitting (40° to 61°) approaches. The volar approach produced the greatest flexion and the greatest extension deficit. The mean Michigan Hand Outcomes Questionnaire scores at baseline and 2 years were 45 and 74 (volar), 45 and 66 (Chamay), and 41 and 75 (tendon splitting), respectively. Seven patients in the Chamay group and two in the volar group required reintervention, which consisted of teno-/arthrolysis. Compared with the volar and Chamay approaches, the tendon-splitting approach showed a tendency to produce the best results, which were associated with fewer complications [60].

SRA has been used with or without cement and its results have been examined. Johnstone et al. in a long-term retrospective study found no difference in pain score or range of motion, although cemented implants had a higher revision rate (26% vs. 8%) and uncemented components had a higher rate of radiographic loosening of the implant [61]. Murray et al. reported no difference in clinical or radiographic outcomes between cemented and uncemented PIP-SRA implants [62].

Many surgeons avoid the use of cement since revisional surgery becomes more difficult and heat released during cement curing may negatively affect bone and soft tissues [42].

Other possible complications are tendon adhesions, joint instability, swan neck deformity, boutonniere deformity, intraoperative fracture, malalignment, dislocation, and infection [26, 42, 63]. Revision surgery or conversion to arthrodesis is necessary in 9.1%–27% [26, 42, 61].

20.3.3 Complications After Surface-Replacing and Silicone PIP Arthroplasty

In 2021, Helder et al. analyzed complications after surface-replacing and silicone PIP joint arthroplasty [64]. They studied complications, reoperations (subsequent intervention without implant modification), and revisions (subsequent surgery with implant modification or removal) in two groups of patients: those operated with a surface-replacing arthroplasty at the PIP joint using the CapFlex-PIP prosthesis and those operated with a PIP silicone implant. In addition, they evaluated radiographs for deviations of the longitudinal axis of the finger. They analyzed 279 surface-replacing implants and 424 silicone implants. The overall complication rate was 20% for surface-replacing implants and 11% for silicone implants ($p \leq 0.01$), with soft tissue-related events being the most frequent in both groups. Reoperations were significantly more frequent after surface replacement (5.4%) than after silicone arthroplasty (0.5%; $p \leq 0.001$); however, revision rates did not differ significantly (4.4% and 3.3%, respectively; $p = 0.542$). Postoperative axis deviations were significantly less frequent in the surface replacement group (19% vs. 58% for silicone arthroplasty; $p \leq 0.001$). Ultimately, Helder et al. recommended using a surface-replacing implant in cases with preoperative axis deviations and a correctable anatomical situation [64].

20.3.4 Lateral Stability in Healthy PIP Joints Versus Surface Replacement and Silicone Arthroplasty

In 2020, Hensler et al. attempted to quantify the lateral stability of healthy PIP joints using a three-dimensional motion capture system and to compare it to affected joints after surface replacement or silicone arthroplasty [65]. The three study groups were healthy individuals, patients with osteoarthritis of the PIP joint treated with a surface-replacing implant (CapFlex-PIP), and patients with osteoarthritis treated with silicone arthroplasty. All participants were matched for gender and digit, and the two groups of patients were also matched for duration of follow-up. An optical tracking system was used to measure lateral stability. Radial and ulnar stability of the PIP joint were measured as the maximal lateral deviation angle of the middle phalanx under loads of 40 g, 90 g, and 170 g at 0°, 20°, and 45° of PIP joint flexion. Thirty joints were evaluated (5 index and 5 middle fingers in each of the three study groups). Lateral deviation increased proportionally with the applied load. Silicone arthroplasty joints had a higher mean lateral deviation angle (5.18) than healthy joints (3.08) and surface replacement joints (3.38) at 45° flexion and under a 170-g load. After PIP joint arthroplasty, the lateral stability of the PIP joint was highly variable in both healthy participants and patients. Surface replacement PIP joint arthroplasty showed a tendency to provide better anatomical stability than flexible silicone implants [65].

Despite favorable reports with SRA implants for RA of the PIP joint, some authors prefer the use of silicone in this patient group [20].

20.3.5 Pyrolytic Carbon PIP Arthroplasty

Pyrocarbon is biologically inert, has elastic modulus similar to that of bone, and its implant stem has no bony ingrowth. PCA for PIP joint was developed to provide patients with an alternative to silicone and SRA. The primary indication for PIP arthroplasty is pain. Literature suggests that PCA has been relatively successful in improving pain, shows low complications, and presents reasonable implant survival [27, 66–70].

However, other studies have demonstrated high rates of complications and revision surgery. Pyrocarbon implant is vulnerable to dislocation, implant migration, contracture, and squeaking. Sweets and Stern found a gradual decrease in motion over time, high rate of revision surgery, dislocation, stiffness, and implant fracture [25]. Due to the lack of bony ingrowth, pyrocarbon rates of migration and loosening have been high (64%) [25, 68]. A meta-analysis reported higher rates of complications associated with the use of pyrocarbon (30%) versus silicone implant (8%) and the authors have abandoned this technique [71].

In 2020, Mora et al. stated that the use of pyrolytic carbon arthroplasty (PCA) for the proximal interphalangeal (PIP) joint is still controversial [72]. They conducted a prognostic study (grade IV evidence) to evaluate the midterm clinical and radiographic outcomes of PCA of the PIP joint. Patients were assessed after a mean of 6.4 years. Evaluation included grip and pinch strength and digital range of motion (ROM). The study included 29 PIP joint PCAs implanted in 23 hands of 19 patients. Seven implants required further surgical procedures. Three implants were removed and revised by silicone implants due to two dislocations and one implant migration. One was revised with a larger distal component. Three required soft tissue surgical revisions in which the implant was retained (one flexor digitorum superficialis tenodesis and two capsulectomies). At the end of follow-up, the survival of the original implant was 86.2%. Final radiographic review of the remaining 26 implants showed two swan neck deformities and two implant migrations. Postoperative grip strength (38.4 lb) and postoperative pinch strength (13.8 lb) were 92% and 91% of nonsurgical grip and pinch strength, respectively. The final mean ROM for the MCP joint was 82.1° and for the PIP joint was 60.6°. Mean outcome scores were visual analog scale, 1.6; Michigan Hand Outcomes Questionnaire, 71.6; and Disabilities of the Arm, Shoulder, and

Hand, 24. Ultimately, midterm follow-up (mean 6.4 years) of 29 PCA implants in 19 patients revealed a surgical revision rate of 24.1%. Of the 29 implants, 13.8% were removed after a mean of 4.6 years. Strength, ROM, and pain relief were satisfactory [72].

The indications of pyrocarbon implant arthroplasty are young patients with posttraumatic arthritis, no angular deformity, and adequate soft tissue coverage [28] and its use should be avoided in the rheumatoid hand secondary to progressive destruction of capsuloligamentous support.

20.4 Autologous Tissue for Small Joint Arthroplasty

Autologous tissue transfer affords complete biocompatibility and the opportunity for composite reconstruction. The first island, vascularized joint transfer was performed by Buncke in 1967 [73] and subsequent studies of vascularized joint transfer have shown both maintenance of hyaline cartilage and preservation of the joint space [74].

A systematic review of outcomes after vascularized toe joint transfer, silicone implant arthroplasty, and pyrocarbon arthroplasty found that vascularized joint transfer for posttraumatic PIP joint reconstruction had worse arc of motion (37 ± 11°) than either silicone (44 ± 11°) or pyrocarbon arthroplasty (43 ± 11°). Despite limited improvement in arc of motion, relatively higher major complication rates, and need for secondary surgery, vascularized joint transfer is the only procedure that allows future growth [75].

Another treatment option is perichondrium grafting. In 2020, Muder et al. compared the long-term results of perichondrium transplantation and those of two-component surface replacement (SR) implants to the MCP and PIP joints (therapeutic study with level III evidence) [76]. They evaluated 163 joints (in 124 patients), divided into 138 SR implants (in 102 patients) and 25 perichondrium transplantations (in 22 patients). The primary outcome was any revision surgery of the index joint. The mean follow-up was 6 years for SR implants and 26 years for perichondrium transplantations. Patient age at the time of surgery was 64 years for SR implants and 45 years for perichondrium transplantations. MCP joint survival was slightly better in the perichondrium group (86.7%) than in the SR implant group (75%), but not statistically significant. PIP joint survival was also slightly better in the perichondrium group (80%) than in the SR implant group (74.7%), but below the threshold of statistical significance. Ultimately, resurfacing of finger joints using transplanted perichondrium is a technique worth considering, as its low midterm revision rates were similar to those of SR implants [76].

Another technique to avoid silicone or pyrocarbon arthroplasty is to perform arthroplasty using cadaveric meniscus for osteochondral defects in hand joints. The cadaveric meniscus provides resurfacing of the affected bone and serves to maintain the articular space. Hoang et al. reported improvement in both ROM and pain relief, no complications occurred, and only two patients (14%) required postoperative revision surgery for tenolysis and capsulotomy [77].

The development of biotechnology and the application of stem cells to degenerated articular surfaces may render implant arthroplasty obsolete in the future. However, for the time being, it is necessary to continue improving the design and longevity of implants.

20.5 Prevalence of Complications and Cost of Small Joint Arthroplasty for Hand Osteoarthritis and Posttraumatic Arthritis

In 2020, Billig et al. stated that osteoarthritis of the hand is commonly treated by implant arthroplasty [78]. However, despite the increasing prevalence of hand OA, data on the complications and associated cost of patients undergoing PIP joint and MCP joint arthroplasty were lacking. Therefore, they evaluated the complications and cost of PIP joint and MCP joint arthroplasty in patients undergoing such interventions after a 2-year follow-up (prognostic study with level II evidence). They analyzed insurance claims from

2009 to 2016 using Truven MarketScan databases for adult patients undergoing PIP and MCP arthroplasty after a diagnosis of OA or posttraumatic arthritis. They analyzed 2859 patients, of whom 36% had received an MCP arthroplasty and 64% had received a PIP arthroplasty. The mean complication rate was 35%. PIP arthroplasty patients were more likely to suffer a prosthetic fracture than MCP arthroplasty patients (3.4% vs. 1.5%, respectively). Each complication resulted in an additional cost of $1076 [78].

20.6 Conclusions

Arthritis of the hand (proximal interphalangeal [PIP] and metacarpophalangeal [MCP] joints) is frequent and can result from osteoarthritis (OA), inflammatory arthritis, or posttraumatic arthritis. The main clinical presentation is pain and loss of range of motion. Initial treatment is conservative, including splinting, oral analgesics, and sometimes local injections. Cases where pain persists despite conservative treatment warrant surgery. Continued pain is considered the main indication for arthroplasty of MCP and PIP joints. Other surgical indications are deformity, stiffness, and joint incongruity. Surgical options are debridement of painful osteophytes, arthroplasty, and arthrodesis. Improvements in implant materials and developments in MCP and PIP joint arthroplasty have provided physicians and patients more options in treating these joints. Several designs of primary MCP joint arthroplasty are available: unconstrained pyrocarbon has shown good results in OA, silicone implant is the gold standard for RA, and little can be said about surface replacement arthroplasty (SRA) for the MCP joint. Primary PIP joint arthroplasty with silicone implants remains the gold standard for OA. The use of a pyrolytic carbon implant is controversial because of its high reoperation rate compared to silicone and surface-replacing implants. The SRA implant for PIP joint has shown good clinical and survival results at medium follow-up. However, silicone prostheses are often preferred for the PIP joint. Early results have demonstrated improvements in pain and ROM, but lower rates in complications and long-term follow-up studies are required. Nowadays, there is no clear consensus in the arthroplasty option.

References

1. Mercer D, Imada AO. Arthrodesis and arthroplasty of the small joints. Oper Tech Orthop. 2020;30:100832.
2. Kirschenbaum D, Schneider LH, Adams DC, Cody RP. Arthroplasty of the metacarpophalangeal joints with use of silicone-rubber implants in patients who have rheumatoid arthritis: long-term results. J Bone Joint Surg Am. 1993;75:3–12.
3. McArthur PA, Milner RH. A prospective randomized comparison of Sutter and Swanson silastic spacers. J Hand Surg Br. 1998;23:574–7.
4. Bogoch ER, Escott BG, Ronald K. Hand appearance as a patient motivation for surgery and a determinant of satisfaction with metacarpophalangeal joint arthroplasty for rheumatoid arthritis. J Hand Surg Am. 2011;36:1007–14.
5. Waljee JF, Chung KC. Objective functional outcomes and patient satisfaction after silicone metacarpophalangeal arthroplasty for rheumatoid arthritis. J Hand Surg Am. 2012;37:47–54.
6. Chung KC, Nellans KW, Burns PB, Wilgis EFS, Burke FD, Fox DA, et al. Patient expectations and long-term outcomes in rheumatoid arthritis patients: results from the SARA (Silicone Arthroplasty in Rheumatoid Arthritis) study. Clin Rheumatol. 2015;34:641–51.
7. Chung KC, Kotsis SV, Burns PB, Burke FD, Wilgis EFS, Fox DA, et al. Seven-year outcomes of the Silicone Arthroplasty in Rheumatoid Arthritis Prospective Cohort Study. Arthritis Care Res (Hoboken). 2017;69:973–81.
8. Goldfarb CA, Stern PJ. Metacarpophalangeal joint arthroplasty in rheumatoid arthritis: a long-term assessment. J Bone Joint Surg Am. 2003;85:1869–78.
9. Bass RL, Stern PJ, Nairus JG. High implant fracture incidence with Sutter silicone metacarpophalangeal joint arthroplasty. J Hand Surg Am. 1996;21:813–8.
10. Williams NW, Penrose JM, Hose DR. Computer model analysis of the Swanson and Sutter metacarpophalangeal joint implants. J Hand Surg Br. 2000;25:212–20.
11. Trail IA, Martin JA, Nuttall D, Stanley JK. Seventeen-year survivorship analysis of silastic metacarpophalangeal joint replacement. J Bone Joint Surg Br. 2004;86:1002–6.
12. Swanson AB. Flexible implant arthroplasty for arthritic finger joints: rationale, technique, and results of treatment. J Bone Joint Surg Am. 1972;54:435–55.
13. Moller K, Sollerman C, Geijer M, Kopylov P, Tagil M. Avanta versus Swanson silicone implants in the MCP joint—a prospective, randomized comparison

of 30 patients followed for 2 years. J Hand Surg Br. 2005;30:8–13.
14. Delaney R, Trail IA, Nuttall D. A comparative study of outcome between the Neuflex and Swanson metacarpophalangeal joint replacements. J Hand Surg Br. 2005;30:3–7.
15. Parkkila T, Belt EA, Hakala M, Kautiainen H, Leppilahti J. Comparison of Swanson and Sutter metacarpophalangeal arthroplasties in patients with rheumatoid arthritis: a prospective and randomized trial. J Hand Surg Am. 2005;30:1276–81.
16. Pettersson K, Wagnsjo P, Hulin E. NeuFlex compared with Sutter prostheses: a blind, prospective, randomised comparison of silastic metacarpophalangeal joint prostheses. Scand J Plast Reconstr Surg Hand Surg. 2006;40:284–90.
17. Escott BG, Ronald K, Judd MG, Bogoch ER. NeuFlex and Swanson metacarpophalangeal implants for rheumatoid arthritis: prospective randomized, controlled clinical trial. J Hand Surg Am. 2010;35:44–51.
18. Tagil M, Geijer M, Malcus P, Kopylov P. Correlation between range of motion and implant fracture: a 5 year follow-up of 72 joints in 18 patients in a randomized study comparing Swanson and Avanta/Sutter MCP silicone prosthesis. J Hand Surg Eur. 2009;34:743–77.
19. Weightman B, Simon S, Rose R, Paul I, Radin E. Environmental fatigue testing of silastic finger joint prostheses. J Biomed Mater Res. 1972;6:15–24.
20. Srnec JJ, Wagner ER, Rizzo M. Implant arthroplasty for proximal interphalangeal, metacarpophalangeal and trapeziometacarpal joint degeneration. J Hand Surg Am. 2017;42(10):817–25.
21. Dickson DR, Badge R, Nuttall D, Watts AC, Talwalkar SC, Hayton M, Trail IA. Pyrocarbon metacarpophalangeal joint arthroplasty in noninflammatory arthritis: minimum 5-year follow-up. J Hand Surg Am. 2015;40:1956–62.
22. Wall LB, Stern PJ. Clinical and radiographic outcomes of metacarpophalangeal joint pyrolytic carbon arthroplasty for osteoarthritis. J Hand Surg Am. 2013;38(3):537–43.
23. Aujla RS, Sheikh N, Divall P, Bhowal B, Dias JJ. Unconstrained metacarpophalangeal joint arthroplasties: a systematic review. Bone Joint J. 2017;99-B:100–6.
24. Branam BR, Tuttle HG, Stern PJ, et al. Resurfacing arthroplasty versus silicone arthroplasty for proximal interphalangeal joint osteoarthritis. J Hand Surg Am. 2007;32A:775–88.
25. Sweets TM, Stern PJ. Pyrolytic carbon resurfacing arthroplasty for osteoarthritis of the proximal interphalangeal joint of the finger. J Bone Joint Surg Am. 2011;93(15):1417–25.
26. Daecke W, Kaszap B, Martini AK, et al. A prospective, randomized comparison of 3 types of proximal interphalangeal joint arthroplasty. J Hand Surg Am. 2012;37(9):1770–9.
27. Ono S, Shauver MJ, Chang KW, et al. Outcomes of pyrolytic carbon arthroplasty for the proximal interphalangeal joint at 44 months' mean follow-up. Plast Reconstr Surg. 2012;129(5):1139–50.
28. Drake ML, Segalman KA. Complication of small joint arthroplasty. Hand Clin. 2010;26(2):205–12.
29. Swanson AB. Implant resection arthroplasty of the proximal interphalangeal joint. Orthop Clin North Am. 1973;4(4):1007–29.
30. Murray MP. New-generation implant arthroplasties of the finger joints. J Am Acad Orthop Surg. 2003;11(5):295–301.
31. Chung KC, Burns PB, Kim HM, Burke FD, Wilgis EFS, Fox DA. Long-term followup for rheumatoid arthritis patients in a multicenter outcomes study of silicone metacarpophalangeal joint arthroplasty. Arthritis Care Res. 2012;64:1292–300.
32. Neral MK, Pittner DE, Spiess AM, Imbriglia JE. Silicone arthroplasty for nonrheumatic metacarpophalangeal joint arthritis. J Hand Surg Am. 2013;38(12):2412–8.
33. Hansraj KK, Ashworth CR, Ebramzadeh E, et al. Swanson metacarpophalangeal joint arthroplasty in patients with rheumatoid arthritis. Clin Orthop Relat Res. 1997;342:11–5.
34. Olsen I, Gebuhr P, Sonne-Holm S. Silastic arthroplasty in rheumatoid MCP-joints 60 joints followed for 7 years. Acta Orthop Scand. 1994;65(4):430–1.
35. Chetta M, Burns PB, Kim HM, Burke FD, Wilgis EFS, Fox DA, Chung KC. The effect of swan neck and boutonniere deformities on the outcome of silicone metacarpophalangeal joint arthroplasty in rheumatoid arthritis. Plast Reconst Surg. 2013;132:597–603.
36. Boe C, Wagner E, Rizzo M. Long-term outcomes of silicone metacarpophalangeal arthroplasty: a longitudinal analysis of 325 cases. Journal of Hand Surgery (European Volume). 2018;43:1076–82.
37. Zhu A, Rahgozar P, Chung KC. Advances in proximal interphalangeal joint arthroplasty: Biomechanics & Biomaterials. Hand Clin. 2018;34(2):185–94.
38. Morrell NT, Weiss A-PC. Silicone metacarpophalangeal arthroplasty for osteoarthritis: long-term results. J Hand Surg Am. 2018;43:229–33.
39. Iwamoto T, Ishii K, Suzuki T, Kimura H, Matsumura N, Sato K. Risk factors contributing to early implant fracture in silicone metacarpophalangeal joint arthroplasty for patients with rheumatoid arthritis. J Hand Surg Am. 2021;46(243):e1–7.
40. Squitieri L, Chung KC, Hutton DW, Burns PH, Kim HM, Mahmoudi E. A 5-year cost-effectiveness analysis of silicone metacarpophalangeal arthroplasty in patients with rheumatoid arthritis. Plast Reconstr Surg. 2015;136:305–14.
41. Estermann L, Marks M, Herren DB, Schindele S. Determinants of long-term satisfaction after silicone MCP arthroplasty in patients with inflammatory diseases. Hand Surg Rehabil. 2020;39:545–9.
42. Linscheid RL, Murray PM, Vidal MA, Beckenbaugh RD. Development of a surface replacement arthroplasty for proximal interphalangeal joints. J Hand Surg. 1997;22(2):286–98.

43. Claxton MR, Wagner ER, Rizzo M. Long-term outcomes of MCP surface replacement arthroplasty in patients with rheumatoid arthritis. Hand. 2020:1–7.
44. Wagner ER, Houdek MT, Packard B, Moran SL, Rizzo M. Revision metacarpophalangeal arthroplasty: a longitudinal study of 128 cases. J Am Acad Orthop Surg. 2019;27:211–8.
45. Walker KL, Johnson AJ, Marchessault JA. Dorsal capsule interpositional arthroplasty of the metacarpophalangeal joint. Hand. 2020:1–6.
46. Ikavalko M, Skytta ET, Belt EA. One-year results of use of poly-L/D-lactic acid joint scaffolds and bone packing in revision metacarpophalangeal arthroplasty. J Hand Surg (European Volume). 2007;2E(4):427–33.
47. Tiihonen R, Honkanen PB, Belt EA, Ikävalko M, Skyttä ET. The mean seven years' results of the use of poly-L/D-lactic acid (PLDLA) interposition implant and bone packing in revision metacarpophalangeal arthroplasty: a prospective cohort study. Scand J Surg. 2012;101:265–70.
48. Notermans BJW, Lans J, Arnold D, Jupiter JB, Chen NC. Factors associated with reoperation after silicone metacarpophalangeal joint arthroplasty in patients with inflammatory arthritis. Hand. 2020;15:805–11.
49. Lin HH, Wyrick JD, Stern PJ. Proximal interphalangeal joint silicone replacement arthroplasty: clinical results using an anterior approach. J Hand Surg. 1995;20(1):123–32.
50. Asworth CR, Hansraj KK, Todd AO, et al. Swanson proximal interphalangeal joint arthroplasty in patients with rheumatoid arthritis. Clin Orthop. 1997;342:34–7.
51. Takigawa S, Meletiou S, Sauerbier M, Cooney WP. Long-term assessment of Swanson implant arthroplasty in the proximal interphalangeal joint of the hand. J Hand Surg. 2004;29(5):785–95.
52. Bales JG, Wall LB, Stern PJ. Long-term results of Swanson silicones arthroplasty for proximal interphalangeal joint osteoarthritis. J Hand Surg. 2014;39(3):455–61.
53. Swanson AB. Flexible implant arthroplasty in the proximal interphalangeal joint of the hand. J Hand Surg Am. 1985;10:796–805.
54. Conolly WB, Rath S. Silastic implant arthroplasty for post-traumatic stiffness of the finger joints. J Hand Surg Edinb Scotl. 1991;16(3):286–92.
55. Adamson GJ, Gellman H, Brumfield RH, Kuschner SH, Lawler JW. Flexible implant resection arthroplasty of the proximal interphalangeal joint in patients with systemic inflammatory arthritis. J Hand Surg. 1994;19(3):378–84.
56. Laurent R, El Rifai S, Loisel F, Lepage D, Obert L, Pluvy I. Functional evaluation following emergency arthroplasty of the proximal interphalangeal joint for complex fractures with silicone implant. Hand Surg Rehabil. 2020;39:423–30.
57. Foliart DE. Swanson silicone finger joint implants: a review of the literature regarding long-term complications. J Hand Surg Am. 1995;20:445–9.
58. Jennings CD, Livingstone DP. Surface replacement arthroplasty of the proximal interphalangeal joint using the PIP-SRA implant: results, complications, and revisions. J Hand Surg Am. 2008;33(9):1565e1–1565e11.
59. Stoecklein HH, Garg R, Wolfe SW. Surface replacement arthroplasty of the proximal interphalangeal joint using a volar approach: case series. J Hand Surg Am. 2011;36(6):1015–21.
60. Bodmer E, Marks M, Hensler S, Schindele S, Herren DB. Comparison of outcomes of three surgical approaches for proximal interphalangeal joint arthroplasty using a surface-replacing implant. J Hand Surg (European Volume). 2020;45:608–14.
61. Johnstone BR, Fitzgerald M, Smith KR, et al. Cemented vs uncemented surface replacement arthroplasty of the proximal interphalangeal joint with a mean 5-year follow-up. J Hand Surg Am. 2008;33A:726–32.
62. Murray PM, Linscheid RL, Cooney WP III, Baker V, Heckman MG. Long-term outcomes of proximal interphalangeal joint surface replacement arthroplasty. J Bone Joint Surg Am. 2012;94(12):1120–8.
63. Luther C, Germman G, Sauerbier M. Proximal interphalangeal joint replacement with surface replacement arthroplasty (SR-PIP): functional results and complications. Hand. 2010;5(3):233–40.
64. Helder O, Marks M, Schweizer A, Herren DB, Schindele S. Complications after surface replacing and silicone PIP arthroplasty: an analysis of 703 implants. Arch Orthop Trauma Surg. 2021;141:173–81.
65. Hensler S, Behm P, Wehrli M, Marks M, Ferguson SJ, Herren DB, Schindele S. Lateral stability in healthy proximal interphalangeal joints versus surface replacement and silicone arthroplasty: results of a three dimensional motion analysis study. Hand Surg Rehabil. 2020;39:296–301.
66. Tagil M, Geijer M, Abramo A, Kopylov P. Ten years' experience with pyrocarbon prosthesis replacing the proximal interphalangeal joint. A prospective clinical and radiographic follow-up. J Hand Surg Eur. 2014;39(6):587–95.
67. Watts AC, Hearnden AJ, Trail IA, Hayton MJ, Nuttall D, Stanley JK. Pyrocarbon proximal interphalangeal joint arthroplasty: minimum two-year follow-up. J Hand Surg Am. 2012;37(5):882–8.
68. Herren DB, Schindele S, Goldham J, Simmen BR. Problematic bone fixation with pyrocarbon implants in proximal interphalangeal joint replacement: short-term results. J Hand Surg Edinb Scotl. 2006;31(6):643–51.
69. Wijk U, Wollmark M, Kopylov P, Tägil M. Outcomes of proximal interphalangeal joint pyrocarbon implants. J Hand Surg. 2010;35(1):38–43.
70. Storey PA, Goddard M, Clegg C, Birks ME, Bostock SH. Pyrocarbon proximal interphalangeal joint arthroplasty: a medium to long term follow-up of a single surgeon series. J Hand Surg Eur. 2015;40(9):952–6.
71. Chan K, Ayeni O, McKinght L, Ignacy TA, Farrokhyar F, Thoma A. Pyrocarbon versus silicone

proximal interphalangeal joint arthroplasty: a systematic review. Plast Reconstr Surg. 2013;131(1):114–24.
72. Mora AN, Earp BE, Blazar PE. Midterm clinical and radiographic follow-up of pyrolytic carbon PIP arthroplasty. J Hand Surg Am. 2020;45(253):e1–6.
73. Buncke HJ Jr, Daniller AI, Schultz WP, et al. The fate of autogenous whole joints transplanted by microvascular anastomoses. Plast Reconstr Surg. 1967;39(4):333–41.
74. Ellis PR, Hanna D, Tsai TM. Vascularized single toe joint transfer to the hand. J Hand Surg Am. 1991;16(1):160–8.
75. Squitieri L, Chung KC. A systematic review of outcomes and complications of vascularized toe joint transfer, silicone arthroplasty and pyrocarbon arthroplasty for posttraumatic joint reconstruction of the finger. Plast Reconstr Surg. 2008;12(5):1697–707.
76. Muder M, Hailer NP, Vedung T. Two-component surface replacement implants compared with perichondrium transplantation for restoration of metacarpophalangeal and proximal interphalangeal joints: a retrospective cohort study with a mean follow-up time of 6 respectively 26 years. BMC Musculoskelet Disord. 2020;21:657.
77. Hoang D, Chen VW, Gould DJ, Cohen MJ, Kulber DA. Successful arthroplasty using cadaveric meniscus for osteochondral defects in the wrist and hand joints. Plast Reconstr Surg Glob Open. 2017;5(e1257):1–9.
78. Billig JI, Nasser JS, Chung KC. National prevalence of complications and cost of small joint arthroplasty for hand osteoarthritis and post-traumatic arthritis. J Hand Surg Am. 2020;45:553.e1–e12.

GPSR Compliance

The European Union's (EU) General Product Safety Regulation (GPSR) is a set of rules that requires consumer products to be safe and our obligations to ensure this.

If you have any concerns about our products, you can contact us on ProductSafety@springernature.com

In case Publisher is established outside the EU, the EU authorized representative is:

Springer Nature Customer Service Center GmbH
Europaplatz 3
69115 Heidelberg, Germany

Batch number: 10732801

Printed by Printforce, the Netherlands